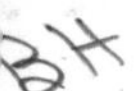

AF541236

NURSING SERVICES IN HOSPITALS

NURSING SERVICES IN HOSPITALS

(Encyclopaedia of Hospital Management—5)

DR. S.L. GOEL

Professor of Public Administration (Retd.),
Panjab University, Chandigarh
Editor, Indian Journal of Public Administration, IIPA, New Delhi
Former Member, UGC, Former Member Distance Education Council
Former Member All India Board of Management, AICTE
Member, Executive Council, IIPA, New Delhi.
Former Vice-President, IIPA, New Delhi.
Emeritus Fellow, University Grants Commission
Former Director, State Bank of India (Local Board) Chandigarh
Former Director, National Horticulture Board, Ministry of Agriculture,
Government of India, New Delhi.

and

DR. R. KUMAR

MBBS, MS, Ex. PGI
President, Chandigarh Ophthalmological Society, 2000-01,
Columnist on Health Education and Management,
Advisor on Health Care and Medical Tourism,
Member Tourism Advisory Forum,
Chandigarh Administration, Chandigarh

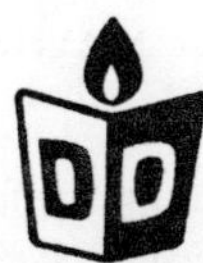

DEEP & DEEP PUBLICATIONS PVT. LTD.

F-159, Rajouri Garden, New Delhi-110027

NURSING SERVICES IN HOSPITALS
(Encyclopaedia of Hospital Management—5)

ISBN 978-81-8450-220-6

Typeset by S.S. COMPOSERS
3190, Mohindra Park, Shakur Basti, Delhi-110034.

Printed in India at MAYUR ENTERPRISES
WZ Plot No. 3, Gujjar Market, Tihar Village, New Delhi-110018.

Published by DEEP & DEEP PUBLICATIONS PVT. LTD.
F-159, Rajouri Garden, New Delhi-110027.
Phones: 25435369, 25440916
E-mail: ddpbooks@yahoo.co.in • ddpubs@gmail.com
Showroom:
2/13, Ansari Road, Daryaganj, New Delhi-110002 • Telefax: 23245122

Contents

Contents

Preface

The nursing profession is crucial to the functioning of hospitals as they are directly involved with the patients and their relatives. That is why nurses are considered by the society as sisters. A nurse must combine scientific and technical knowledge along with communication, observation and clinical skills. In addition, she must possess personal qualities like sympathy, perseverance and skill of interpersonal relations. Other essential attributes are: compassion, passion, integrity, tolerance of ambiguity, willingness to play with ideas, knowledge and inquiry, committed to viewing the social world from the viewpoints of people being studied, valuing of detail, willingness to inject something of themselves into the CARE process and hence into the outcomes. This combination makes nursing a challenging as well as a fascinating occupation. The nursing profession gives a sense of satisfaction that comes from knowing that you have made a difference in another person's life. This satisfaction is priceless and serves as a source of inspiration to the nurses to do their best.

Nurses may work in a variety of settings ranging from large institutional settings to patient homes. The hospital, nursing homes, and extended care facilities employ most of the nurses. A new dimension of nursing is public health nursing employed in primary health services, which is the pillar of sound health infrastructure. The type of work nurses does vary greatly depending on where they work. The medical and surgical wards involve the care and assessment of patients with diseases, injuries, and those who are waiting for or recovering from operations. Nurses on these wards should have from four to five patients to care for each day depending on the facility. The broad range of medical problems and the frequent use of nursing skills make this a good unit for new nurses to begin their careers. However, in Indian set-up a nurse may have to care many more patients that may affect quality of care. The intensive care/critical care unit should involve the care of no more than three seriously ill patients, since this unit involves special skills and more intense assessment. These nurses are supposed to attend further training to attain critical care skills.

There are different specialties in nursing services for which they are trained in nursing colleges. Pediatric nurses care for children aged twelve and under. Some of the larger hospitals have special newborn units that involve the care of newborns and include their parents in that care. Maternity (also called obstetrical or OB) nurses assist mothers through the childbirth process. They teach mothers and families to care for their infants. They also do some of the prenatal (before birth) testing to make sure the unborn baby is healthy. Psychiatric nurses care for patients with emotional problems and thought disorders. This occupation requires patience and the ability to understand and accept the patient's thoughts and feelings. Emergency care nurses care for patients in life threatening situations. They must be able to evaluate which patients need immediate care and which ones can wait. The nurse in this unit must be able to assess patients and make decisions quickly. Community health nursing is another dimension, where nurses are to take care of the community through primary health care.

Some of the other places where nurses work are; extended care facilities or nursing homes, doctor's offices, businesses, schools, patient homes and clinics. Nursing homes and extended care facilities employ registered nurses, licensed practical nurses, and certified nursing assistants to take care of the residents. Because extended care facilities operate constantly their employees must be willing to work some weekends and some day, evening, and night shifts. Nurses working in doctor's offices administer medications, assess patients, do paperwork, assist the doctor, and do some of the office procedures such as throat cultures and simple urine tests. Some businesses are employing occupational health nurses. The job of these nurses is to educate staff and develop programs that will help prevent sickness and injury. Schools in some states are required by law to employ nurses to deal with the injuries and illnesses of the students. They are also responsible for preventive health care that includes health screening, immunizations, and education. Private duty nurses may be hired to care for the health needs of one person. These nurses work in the patient's home. Home care nurses have several patients that they will visit as needed. These nurses do patient education, wound care, give medications, and get an overall idea of how the patient is doing and what the patient may need.

Most of the observations made in the text are based on personal experience of the authors. One of the authors Dr. S.L. Goel has been engaged in teaching M.Sc. and B.Sc. nursing classes at PGI, Chandigarh for the last 25 years. While the other author Dr. R. Kumar, who earlier worked at PGI and then in private sector hospitals, has been interacting with the nurses on duty, for the last 30 years. Both the authors have jointly penned several books on topics of health administration, notable being Hospital Administration and Management in 3 volumes in the year 1991 and Management of Hospitals in 4 volumes in the year 2001.

Nurses are constantly using their knowledge, energy· and skills to make a difference in the lives of patients, giving an immense satisfaction. Every day they come across a new opportunity for teaching and/or learning something new. Working as a nurse is never boring. Being a Nurse is a career by which they can feel satisfied spiritually, emotionally and financially. A special person with qualities such as empathy, compassion, intelligence and above all patience should only decide to become a nurse. During nursing career they will encounter many wonderful and terrible experiences from a death to a birth. It is a paradox of sweet and sour. Nurses must have the ability to manage emotions during these extreme times and be able to perform with confidence and accuracy. A true nurse will assume the role of patient advocate; at times she will be the only voice they have.

As per the Xth Plan of Govt. of India, around 7.37 lakh nurses have been registered in the various state nursing councils in the country; it is estimated that only about 40% are in active service. About 1.5 lakh nurses are employed in the government sector. Out of the 654 general nursing-midwives training schools in the country, private/voluntary/missionary institutions run 465. Around 20,000 trained nurses become available in the country annually. The current capacity being just adequate to fill the vacancies in the government sector. There is a growing demand of the specialized nurses, which has to be met.

What is required is: (a) To set-up excellent nursing institutions attached to post-graduate medical institutions wherein all facilities are available. (b) The faculty of nursing must be given UGC grades and the positions of professors must be created to improve teaching and skills. (c) The head of the nursing institution should be given the authority and powers so that she is able to work efficiently and not have to look up towards higher ups for small things. (d) A lot of innovation through projects and Ph.D. guidance is required. (e) Research which is very hollow at present, needs upgradation. (f) Nurses may be trained in clinical work so that they can take up independent positions for minor and repetitive ailments. (g) B.Sc. nurses with 5 years' experience may be admitted to MBBS against 5% reserve seats. (h) There must be refresher courses to update their knowledge.

However, being a nurse is no bed of roses. Working in an emergency room is hectic. Often there are no lulls. A hall full of ailing, irritable people that have over-flowed from the waiting room greet you at the beginning of each shift. Every frantic minute of the day is spent racing from one task to the next. Nurses have to learn to deal with a hysterical mother whose child has a fever while nurses are titrating drugs and monitoring a patient who has just suffered a heart attack. This type of work environment takes a toll on them, physically, mentally and emotionally. It also takes a toll on their family when they come home too tired and are miserable to play with their children. Or when they have to work weekends and holidays, or during the school play. Also, one of the most stressful things is to know that a mistake could hurt their patient or cost them their life. Even when your work is flawless, there is always the threat of a lawsuit. Nursing is suffering. Often doctors view them not as equals, but as helpers. Their knowledge and skills are highly overlooked. Another problem facing nursing is themselves. Too often are nurses unfriendly and unwilling to assist one another that they make their jobs even less pleasant. Nurses are pushed to take out aggression and hostility amongst themselves because they do not do so with patients or physicians.

Set of Challenges

Nursing profession is passing through a number of challenges that need the attention of policy-makers, planners and decision-makers to make it fit for discharging the arduous and difficult functions entrusted to their care. The first is a challenge of condition of services, which need analysis review keeping in view their condition of work. The grades need revision. Secondly, the avenues of promotion are limited, which must be at par with other professions, i.e. automatic promotions-time scale. Thirdly, the number of patients per nurse must be lessened to improve efficiency. Fourthly, there should be leadership positions at the top level in hospital hierarchy, e.g. Deputy Medical Supdt., Store Officer, etc.

The nurses need to stay strong and show physicians and patients that they are educated and skilled workers who possess the training and critical thinking skills to care for patients and collaborate in their care planning. Whereas once a big heart was enough to get a nurse through, nursing today presents a whole different set of challenges. Nurses need to be self-respecting, highly motivated and confident workers. Only then, will they get the respect they so deserve. Imagine after getting through nursing school, only to find it was "much harder" than you imagined to work in Nursing. It's a given fact that as a nurse, you're on a daily basis exposed to hostile families and patients, deadly diseases, abuse from doctors, families and other nurses. This is unfortunate. When Nursing Staff in hospitals and Nursing homes are not adequate, patients get sicker and die needlessly.

Those who enter Nursing because it's lucrative and in most places high paying, they often burn out, leave or move on. These nurses often become overwhelmed by the amount of work that's involved in providing adequate patient care. It's a profession that requires you to "get your hands dirty." A good comparison for nursing is plumbing. It's a trade that pays well and requires hard labour and skills. It also requires you to kneel down and reach into places that the average person would balk at. A hospital cannot function without adequate Nursing staff. To do so means compromising the quality of care patients receive.

Why are nurses leaving this noble profession? The main complaints of nurses are long hours; many health care facilities require nurses to work 12-hour shifts, overtime, and days-off to insure adequate staffing of nurses in order to care for patients and/or residents. Other factors include low pay scale, inadequate employee benefits, requirements to work most weekends, holidays, and being on call should another nurse falls out sick. Nurses are expected to be quick learners, exhibit good people skills, and perform increasing complex nursing duties. Nurses are required to attend mandatory continuing education classes and/or in-services to renew their nursing licenses. Nurses must be prepared to expect that this may interfere with their personal time normally spent with family, loved ones, and/or friends. Dealing with unruly and combative patients is another drawback that nurses are routinely faced with as well as the hard to read physician's handwriting that accounts for many medication errors. Nurses face enormous emotional stresses and physically demanding lifting, bending, and carrying activities that are required in giving good nursing care. Nurses can expect to work shorthanded of other nurses and nurse's aides, which only increases the stress levels on Nurses and their Nursing Aides. Nurse's greatest complaints are the feelings that are not appreciated by nursing administrators, physicians, and patients. Nurses often hear complaints and insults.

The plan, Nursing's Agenda for the Future, in US focuses on strategies that will move the profession forward in quantum leaps, thereby ensuring that consumers have access to high quality nursing care. The plan is organized around 10 key domains, including: leadership and planning, economic value, delivery systems/nursing models, work environment, legislation/regulation/policy, public relations/communication, professional/nursing culture, education, recruitment/retention and diversity.

Job Satisfaction

Evidence in the literature suggests job satisfaction can make a difference in keeping qualified workers on the job, but little research has been conducted focusing specifically on nursing faculty. These factors include professional autonomy, leader role expectations, and organizational climate, perceived role conflict and role ambiguity, leadership behaviors, and organizational characteristics.

We may reiterate that the union and state governments must come out with new package of working conditions for nurses—good pay scales, promotion, retirement benefits, fringe benefits seeing their qualifications and work hazards. In turn nurses may keep intact the qualities of Florence Nightingale viz., devotion, dedication, professionalism, love, affection and care to ensure excellence. Only then she will enjoy respect in the hospital team on the one hand and the community on the other.

Nursing educators who nurture, motivate, and listen and give personal attention to students who are entering nursing education programs are appreciated. To compete with other career options and address the global nursing shortage, nursing education must be considered a collaborator. Ageing faculty and declining faculty numbers increase the challenges related to recruiting and retaining the emerging workforce in nursing professions. Characteristics about the nursing profession influencing career decisions are care and concern for others, job security, and variety of work settings. Because health care delivery increasingly requires timely information for effective decision-making, information technology must be integrated into nursing education curricula for all future nurse clinicians and educators.

It is hoped that this book on "Nursing Services in Hospitals " would make a modest contribution to the knowledge and existing literature on this expanding field. Besides, this would help the academicians, national health officials, public health administrations, medical research workers and the policy-makers and planners in the proper understanding of health care delivery system. We will consider our labour well rewarded if the findings of the study are translated to provide decent health care to the millions of people living in rural areas, urban slums and tribal areas. Comments and suggestions from the readers would always be welcome.

The authors have summed up their observations and knowledge in the following chapters:

1. Challenges of nursing services and administration, 2. Nursing services and hospital administration, 3 Classification of Nursing Personnel and Nature of duties in hospitals, 4. Planning Nursing Organization, 5. Decision-making, 6. Nursing Leadership, 7. Nurse-Patient Relationship, 8. Nurse and doctor; relationships, and 9. Health education and nurse.

Chandigarh

S.L. GOEL
R. KUMAR

1

Challenges of Nursing Services and Administration in Hospitals in New Millennium

New Millennium is going to be different as the health problems would change with the change in other aspects of life. We mention here the challenges of Nursing in New Millennium and suggest solutions to meet the Challenges.

I. NEED OF BROAD BASED NURSING SERVICES AND HOLISTIC APPROACH

Nursing is a service to individuals and to families; therefore to society. It is based upon an art and science which mold the attitudes, intellectual competencies, and teaching skills of the individual nurse into the desire and ability to help people, sick or well, cope with their health needs, and may be carried out under general or specific medical direction.

The social nature and the broad purpose of nursing are described by the faculty of the Catholic University School of Nursing in the following statement:

Nursing is a social institution with roots in the basic needs of society and as such is characterized by two essential elements: (a) an organized group of people working together toward a common goal directly concerned with the welfare of people; and (b) a way of acting, specific to the group, for the accomplishment of the common goal. The responsibility of nursing includes the prevention of illness, the promotion of health, direct supportive and therapeutic care, and rehabilitation. It is a service to man, arising from his distinctive body-mind spirit unity, his health status, his therapeutic, preventive, or rehabilitative health needs, and his role in society. Nursing encompasses all persons at all ages from every walk of life and correlates its own role with the work of other health disciplines for the welfare of the person being served. Nursing has a need for various types and levels of practitioners who assume the obligation to serve in the area of indentifiable health needs.[1]

Nursing in the past has been understood merely as a help to a doctor or a sister to a patient. But in the new millennium, the cost of health services would increase beyond the capacity of patients and society. Therefore, there is a need of educating nurses in such a way that they can handle routine medical care activities. Advanced countries like USA are depending more and more on nurses to carry out medical and health care. In developing countries nurses are not enjoying much importance. Thus in the New Millennium, we have to raise the status of nurses through education and training.

Nursing, according to Reiter, can be described in two parts:

1. Direct contact with patients

Direct contact with patients and ministrations of nursing care and observation of patient's and his responsibilities to his total therapeutic program as well as to his nursing care, implementing any part of the total therapeutic plan, i.e., medicines, clinical tests, treatments, diet, exercise, emotional support; and teaching the patient and supervising his activities.

2. Indirect contact with patients

Indirect contact with patients—activities carried away from the patient but in his behalf and related to his direct care. It includes preparation of medications and technical equipment for ministration to the patient; recording of observations and communication with: (a) physician and other professional and non-professional persons engaged in patient care, and (b) the patient's family, seeking information which will enhance the care of a patient or a group of patients; planning for continuity of and engaging in conferences for evaluating the care of patients as a basis for further planning; and planning the total program for nursing care and directing and supervising other persons such as practical nurses who may assist in or give the nursing care.[2]

Johnson defines nursing care as that which "is provided to individuals or groups under stress of a health-illness nature, has as its primary purpose to relieve tension and discomfort to the end of restoring or maintaining internal and interpersonal equilibrium.[3]

These definitions are exhaustive and to live upto these definitions, nurses in developing countries, especially India would have to undergo rigrous training and lead a disciplined life.

The Christian concept of love serves the Christian nurse as the basic principle governing her relations with others. Christian love must be universal, embracing all over fellowmen, for through the eyes of faith we perceive that all the children of god, created out of Love, and destined to an eternity of love as members of God's family throughout eternity. Hence all men are brothers. Our relations with each and every one of them must be governed by love.

The professional nurse should see her own role and responsibility in relation to society and to her profession. The nurse not only serves society by her service to the sick and needy but also by promoting the welfare of her profession. She does this by taking a keen and active interest in the development of nursing and of those engaged in it; and she cooperates as a member of an organized profession in trying to secure the best nursing and health care for people. She serves her profession by cooperating in the activities o the community, by respecting authority, both civic and institutional, and by her example teaching others the same respect.

Thus, he nurse serves both society and her profession by taking an active interest in the welfare of the community in all things that tend to the common good. She does this by working for the improvement of both nursing service and nursing education through active members in professional nursing and allied organizations.

Comprehensive Nursing Care based on a Christian Philosophy. In summary, we may say that professional nursing requires that the nurse have an adequate understanding of principles drawn from the humanities, the social sciences, the natural sciences, medical science and nursing which she consciously synthesizes and integrates with her understanding of the dynamics of human relationship in the performance of nursing actions; that she be a real humanitarian, motivated by a love of God as well as of fellow men; for to give such care she must have insight into the patient's physical, emotional, psychological, social, economic and spiritual problems and be equipped to help the patient to solve these problems. At the same time, she must be technically competent, able to teach health and to function as a member of the nursing, the medical and the health team and recognize her responsibilities to God, herself, society and her profession.

2. NEED OF QUALITY HEALTH CARE BY NURSING PERSONNEL

Quality is of great significance to both the providers of health care and the receivers of health care and in the process builds a solid foundation of health care institutions. Press Reports, personal discussions and observation reveal the poor functioning of health services as there is no emphasis on quality health care. Such situations create unnecessary sufferings to people and even become cause of death in many cases. This situation can be improved by injecting quality in health care system rigorously and meticulously. Talveen Singh in an Article, "What is wrong with Indian Hospitals" in the *Daily Tribune,* May 6, 2000, rightly observes, in India I notice that we are very far from world standards even when it comes to basic things like cleanliness. My room is cleanish but there are visible layers of dust encrusted on the Venetian blind and the window panes and the bathroom is less clean than those you find these days. A friend's mother had been taken to the intensive care unit of a smaller

Mumbai hospital and I had gone to see her only to find myself in a place of dark, dirty corridors and wards that looked more like prison cells than places of healing. Garbage lay uncollected amid piles of old furniture in forgotten corners. It is also true that you put your life at risk when you go into an Indian hospital for treatment. In Delhi I know personally at least two women who went into hospital for minor gynaecological problems and carne out with hepatitis C. I know of a young boy who went into hospital with a broken arm and ended up nearly dying of septeicemia. I know of heart patients at the best hospitals in India who worry not about whether the surgeon will be able to perform their bypass properly but about whether they will survive the aftercare. ORA, AI-Assaf, WHO consultant, defines the concept of quality health care as:[4]

Quality is doing the right thing right the first time and doing it better the next, and that quality is simply the process of incremental improvements. Quality in health care should also be client focused and should emphasize meeting the clients' needs and expectations in the most effective and efficient manner. Quality, however, does not have to be luxurious or expensive. It should also be the responsibility of everyone involved and should be based on a learning environment rather than a disciplinary environment. Quality is simply a process of continuous improvement of the *status quo.*

Quality is described as having eight dimensions: effectiveness, efficiency, interpersonal relationships, safety, technical competency, access, continuity, and amenities. Each of these dimensions should be met at least minimally to meet the definition of quality.

The concept of quality has been defined as "The totality of features and characteristics of a product or service that bear on the ability to satisfy stated or implied needs." The features or characteristics may be: (1) Meeting well defined purposes; (2) Satisfying patients and job satisfaction to health personnel; (3) Complying with applicable standards; (4) Reliability of products/services; (5) Excellence; (6) Complying with safety requirements; (7) Complying with Environment requirements, and (8) Improving health status.

Quality is not obtained by chance. Efforts must be made by everybody at every level and at various phases of health care delivery system. In this context, the concept of total quality management (TQM) which is being adopted by almost all excellent institutions throughout the world appears to be the only hope for establishing quality standards.

TQM may be thought of as a way of organising and involving the whole health institution—every department, every activity and every single person at every level towards achieving excellence, high quality health care and research, growth of institution, patient satisfaction, and finally, moulding doctors of highest calibre. TQM can work well where culture and environment in the institution reflects academic quality as a way of life for all its employees.

Sri R. Venkatraman, former President of India, delivered the

Convocation Address at the sixteenth convocation of Gandhigram Rural Institute, Gandhigram. He said,[5] "A quality conscious system has been described as one which produces people who have the attributes of mental agility, efficacy and reliability and, above all, the capability to take initiative and innovative measures to meet situations."

Quality control is essential to make the efficiency of health institutions possible through:[6]

(a) Improvement of existing obsolete processes and procedures.
(b) Improved layout of office and working environment.
(c) Economy in human effort.
(d) Suggesting the best use of money and material.
(e) Improved design of the goods or services provided by the organization.
(f) Improved performance.
(g) Job satisfaction.
(h) Improved flow of work.
(i) Standardisation of processes and products.

In brief, it aims at optimisation of resources, which are:

- *Manpower*: Brain, skill, morale and effort.
- *Materials*: Inventory, Quality, Standards.
- *Equipment*: Design and Operation.
- *Services*: Communication and Information systems.
- *Space and Building*: Availability, design, utilisation.

3. ENVIRONMENT OF QUALITY CONTROL

(a) An urge and Desire on the part of the Personnel in the Health Organisation to Find Better Methods of Quality Health Care through Analaysis of Existing Practices.
(b) Need of Requisite Skill, Attitudes, and ability in the Persons Engaged in quality control.
(c) Need of vision among Medical Professionals to Inject Quality.

The Nursing council of India (NCI) is all set to start a pilot project —Quality Ensurance Model for Nursing Practice (QEMNP) that aims at enhancing the quality of patient care in the hospital.

According to NCI president Daleep Kumar, who is also nursing advisor to the Government of India, the pilot project will start at PGI and Ram Manohar Lohia Hospital, New Delhi, to ensure the quality of patient care and nursing services in the hospitals.

Giving details o the project, which is being sponsored by the World Health Organization (WHO). "In the end, the project would standardise nursing needs of patient in the hospital with an optimum patient-nurse ratio."

Ensuring the nursing needs in the public health, the curriculum for the public health nursing would be revised to make it more responsive to the community nurse would head all nursing department.

In its endeavour to improve nursing care through better interaction between nurses and patients families, the Indian Nursing Council (INC) will be launching a quality assurance programme. The nurses would be given short-term training to assess the needs of the patient so that comprehensive individualised care can be provided. Under the project, special focus would be laid on proper documentation and evaluation of patient care. "One of the most important aspect of the project would be better inter-personal relationship between nurses, patients and their families, so that a congenial environment can be created."

The need is for having more research-oriented education for nursing students. "There is an urgent need to improve the image of nurses in the eyes of the public and create higher positions for clinical nurses. Ms. M. Prakashanme and others in their article, "Quality Nursing Cares Myth or Reality states that just as precision is given importance in pure sciences, so is quality in the behavioural professions. A surgeon or mechanic may need precision and expertise in technical and mechanical skills to produce a work of art, but nurses who deal with interacting people need much more than skills—they are expected to give quality care.

The reasons for poor quality could be divided into five those related to the nurse, materials allied workers, society, and the nursing department. The actors related to the nurse could be subdivided into:

(a) *Conceptual factors*: One finds an absence of a clearcut professional concept of roles and responsibilities. Since nurses are not fully aware of their duties, many other activities are done by them and some important nursing functions are neglected.

(b) *Lack of interest to nurse is another reason for poor quality*: Many nurses enter the profession not with the idea of helping others in need but for personal gain and so a lot of time is spent in concentrating on working hours, remuneration, and other personal and family affairs.

(c) In the preparation of the nurse one finds shortages in that education does not prepare nurses to work in reality. There are inter-state and inter-insti- tutional discrepancies in the preparation of the nurse.

(d) Deficient nursing manpower poses a threat to nursing quality as manpower needs are not being met and we are very far from the accepted standards. The nurse-patient ratio being 1:25 in some teaching hospitals and 1:5 in critical care units. Instead of the required three nurses to every doctor we ironically have 2.4 doctors to every nurse.

Materials comprise an important aspect in the delivery of quality nursing care. Take the example of linen, the deficiency of which leads to use of dirty linen which harbours bacteria spreads infection, and demoralizes patients. In many hospitals it is common to see patients either lying on dirty linen or directly on the mattress. Even in places where adequate materials, equipment and supplies are available they are not used for fear of losses.

Many allied workers do not clearly understand the role of the nurse and nurses blindly accept activities which belong to others and perform them badly as they have not been adequately prepared to undertake them. By its lethargy and disinterest the Nursing department promotes poor quality.

How can Quality be Improved? Provision of quality nursing care need not become a myth fading away from reality. There is a gradual increase in awareness of the necessity for better care. Nurse researches and theorists are delving into newer methods and concepts with inbuilt quality assurance. Progressive Patient Care is one method in which there is reorganization of the complex system of health care delivery into systematic methods based on structure and functions. Patients are grouped into units based on their needs and physical and manpower resources are arranged to meet these needs. Since patients in each unit will be in similar stages of illness and dysfunction it is clear to meet needs and develop outcome criteria.

The Nursing Process with its phases of assessment, planning, intervention and evaluation has quality assurance inbuilt within it. Primary Nursing Care is another method which is adopted to improve quality of the care given. But research and newer methods alone will not suffice without some basic changes. Nurses must fight for manpower without which it is impossible to give quality care. Professional organizations need to strengthen themselves and strive for improvement.

4. NEED OF INJECTING ETHICAL VALUES IN NURSING CARE

Nurses were subjected to rigorous ethical practices whether it may be duty hours or dress or marriage. All these are being relaxed as nurses are human beings and part of the society and not angles.

However, they must be loyal and committed to patient care. The New Millenium would not tolerate those nursing personnel who are negligent and do not take their profession seriously J.S Neki in his Article, Medical Ethics—A viewpoint from the Developing world" in world health, July 1979, states behind medical ethics must stand such cardinal virtues as wisdom, justice, temperance, courage and benevolence. In other words, medical ethics has its locus standi only in the setting of general ethical principles to which it cannot run counter.

For centuries, medicine hardly advanced beyond the stage of folklore. The comparative suddenness with which the advent of modern science has transformed this ancient professional art is a remarkable phenomenon. Traditional medical ethics is already proving rather narrow for the horde of new ethical problems released by this phenomenon. A purely juridical approach gives a false and one-sided impression of the meaning of our ethical codes. To help, to heal, to reconstruct, to comfort—and all along the line to act with compassion—all these bear testimony to the moral consciousness of the doctor. Whatever the new strains imposed upon medical ethics, this structure will survive and continue to guide doctors in their professional conduct.

Doctors/nurses are human beings. They also have human appetites, ambitions and infirmities. However, when a doctor enters the sick room of a gravely ill patient, the latter endows him with divine or near-divine powers over life and death. This exposes the doctor Nurse to the temptation of considering himself above other men; to fall into the sin of self-glorification. Against this, doctors Nurses need to guard themselves studiously whether they may belong to the developed world or to the developing one. Legal and juridical obligations they have, of necessity, to fulfil. But these are not genuine ethics, Genuine ethics has to be ingrained into character and does not have to depend upon external controls.

Nurses in New Millenium must follow the professional ethics to raise the status of the profession which was at its glory during initial times. Degradation in nursing profession must be checked to brighten the image of nursing profession and status of nursing personnel.

Vijay Kanase rightly feels that both legally and professionally, Nurses are unequivocally accountable for their practice to various parties and in many arena. If a patient dies as a result of a Nurse administering the wrong drug under the orders of a doctor, the Nurse could be liable for civil action since she/he failed to deliver a reasonable standard of care expected of a Nurse.

Such Nurses could also face disciplinary proceedings before the Nursing Council and their line managers because they failed to use due care and skill in carrying out their contract of employment. Additionally they would probably have to appear in the coroners courts and might also face criminal proceedings. The contrast with the medical profession is tremendous. Nowhere in doctor's code does the word 'Accountability' appear.

It is for this reasons Nurses are placed in an invidious positions. The nursing profession is often accountable to the medical profession which arrogantly sees itself as "Accountable to None."

5. PROFESSIONAL COMPETENCE

According to Lorreta E. Heidgerken: A nurse who meets the requirements for professional nursing practice means that:

1. She possesses a body of selective knowledge, relevant to the health sciences and (a) drawn from the biologic, the physical and the psychological basic sciences and selected medical

science knowledge—etiology, pathology, symptomatology, treatment and prevention of disease, and (b) nursing knowledge gained from nursing information, facts, principles and clinical nursing experience merging through continued study into unified whole. This total body of knowledge is based on and keeps pace with general scientific advancements. It forms the basis on which the nurse makes clinical judgements regarding nursing intervention.

2. She is able to apply this knowledge in (a) evaluating behavior and situations readily and to function intelligently in response to these variations; (b) recognizing physical symptoms of illness commonly identified with organic changes, as well as manifestations of illness, such as anxieties, conflicts and frustrations which have a direct influence on organic changes; (c) diagnosing, planning and meeting nursing needs on the basis of the medical care and the health plans for the patient, whether they be palliative, symptomatic, restorative, rehabilitative or preventive, and observing and evaluating the patient's response to the total regimen; and (d) coordinating the nursing aspect of the patient's regimen through all the states of care-acute, convalescent, ambulatory, chronic and home care.
3. She is able to carry through nursing actions, whether they be simply those of helping the patient in meeting personal daily living needs, such as hygiene, nutrition, etc., or those involving complex technical operations, such as resuscitating a patient following surgery.
4. She is able to assume responsibility for a clean, sanitary and safe environment for the patient. She knows the principles of sanitary service and applies these principles to promote health and to control disease.
5. She understands the meaning of scientific method, its relation to practitioner activities and to research and to science. She is able to use scientific problem-solving activities in her own practice. She has interest in research and is able to make application of research findings to her own practice. She is interested and participates in accordance with her research ability in the research programs for improvement of nursing practice and nursing education. She participates with other allied workers in medical-care and health-care programs. This she may do as a team leader in the nursing team or as a member of a health team, a therapeutic team or a medical care team.

In summary then, the professional nurse is able to make critical, reasoned judgements based on her clinical knowledge—scientific, medical and nursing in determining the manner, the timing and the appropriate nursing action; she carries this action through with safety, accuracy, speed, gentlesness, human warmth and charity as she fulfils the role functions of processional nursing.

However this will not be sufficient in New Millenium. They must upgrade their clinical skill and learn advance technique made possible through modern science and technology. Since the introduction of B.Sc and M.Sc. Nursing, nurses must be engaged on higher duties and responsibilities. They must now come foreward for managing new instruments and techniques. They must depict their professional knowledge through application in patient care.

We suggest here the need of career development planning for nurses. A career system is one in which a hierarchically organised group includes posts at different levels. The whole professional life of the employee under this system is utilised profitably from one level to another. In contract or position system, an official is recruited for a particular job, which he/she will occupy throughout his/her stay in the organisation. Many commissions in different countries favoured the adoption of the career system. No nursing personnel can hope to survive long if it fails to compensate adequately through reasonable career prospects, those of its staff who have served it for long periods conscientiously and with dedication. Career system is a guarantee of efficiency and integrity and a shield against patronage and political pressure.

In essence, a career system may comprise careful selection of able nurses with the requisite qualifications and necessary attributes of character and motivation. Such nurses maybe carefully trained later on in those aspects of the organisation which cannot be acquired before-hand and their attitudes continually tested by assigning them a variety of tasks during a period of probation, after which nurse may be retained on a career basis or released. Moreover, forward planning of their assignments may be made to ensure the maximum utilisation and proper development of their aptitudes. Constant in service training courses may be provided to keep them abreast of the latest developments and to prevent them from becoming stagnant. This may be followed by an open system of promotion, permitting the ablest nurses to serve at the highest posts. The career status should not prevent the management from releasing nurse ineffective or who lose their effectiveness.

Benefits of Career Development to the Nurses

(a) It helps the nurses to discover his/her own talents, needs and motives related to work (through performance appraisal, career counselling and planned work assignments and training);

(b) It helps fulfil the nurses need to know that his/her position and future in the organisation will be (by providing realistic information and feedback related to career expectations);

(c) It provides a sense of affiliation with the organisation and a feeling that the organisation is interested in the nurse's development;

(d) It provides greater opportunity for the nurse to obtain optimal return for his/her personal investment (contribution of talents, time, energy, etc.) in the organisation;

(e) It provides the nurse with a greater awareness of his/her work environment and hence promotes more intelligent decision-making with respect to careers and avoids frustration caused by lack of career information;

(f) It helps fulfil the nurses need to retain a sense of control over his/her personal destiny in the increasingly complex and impersonalised modern industrial society;

(g) It provides greater opportunities for change in the working environment that would otherwise lead to boredom;

(h) It is conducive to job satisfaction by providing assignments most suited to the individual's needs and talents; and

(i) It leads to optimal personal development by developing abilities and aptitudes to the full.

6. NEED OF DEVELOPING SKILLS IN INTERPERSONAL RELATIONS

Hospitals consist of individuals, who work in relation to one another in different capacities, to produce results. Only a coordinated effort among individual, i.e. doctors, nurses, paramedicals, etc. can sustain the efficiency of an organization. Else a major effort would be wasted in misunderstandings, jealousies, etc. Today, most of the hospitals are plagued by poor interpersonal relations, resulting in lack of interactions, team work, harmony and resultant low output. Only effective interpersonal relations can lay the foundation of a sound organisation, otherwise it would lead to disparate elements working in different directions, causing great harm to the efficiency of the organization.

The nurse who meets the requirements for the giving of professional nursing care means that she has a sound understanding of and skill in effective human relations. The nursing act is described by Henle as an activity which takes place within the context of a complex of interpersonal human relationship which involves not only the act itself but also the awareness of a psychological and personal interchange not called for in any other act. The Christian concept of love serves the Christian nurse as the basic principle governing her relations with others. "Christian love must be universal, embracing all our fellowmen, for through the eyes of faith we perceive that all are children of God, created out of Love, and destined to an eternity of love as members of God's family throughout eternity. Hence all men are brothers. Our relations with each and every one of them must be governed by love.

Health activities involve multi-dimensional aspects carried out by different functionaries. Therefore, it is essential to make all of them appreciate the intentions of health programme. Let us take the case of malaria control programme. It involves doctors, paramedical people, spray men, etc. To make the programme successful, all must communicate among themselves.

Communication is an integral part of every function of health administration "and that is why it is said to be the bloodstream of an organisation." It is a two-way process between people. In communication a message is transmitted and received.

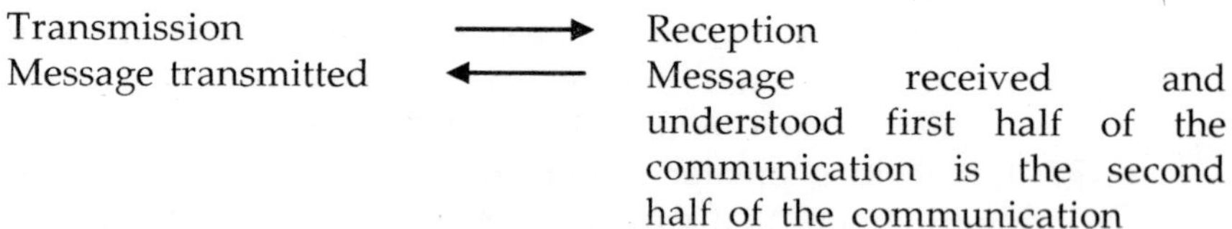

The art of effective communication is one of the key factors dictating the The art of effective communication is one of the key factors dictating the quality of human relations and also the professional performance level. Communication can be transmitted through audio, visual and audio-visual means. Communication plays theme role as the nervous system in a body. Norbert Wiener has rightly observed that "communication is the cement that makes an organisation." Communication is central to the exercise of authority in an organisation. In the words of Ordway Tead, . . . Communication is the touching of mind by mind, of person with person, whether it be one man, or a thousand. . . . It can include conversation, interview, dialogue, visual technique carefully used.

Team work can also facilitate good inter-personnel relations

Team-building represents an approach to enhance the overall performance of the work group of which Nurses are important. The primary emphasis is on providing insight to the group rather than to individuals. Attempt is made to assess critical variables known to be relevant to the group operations and feeding this information back to the team to permit it to develop plans to resolve identified problems.

Therefore, team-building is a facilitative strategy through which organisational work group members are able to gain additional insight into themselves and their work group.

The performance of health teams depends upon critical variables like:

- Team goals
- Role definition
- Decision-making practices
- Communication patterns
- Leadership
- Group norms

The advantages of health team to Nurses are:

- Greater work productivity.
- Increased clarity of roles and improved supervisory practices.
- More participative and flexible decision-making.
- More interaction and shared work among team members.

Thus team building can improve the overall performance of a health team.

7. NEED OF HOSPITAL MAINTENANCE

Need of Maintenance and Beautification

A visit to hospital is horrifying. Stinking smell, dirty walls, broken furniture, dirty rooms of wards. Nurses are the main persons who can ensure cleanliness and beautification.

The first impression of the visitors to the hospital depends upon the proper upkeep of buildings, equipment water-supply, electricity supply, etc. A visit to a number of hospitals revealed the following which should be taken care of in the new millennium:

(i) The surroundings of the hospitals are covered with congress grass and is full of dirt. Even in many hospitals there are no boundary walls. It is suggested that green grass and plants should be grown to make the hospitals clean and greener.

(ii) Buildings of the hospitals are in bad shape. Because of the shortage of funds, these are not maintained properly. These become the breeding ground of insects and cause infection. In the hospitals, buildings must be maintained properly at regular intervals of time to avoid deterioration.

(iii) Sweepers and ward boys must be encouraged to keep the hospital clean. They must be told that cleanliness is very important for the recovery of patients.

(iv) Lavotaries are in bad shape and even stinking. Hospital authorities must attend to it seriously otherwise the foul smell make the whole environment of the hospital unpleasant.

8. NURSING EDUCATION OUT DATED: NEED OF REVIEW FOR UPGRADATION TO SUIT THE NEEDS OF NEW MILLENNIUM

Nursing Education at present is based on outdated syllabus which do not build confidence, qualities of leadership and professional competence. The syllabi need revision to suit modern times. Education should make nurses to take new challenges seriously and positively. The professional nurse should see her own role and responsibility in relation to society and to her profession. The nurse not only serves society by her service to the sick and needy but also by promoting the welfare of her profession. She does this by taking a keen and active interest in the development of nursing and of those engaged in it; and she cooperates as a member of an organized profession in trying to secure the best nursing and health care for people. She serves her profession by cooperating in the activities of the community, by respecting authority, both civic and institutional, and by her example teaching others the same respect.

Thus, the nurse serves both society and her profession by taking an active interest in the welfare of the community in all things that tend to the common good. She does this by working for the improvement of both nursing service and nursing education through active membership in professional nursing and allied organizations.

Comprehensive Nursing Care Based on a Christian Philosophy

In summary, we may say that professional nursing requires that the nurse have an adequate understanding of principles drawn from the humanities, the social sciences, the natural sciences, medical science and nursing which she consciously synthesizes and integrates with her understanding of the dynamics of human relationship in the performance of nursing actions that she be a real humanitarian, motivated by a love of God as well as of fellow men; for to give such care she must have insight into the patient's physical, emotional, psychological, social, economic and spiritual problems and be equipped *to* help the patient to solve these problems. At the same time, she must be technically competent, able to teach health and to function as a member of the nursing. the medical and the health team and recognize her responsibilities *to* God, herself, society and her profession.

9. NURSING EDUCATION DO NOT PROMOTE RESEARCH: NEED OF DEVELOPING RESEARCH POTENTIAL

Nurses and their associations should emphasize research and come out with nursing issues clearly. The nursing council and Nursing association can take up project to produce literature on nursing based on the needs of India. Such literature can be made available to the Nursing students. The nurses may not use those books only which were written long back.

There is a need for conducting systematic research on many aspects of health care administration. By using operational research methods and techniques one can assess the extent to which scientific knowledge is utilised for bringing about improvement in the health level of the bulk of the people at the lowest cost. Research in health administration is concerned with administrative, economic and organisational aspects of the delivery of health and medical services. Success of health care administration depends not only on research investigations in the medical field but also on the researches in other allied fields and particularly on the application of the procedures and practices as evolved in these fields. It may be stressed that operational research has special relevance to health administration in India because of inadequacy of organizing health services as well as of several shortcomings of policy-making. However, nothing much can be achieved without providing the necessary training to personnel engaged in public health programmes and activities. The Central and the state ministries of health and family welfare have to play a special role in this regard. There is a definite need for studying the patterns of utilization of health services both in the rural and urban areas. By identifying factors affection delivery of health care services, they can possibly plan to overcome them.

10. MEDICAL EQUIPMENT AND ITS MAINTENANCE IN A BAD SHAPE: NEED OF PREVENTIVE MAINTENANCE APPROACH BY NURSES AND OTHER STAFF USING THESE EQUIPMENTS

Medical institution requires utilisation of wide variety of equipment ranging from the simplest to the most complicated for diagnostic, therapeutic and research purposes and it is becoming complex day by day because of the scientific and technological revolution. However, sophisticated equipments are acquired in most of the hospitals without prior assessment of the availability of technical knowledge and facilities for maintenance and repair. Besides, the hospital authorities purchase equipment from dubious sources of low quality. Such equipments go out of order soon.

Nurses frequently use equipment, therefore there is a need of intensive training in preventive maintenance. Preventive maintenance is a continuous maintenance procedure wherein the condition of the equipment is watched through a systematic inspection mechanism and preventive action taken to reduce the incidence of breakdown. The necessity for either major or minor repairs is determined to prevent unscheduled interruptions or deterioration of equipment. The fundamental activities of preventive maintenance are:

(a) Periodical inspection of the equipment to discover conditions of deterioration.
(b) Upkeep of equipment to remove or repair such conditions while they are still in a minor stage.

The salient advantages of such a system have been identified as:

(a) Continuous availability of equipment
(b) Increased life of the equipment
(c) Prolonged service
(d) Timely replacement of spares
(e) Timely availability
(f) Satisfactory quality of services
(g) Sagety of operation
(h) Savings in costs of repairs.

11. MODERNIZING NURSING ADMINISTRATION

People of advanced countries get their health services as much for granted as the essential utility services like water, electricity, public transport, etc. Despite the magic bullets of the modern medicine, the health services in the developing countries are far from satisfactory. The people living in the developing world, and especially 70 per cent of them living in rural areas, have little or no access to modern medical and health care resulting in high rates of morbidity and mortality from diseases which are preventable. If we want to reach the objective of providing decent quality health care to all by the first quarter of 21st century. We will have to introduce innovations in technical and administrative fields. It has been recognized by health experts in all the countries that the difficulties in meeting the health needs of the community are largely dependent upon the capabilities to design and manage the health care delivery system. The management of health care system can help in the greater achievement of goals through the optimum utilization of resources available—men, money and material. Indian rank in Human Development index is 128 as per Human Development Report 2000. To quote Dr. Chi-Yuen Wu of UNDP:

> "To create administrative capabilities, commensurate with requirements, developing countries must be able among other things, to use modern management techniques more, effectively than in the case of the industrially advanced countries."

Strategies and Policies in Administrative Improvement

As stated in a UN publication, the following strategies and policies are necessary to bring about administrative improvement:

(a) Improvement work must be a systematically planned organised activity with specific work programmes, a continuous activity, and it should be based on long-term planning and development.

(b) Classification of objectives and goals is necessary to be able to measure or evaluate the effectiveness and manage the improvement work.

(c) Improvement work must be recognised as a responsibility of the management; and in planning and organising improvement projects, participation and involvement of management in the organizations affected by possible changes are of great importance.

(d) Special resources must be allocated to the improvement projects including the support of professional staff of high quality with special qualifications in the management fields.

(e) Improvement work must be based on the concept or the organization as a socio-technical system where human and social factors are of primary importance.

(f) Training and development of the members of organizations-both management and staff, usually constitute one of the most important parts of improvement work.
(g) Improvement projects should from the beginning be oriented towards implementation and change, step by step, and not only towards writing reports and giving recommendations. Such projects should include specific implementation plans.
(h) As a rule, there is need for both centralised and decentralised (though coordinated) improvement programmes. It is advisable first to build up a strong, central activity.
(i) An improvement work programme should be formalised as an obligation for the public administration institutions and tied with long-term development plans, and budgeting and accounting control procedures.
(j) The improvement project organization should be flexible. A task force, under a responsible project leader and a Steering Committee, is often a usual type of organization.
(k) In larger projects, pilot studies of the implementation of new organizational structures in a limited part of the administration are often necessary and useful to demonstrate effects and results.
(l) Improvement projects must be planned in terms of activities, time and resources. The setting of deadlines or time-limits in the work programmes has frequently proved most helpful in the effort to obtain a high level activity and results.

12. NEED OF DEVELOPING EMERGENCY NURSING—SWAPNA NASKHAR WILLIAMSON IN HER ARTICLE "EMERGENCY NURSING"

The need for "Clinical Specialization" states that Emegency nursing is the term used to describe the level of care that includes prompt action, continuous, observation, monitoring, investigation, the treatment required to support and manage any emergency and life-threatening and manage any emergency and life threatening and critical conditions. Nurses play an important role in the emergency department. They assume leadership functions in organizing and directing services for emergency victims and their relatives. Therefore, a speciality nursing education in emergency nursing will ensure that the existing competencies of Nurses are further developed and new competence required are introduced. Nurses, who have undergone a speciality course in emergency nursing, would possess superior expertise and competencies and could assume more responsibility and accountability in order to adopt multiple roles such as practitioner, educator, manager and change agent. Thus, it is expected that emergency Nurses with advanced training will be high level practitioners and these practitioners of nursing will attain teacher competencies as well.

In India, emergency medical care, a much needed medical speciality, is moving into the realm of high technology, costly medications and equipment. In this milieu, there is an absolute need for qualified and competent emergency Nurses as well as physicians in order to provide a high quality of care to the emergency victims and also to their relatives. Anantharaman (2000) clearly stated that there cannot be progress in the care of emergency patients if emphasis is laid down on the training of doctors in emergency medicine, as Nurses are equally important members of an emergency care team.

Emergency care areas are highly sensitive and specialized where prompt action, continuous observation, skilled and competent care is essential. Nurses must be adequately equipped with the requisite competencies in order to be able to work efficiently and effectively in the emergency care areas. Thus, the benefit of specialization would accrue through the saving of doctor's precious times and also from patients' special needs bring better served. The potential of Nurses should be utilized to the optimum level. Nurses with specialized training, possessing superior expertise and competence will be more capable of meeting specialty care needs of the patient in a cost-effective and holistic manner.

13. DISASTER PREPAREDNESS

Nurses can play a major role in restoration of health.

Pre-Disaster Planning and Training

(i) The role of Nurses and Nursing in relation to community or a hospital disaster preparedness plan this should include training in immediate care, casualty evacuation, emergency treatment in hospital, psychological assistance to community and provision of safe water and sanitation.

(ii) The Identification of the type of organisations which will enable the Nursing staff to function most effectively puring a disaster.

(iii) Special preparation that Chief Nurses, Supervisors and Head Nurses will need to assume leadership roles.

(iv) The kind of training that should be given to non-professional members of Nursing service who are directly or indirectly involved in patient care.

(v) First Aid training at the grass-root level especially in disaster-prone areas. In real life situations it is often the only way to save lives.

(vi) Creating awareness in the school children and their teachers as they are some of the most receptive groups to disaster preparedness education and training. Recognising the value of school children as 'multipliers' of disaster information: tapping this potential prove its long effectiveness.

(a) Participate in committees or bodies established to prepare, coordinate and supervise programmes for the control and prevention specific health hazards during disasters.

(b) Define their position in relation to the management of the major health problems and solicit the cooperation of government, the community and voluntary organization for the adoption of preventive measures and development of the needed services.

(c) Initiate and participate in research relating to determining the magnitude and nature of the priority areas, appropriate measures to be taken, practices and techniques which enable people to cope with such situation, and prevention of disasters.

(d) Ensure that sufficient number of Nurses receive the specialized preparation required to work with particular groups.

(e) Support the international measures against those problems requiring international co-cooperation (provision of adequate nutrition, control of drug traffic, pollution control, etc.)

(f) Work for bringing about necessary changes in Nursing Education to ensure adequate preparation of Nurses in order to carry out their responsibilities effectively in combating disaster

14. EFFECTIVE PLANNING OF HEALTH SERVICES

While planning health services, we have to take care of every component in a hospital or community health, i.e. doctors of all categories nursing services of all categories, and other staff. It has been seen that nursing services are not attended to properly. The nursing superintendent matron and other senior level functionaries must attend to planning nursing services.

Planning of community health services means the careful analysis, intelligent interpretation and orderly development of these services, in accordance with modern knowledge, techniques, and experience, to meet the health needs of an area or hospital within its resources. A health plan is a predetermined course of action that is firmly based on the nature and extent of health problems, from which are devised priority goals. Health planning is an aid to doctors and nurses to decide how health services can be modernized and improved to provide effective and decent health care to the community. Health planning is not an independent exercise. It is an integral part of the overall socio-economic development. Health planning has been defined as "the orderly process of defining community health problems, identifying unmet needs and surveying the resources to meet them, establishing priority goals that are realistic and feasible and projecting administrative action to accomplish the purpose of the proposed programme. Planning is essentially a process of making choice between available alternatives at all levels of decision-making. Planning is essentially a process of making choice between available alternatives at all levels of decision-making. Planning is the exercise of intelligence to deal with facts and solutions as they are and find a way to solve problems. Planning is, in essence, an organised, conscious and continual attempt to select the best available alternatives to achieve specific goals. As expressed by Ackoff (1970, p.1):

Planning is one of the most complex and difficult intellectual activities in which man can engage. Not to do it well is not a sin, but to settle it for doing it less than well is.

According to Dr. Montoya:

Health Planning is the phase of the total process which leads from the policy statements to the concrete identification of the populations whose needs and demands will be served; the indication of the types of activities that will be performed for those populations, with their general attributes, and the specification of the type of instruments that will be required to carry out the activities.

The Nursing administrators lack the competence and personal qualities essential for making successful plans. Planning is a complicated and complex process and Nursing administrators have to convince all the concerned for preparing meaningful plans. There are still a number of problems requiring solutions with regard to co-ordination, communication and interrelationships between the many individuals and organizations involved. To quote the proceedings of the interregional Seminar: "Planning for administration is not only a desirable but a necessary part of development planning and the absence of it substantially limits the achievement of the social and economic goals emphasized in the development plan."

Planning methodologies need refinements to suit the social, political and economic environment prevailing in the country. The understanding of planning process and methodology in different areas will equip the administrators with a broader horizon of planning. There is still plenty of room for innovation and variety of approaches. The administrators should not blindly adopt any approach which may have been successful in some other countries. They must find out the methodologies most suitable to macro-environment prevailing in their own countries.

Planning is based on Institutional Requirements: Plan for people's Needs

The planning should be based on the needs and requirements of the population. A population base, in contrast to an institutional base, is absolutely necessary for objective planning and evaluation. A planner can formulate a practical plan only, if he is familiar not only with internal problems and limitations but also with external forces in the community. Without knowledge of external forces, the administrators risk underestimating what the public desires. This would require the creation of agencies and institutions to enlist public cooperation and involvement. The important agencies in this field would also be the organizations responsible for implementing the programmes.

All measures of productivity and efficiency should be analyzed in terms of the cost and development of the available and potential resources. They should also be considered in the context of outcome measures that reflect the impact of services on the status of populations.

The planning should encourage people's participation. People should from an integral part of planning process. V Subramanian writes, "A people's plan cannot be a people's plan unless it has an in built flexibility so that adjustment and mid-term corrections are possible in the light of several factors and circumstances which come to the fore during the implementation of the programme." Thus, there is a need to kindle the interest of local people in their own welfare.

The success nursing services in a developing country like ours depends upon the degree to which plan strategy has been carried out. The essence of development involves the setting up of a planning machinery with a view to utilizing the resources in an economical and efficient manner, so as to promote the well-being of the people.

At present, we have expanded nursing education not only in quantity but also in quality through the introduction of B.Sc., M.Sc., Ph.D. Nursing in Nursing colleges. However, there is no incentive after obtaining these qualifications resulting into rusting of qualifications. There is a need of proper utilization of nursing personnel so that they can strengthen the hospital services.

Nurses must take part in all these areas to become partners of modernization.

CONCLUSION

Besides, in the new millennium, the hospitals should attend to maintenance of buildings, equipment, dietry services, security services, registration services, etc. to maintain the prestige and dignity of the hospital as well as to ensure quality health care in new millennium. In this great venture, hospital authorities may seek the involvement and co-operation of the people to make the medical services, patient-oriented. Hospitals in the new millennium should provide an environment of extended family where the patients can get professional and expert medical care and homely environment. Patients should be welcomed in this extended family type hospital services, rather than exposed to sullen or greedy or indifferent faces.

A spirit of service and dedication must pervade among the providers of the health care as they are considered second God on earth by the receivers of health care. In the new millennium, we must empower the patients by looking after them carefully and making them feel important.

The progress and achievements of the past 50 years are solid foundations for a healthier and better world. It is already time to build on them. Life in the 21st century could and should be better for all. We can pass no greater gift to the next generation than a healthier future. That is our vision. Together, the people of the world can make it a reality.

NOTES AND REFERENCES

1. The Graduate Curriculum Study, p. 34. Faculty of the School of Nursing, The Catholic University of America, Washington, D.C., 1962.
2. Reiter Frances, The Improvement of Nursing Practice, in Improvement of Nursing Practice Speeches Presented at the American Nursing Association, 1961.
3. Johnson Dororthy: The Nature of a Science of Nursing, Outlook 7: 292, 1959.
4. *Daily Tribune,* May 6, 2000.
5. *University News,* March 11, 1996, p. 14.
6. S.L. Goel, Modern Management Technique, Deep & Deep, New Delhi, 1996, pp. 375-76.

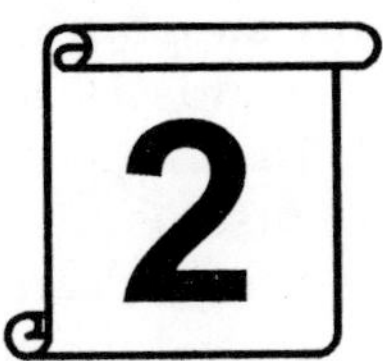

Nursing Services and Hospital Administration

Health Administration is a part of Public Administration and is an important aspect of social welfare activities. The Government of India has a separate Ministry of Health and Family Welfare at the Central level which undertakes the responsibilities of policy formation regarding health, development of new health programmes, provision of financial help and technical assistance to the State Governments, and regulation of health departments of all states. The Ministry of Health and Family Welfare of the Central Government is the nodal agency to look after health services. Nursing Service is an important part of health services. So all its decisions regarding policy matters are taken by the health ministry itself.

Being a unique organ of the vast machinery of health system, nursing service is that devoted profession in the service of mankind, which provides curative, preventive and promotive health services to the individual, family and community irrespective of cast, creed, religion and sex.

India is engulfed with number of problems because of vast geographical area and cultural diversities. The environment of illiteracy, poverty and religious superstitions has kept the status of health at a low level in India. Nursing has a great role to play in National Health Programmes devised to improve and to promote the national health. Considering the importance of Nursing Services, the then Prime Minister of India, Mrs. Indira Gandhi said, "A nurse is not merely an assistant to doctors. She has an independent part to play in many areas where doctors need not necessarily be present . . . ANM who does such valuable field work along with woman health visitor should be given due recognition on the basis of equality and not to be regarded as a lesser member of the profession."[1]

Dr. Mahler, the former Director General of World Health Organisation said, "If the millions of nurses in a thousand different places articulate the same ideas and convictions about Primary Health Care and come together as one force, then they could act as a powerhouse for change. I believe that such a change is coming and that nurses around the globe whose work touches each of us intimately, will greatly help to bring it about. World Health Organisation will certainly support nurses in their efforts to become agents of change in the move towards Health for All."[2]

Nursing is a broad word. The origin of this word is not very old. As per the English Dictionary, 'to nurse' is 'to nourish' and 'to nurture'. The 'nurse' suggests a person who has the care of the young, 'to look after carefully' so as to promote growth and development, to bring up, to train, to feed and tend in infancy.

The genesis of nursing profession is rooted in antiquity. The origin of this profession dates back to the origin of human species. Osler, Sir William writes: " . . . Nursing as an art to be cultivated, as profession to be followed is modern: Nursing as a practice originated in the dim past, when some mother among the cave dwellers cooled the forehead of her sick child with water from the broo . . . "[3]

In the words of Brown, "The professional Nurse will be one who recognises and understands the fundamental (health) needs of a person, sick or well, and who knows how these needs can best be met. She will possess a body of scientific nursing knowledge which is based upon and keeps pace with general scientific advancement and she will be able to apply this knowledge in meeting the nursing needs of a person and community."[4]

Ayurveda gives nursing a significant place by making it one of the four legs on which therapeutics stands.

It means, "The Physician the drugs, the attendant and the patient constitute the four basic factors for treatment. Possessed of required qualities, they lead to the earliest cure of disease."[5] Thus, a nurse was considered as important as the vaidya, the medicine and the patient.

The nursing professionals, working as complementary to the physician have primary responsibilities of 'Caring' the sick by guiding, helping and counselling. This relationship with the patient is continuous and involves both the state of illness as well as state of well being."

The spirit of service combined with the training in the art of nursing makes the woman the proper instrument for the administration of care to the ailing patient. Charaka describes the qualities needed in a nurse thus:

Charaka, the exponent of traditional Indian medicine has defined the attributes of a good nurse which inspired even the west. Charaka makes reference to the attributes of nurse:

(1) Knowledge of the manner in which the drugs should be prepared or compounded for administration;
(2) cleverness;
(3) devotedness to the patient waited upon; and
(4) purity (both of mind and body) are the four qualifications of the attending nurse.[7]

According to Sister Olivia, "Nursing in its broadest sense may be defined as an art and science which involves the whole patient, body, mind and spirit; promotes his spiritual, mental and physical health by precept and by example; stresses health education and preservation, as well as administration to the sick; involves the care of patient's environment—social and spiritual, as well as physical and gives health service to the family and community as well as to the individuals."[8]

The qualities required in a female nurse are well enumerated in the following extract::

> "To become a good nurse, a woman must possess considerable intelligence, good education, healthy physique good manners, an even temper, a sympathetic temperament and deft hands. To these, she must add habits of observation, punctuality, obedience, cleanliness, a sense of proportion and a capacity for and habit of accurate statement. Training can only strengthen these qualities and habits. It can not produce them."[9]

International Council of Nurses refer to Nurse, "as a person who has completed a programme of basic nursing education and is qualified and authorised in her country to supply the most responsible service of nursing nature for promotion of health, prevention of illness and care of the sick"[10]

"Unique function of the nurse is to assist the individual sick or well, in the performance of those activities contributing to health, or its recovery (or to peaceful death) that he would perform unaided if he had the necessary strength, will or knowledge, and to do this in such a way as to help him gain independence as rapidly as possible. This aspect of work, this part of her function, she initiates and controls, of this she is a master."[11]

"Nursing is defined as a process of action, reaction and interaction whereby nurses assist individuals of any age group, to meet their basic human needs, in coping with their health status at some particular point in their life cycle."[12]

The multifarious activities and responsibilities of the nurse has compelled her to streamline her professional activities into three main areas:

(i) Nursing Education;
(ii) Nursing Service; and
(iii) Nursing Administration.

These three areas overlap with each other and they can be distinguished but not separated. Nursing administration has taken all the principles and practices, available, and suitable, from the parent-body of public administration. The principles of public administration are generic and nursing administration is just one field where these generic principles have been applied.

Nursing administration is responsible for giving direction, co-ordination and control of various categories of nursing personnel who work for the objective of giving nursing care to the patient population.

According to Herman Finer: "Nursing Service is that segment of the Administration which actively take part to fulfil the objectives of health programmes and policies to constitute, to serve the patients, with the help of other health workers, to make the services more friendly and effective.[13]

According to Goddard: "Nursing Service Administration at any level is the application of the principles of administration for the ultimate purpose of providing nursing service to the individual. In the overall administration of a nursing service, whether at the national, intermediate or local level, there is the responsibility for forecasting the needs and for estimating the material and human resources required. There is also the responsibility for the adequate training and distribution of staff, and for the organization of the service in order that the staff may maintain the necessary level of efficiency.[14]

Major Responsibilities of Nursing Service Administration:

1. planning for total patient care,
2. selection of personnel and assignment of their activities,
3. organisational and clerical activities of the nursing service office,
4. general supervision,
5. relationships with other departments,
6. public relations, and
7. after-care of patients.[15]

ROLE OF NURSING SERVICES IN THE FIELD OF HOSPITAL ADMINISTRATION

There is a well organised structure of nursing services from top most level to lower most level in the health administration for the successful functioning of the planned health programmes developed for the purpose of promotion of health. The set objectives of the health programmes can be achieved only with the help of nursing personnel. Usually a nursing service personnel is available in each village or town. The personnel working in the rural areas are well aware of the regional geographical condition, cultural heritage, traditions, customs and values. Due to routine contact with the patients they also develop informal personal relations. Nursing personnel can implement the health policies more successfully and effectively because of understanding with the patients, their families and the community. This is reason why even today in the India village, the rural patients prefer to take medical advice from the low level health workers than the employed doctors.

Another reason for the important role of nursing services in the field of health is the continuity of contact of nursing personnel with the patient. Doctors often think that their responsibility is over after prescribing the medicine. Other necessary information regarding treatment, procedures and time and mode of administration of those medicines is completed by nursing personnel only. They very well understand the benefits gained or problems faced by the patients due to medicine or treatment procedures.

Nursing personnel also know and understand the social, psychological and spiritual problems which occur during implementation of health programmes and they suggest the ways and means to overcome them. The success of the family welfare and immunization programmes in practice all over the country depends upon the efficiency, determination and spirit of service of all these workers only. The success of community development programmes launched from 2nd October, 1952, twenty point programme and "Health for All by 2000 A.D." too, depends upon the capability, skill and perfection of these nursing services.

The role played by nursing is portrayed in the following areas:

(i) Prevention of Disease and Promotion of Health

"Prevention is better than Cure." Modern health services follow this saying and provide vaccines and multi-vitamin tablets to the people for the prevention of infectious and deficiency diseases. Good diet and good health habits help to promote health. Health education is provided to the community to develop habits of cleanliness, awareness about diseases and consciousness about health, and the responsibility to do all the above mentioned activities lies on the nursing personnel. It is of utmost importance to complete this work at the primary or lower level in the Indian context especially for the people of remote areas where they still ignore health and believe on superstitions as the cause of diseases.

(ii) Treatment of Diseases

The man has been the target of one or the other disease since the ancient times. He has been continuously developing new techniques to fight against diseases and in search of their treatment. But the situation is becoming so alarming that the new diseases outnumber the new techniques. The development of new techniques does not keep pace with the growth of new varieties of diseases. To fight against these diseases, and for their actual comfortable treatment, efficient nursing services are of utmost importance along with the medical specialists. Surgery done by any skilled surgeon cannot be successful unless and until nursing care is provided to the patient in a scientific way. Therefore, the importance of nursing services is proved to be equal to medical services in the field of health administration.

(iii) Education and Research

With the development of new techniques and methods in the field of medicine, the methods of patient care and treatment are also changing day by day. Similarly, research is being done in the field of nursing. Health education related to family welfare, population control, maternal-child welfare, contagious diseases, habits of cleanliness, spread of diseases, sex education and malnutrition, etc. is being provided through different means of communication or by health workers. Information and broadcasting through electronic communication media is being viewed as revolution these days.

(iv) Service to Humanity

No work is more pious than the service of a helpless person groaning with pain and fighting against illness. This is a noble and memorable job whether it is being carried out by Red Cross, Missionaries of Charity or Government Workers' Administration have well organised nursing service to fulfil the motto of a welfare state. In a country full of diseases like India, the organisation of such services is very important so that suffering and helpless patients can be looked after. This unique service rendered by nursing personnel has no parallel.

ORGANISATION OF NURSING SERVICES

Health care system, like any other enterprise, functions through organisations. Nursing service is one of such organisations. There is a need for the design of sound organisational structures and their continual evaluation in terms of suitability due to inescapable impact of momentous changes in the field of technology and human behaviour on all areas of social activity. It is all the more important for the organisation of nursing services because they deal not with the machines or files, but with the human beings which bring about two-way interaction. Study of the organisational structure of an enterprise is one of the common means of bringing about improvement in corporate performance.

Meaning

Dictionary defines the word 'to organise' as 'to frame and put into working order'. Simply stated, an organisation may be described as a group of people interacting one with another and pooling their efforts towards a common objective. The term 'organisation' lends itself to

(i) the act of designing the administrative structure,
(ii) both designing and building the structure, and
(iii) the structure itself.

Organisation refers to a plan of action to ensure fulfilment of purpose or purposes, which a group of individuals has set for realization and towards the attainment of which they are collectively bending their energies.

According to Gaus Organisation "is the relation of efforts and capacities of individuals and groups engaged upon a common task in such a way as to secure the desired objective with the least friction and the most satisfaction for whom the task is done and those engaged in the enterprise."[16]

Gladden defines it as the pattern of relationships between persons in an enterprise, so contrived as to fulfil the enterpriser's functions.[17]

Dale Yoder states that 'Organisation as a process is purposive and systematic assignment of functions, duties and responsibilities among members of a group or team. It defines the part that each member of an enterprise is expected to perform and the relations among those members.[18]

Edgar H. Schein has defined an organisation as, the rational coordination of activities of a number of people for the achievement of some common purpose or goal, through division of labour and functions and through an hierarchy of authority and responsibility.[19]

Pfiffner and Sherwood, defines organisation as "the pattern of ways in large number of people, too many to have intimate face-to-face contact with all others and engaged in complexity of tasks relate themselves to each other in the conscious, systematic establishment and accomplishment of mutually agreed purposes."[20]

Another definition we acquaint ourselves is that of Amitai Etzioni. According to Etzioni, "Organisations are social units (or human groupings) deliberately constructed and reconstructed to seek specific goals. Corporations, armies, schools, hospitals, churches and prisons are included; tribes, classes, ethnic groups, friendship groups and families are excluded. Organizations are characterized by:

(1) "divisions of labour, power and communication responsibilities, divisions which are not random or traditionally patterned, but deliberately planned to enhance the realization of specific goals;
(2) the presence of one or more power centres which control the concerned efforts of the organisation and direct them toward its goals; these power centres also must review continuously the organisation's performance and re-pattern its structure, where necessary, to increase its efficiency; and
(3) substitution of personnel, i.e. unsatisfactory persons can be removed and others assigned their tasks."[21]

So, we find that organisation is not merely a structure; in fact, it embraces structure as well as the human beings who man and run it in order to realize the preconceived objective. This is dearly borne out in the following observation.

"Organisation is the systematic bringing together of interdependent parts to form a unified whole through which authority, coordination and control may be exercised to achieve a given purpose. Because the interdependent parts are made up also of people who must be directed and motivated and whose work must be coordinated in order to achieve the objectives of the enterprise, organisation is both structure and human beings . . . to try to deal with Organisation merely as frame work and without considering the people who make it up and those for whom its services are intended would be wholly unrealistic."[22]

Hence, Nursing Organisation is the systematic bringing together of different levels of nursing personnel to form the whole nursing services through which authority, co-ordination and control may be exercised to achieve the purpose of provision of best possible nursing care. So, the nursing personnel who constitute the nursing services and the patients for whom nursing services are intended must also be considered along with the structure of nursing organisation.

The function of an organisation is to enlarge the resources and opportunities of those for whom it has been established. In it is implicit the idea of change. "An organisation that ceased to change is Imoribund."[23] According to Dr. Bhandari, "change is a necessary way of life for most organisations. If the change is not brought in time, the organisation becomes stale and stagnant and the opportunity is also lost. The need for change should be anticipated, identified and analysed. It is always better to weigh the pros and cons before implementing a change. Basically, people resist change and greater the proposed change the stronger the resistance. The strategy for change should be selected depending upon the situation, individuals and the time factors."[24] As Simon has stated, it influences the members by:

(i) dividing work among them;
(ii) formulating standard practices;
(iii) transmitting decisions downward, upward and crossways;
(iv) providing a communication system, thereby making known all sorts of information; and
(v) training them."[25]

The principles of organisation are the inductive generalisations as a consequence of keen, informed and continuous observation of administrative phenomena. These principles of organisations are neither rigid nor absolute. Flexibility and capability of adaptation to every need are in the essence of these principles. These have to be applied judiciously in terms of immediate situation and keeping in view the many internal and external pressures exerted on any organised activity by factors like rapidly increasing levels of technology of education and of social consciousness.

Every organisation has some goals or objectives for which it has been established. To achieve these objectives, it is necessary that the members of the organisations should be not only aware of them but should also perceive the relevance of their work to these objectives. The higher the degree of clarity with which an enterprise specifies its objectives the greater is the possibility of their being achieved with optimal utilization of resources. Objectives should indicate in as precise a manner as possible the nature of the desired achievement in terms of quantity, quality, cost and time. They should be periodically reviewed and modified if necessary due to continuous flux of the environment in which it operates.

Goddard has listed the Objectives of Nursing Services as:

(i) "to give the highest possible quality of nursing care in terms of total patient needs (this will involve spiritual, psychological, social, rehabilitative and educational needs as well as the physical);
(ii) to assist the physician in the medical care of the patient, and to carry out such therapy as is prescribed;
(iii) to promote programmes of in-service training; to provide facilities for the clinical instruction necessary for the basic and post-basic preparation of nurses and of auxiliary nursing personnel;
(iv) to promote and encourage nursing studies in order that quality of performance may be improved and maximum utilization of personnel obtained; and
(v) to evaluate the quality of the nursing service."[26]

To attain its prescribed objectives, an organization performs a number of functions. Organizations is essentially the division of functions among all the workers. The distribution of functions and responsibilities is both horizontal and vertical. Vertical distribution creates levels like Top Management, Middle Management or level of Supervision, and the level of Specific Performance. Due to the difference in the qualification and qualities and the difference in the nature of responsibility at these levels and the difference in the salary scales between different levels, superior-subordinate relationship does emerge in the organisation. According to White, "Hierarchy consists in the universal application of the superior subordinate relationship through a number of levels of responsibility reaching from the top to the bottom of the structure."[27] It is called the 'Scalar Process'. Hierarchy provides the much needed channels of communication in the organisation from the top to the bottom and from the bottom to the top. It also facilitates delegation of authority.

Relationship with non-nursing personnel

Nursing personnel have direct relationship with personnel of other departments of the hospital who directly or indirectly contribute towards the achievement of the objectives of the hospital or nursing service administration such as:

- o Medical personnel, i.e. doctors
- o Pharmacists
- o Technologists
- o Physiotherapists

- o Clerical staff
- o Sanitation Staff/Safaiwala
- o Ward servants
- o Dieticians
- o Radiologist
- o Security staff

Equation of Responsibility to Authority

Authority is the right to act and take decision without the obligation to consult others. Authority has two components, i.e. right to command and the power to enforce. Responsibility is accountability for omissions and commissions in carrying out the specified job. It tends to encourage initiative and resourcefulness. It promotes consciousness of the duties and responsibilities inherent in the job and motivates the nurses to discharge them effectively. If authority and responsibility are not properly matched, it will be difficult to achieve harmonious organisational relationships or ensure effective accountability. It is, therefore, necessary that each nursing personnel should be given authority commensurate with her responsibility; responsibility without authority leads to misery; authority without responsibility can lead to tyranny.

Unity of Command

Every worker in any organisation gets instructions or command from their superiors, so as to work orderly, effectively and efficiently. In short, it means that an employee should receive orders from one superior only or in other words, each individual in the enterprise should receive definite instructions whether functional or administrative from one source. Pffifner and Presthus has mentioned that "The concept of unity of command requires that every member of an organisation should report to one and only one leader."[28] This is essential to ensure effective reporting and control, avoid confusion and conflict and maintain the morale of the employees. Further Fayol has added that "should it be violated, authority is undermined, discipline is in jeopardy, order disturbed and stability threatened."[29]

The reality in the modern era in the words of Seckler-Hudson is that "The old concept of one single boss for each person is seldom found in fact in complex governmental situations. Many inter-relationships exist outside the straight line of command which require working with and reporting to many persons for purposes of orderly and effective performance."[30]

Span of Control

Span of control is simply the number of subordinates or the units of work that an administrator or supervisor can personally direct.

According to Dimock, "The span of control is the number and range of direct, habitual communication contacts between the chief executive of an enterprise and his principal fellow-officers."[31]

This is similar to the concept of "Span of Attention" in psychology. As there is a limit to human capacity, a supervisor should have neither too many nor too few subordinates under his minimum control.

If the span of supervision is extended too thinly, the results are unsatisfactory. When an executive controls the work of too large the number of subordinates:

(a) he is left with little or no time for planning, policy formulations and coordination;
(b) he cannot give adequate guidance to the subordinates;
(c) the quality of work suffers; and
(d) there is little or no effective supervision.

There is no unanimity as to the exact number, but there does exist a general agreement that the shorter the span, the greater will be the contact, and consequently, more effective control. When an executive has too few persons to supervise:

(a) there is a possibility of wastage of manpower;
(b) he may do his subordinates work; and
(c) he may exercise too close a supervision amounting to interference which the subordinates may resent.

Seckler-Hudson also points out that, "There are dangers inherent in excessively limited span of control, such as, the risk of detailed supervision of the few reporting; the resultant failure to stimulate subordinates or to fully use the capacities of them. It is possible also that short spans of control mean long chains of command."[32]

The actual fact is that there can be no rigid span of control. The decision regarding the exact span of control of an executive or supervisor depends upon many variable factors such as:

(a) Size of enterprise;
(b) Nature of work;
(c) Personality of the supervisor, i.e. physical and psychological make-up;
(d) Quality of subordinates; and
(e) Geographic dispersion of command.

In the Nursing Service Organisation of any hospital there should be equal span of control at all the levels and in all the shifts to provide quality patient care throughout 24 hours a day.

Delegation of Authority

Centralization stands for concentration of authority at or near the top; decentralization, on the other hand, denotes dispersal of authority among a number of individuals or units.

According to White, "The progress of transfer of administrative authority from a lower to a higher level of government is called 'Centralization', the converse, 'Decentralization'.[33] The essential element in decentralization is the delegation of decision-making functions. According to Avasthi and Maheshwari, "Decentralization signifies the central authority divesting itself of certain powers which are given away to the local authorities which, so to say, become autonomous in the field. Delegation, on the contrary, implies transfer of certain specified functions by the central to the local authority which thereupon acts as the agent of the former which retains the right to issue directives or revise decisions. In brief, what is ceded is merely functions and not authority and responsibility."[34]

As an organisation grows, the decision-making problems become complex and there arises the need for distribution of authority. Operational challenges and problems arising at each level require effective and timely decisions. Delegation is one of the main ways of dividing authority.

The main advantages of delegation are:

(a) effective use of various levels;
(b) development of an increased sense of responsibility in the employees leading to organisational development;
(c) increase in efficient utilization of resources; and
(d) greater effect on use of control.

For delegation of authority to be effective, following are the guidelines:

(a) It should follow well defined procedures and policies.
(b) It should be specific and preferably be written down.
(c) It should be to a post and not to a person.
(d) It should have a proper built in system of reporting.
(e) It should be periodically reviewed.

Ruth Hansten and Marilynn Washburn developed a four step model to illustrate the process of delegation which was essential because nurses need to work with limited resources and to direct less prepared personnel to provide quality care. They proposed the "Four Rights" of delegation. These "Rights" include:

- the right task (the one that can be delegated),
- the right person (the one qualified to do the job),
- the right communication (clear, concise, description of the objective and your expectation), and
- the right feedback (evaluation in a timely manner, during and after the task is completed).[35]

According to Joseph Raj, "Trying to accomplish everything oneself can put an organisation into turmoil and result in loss of opportunities. Moreover, demotivated subordinates will cease to give their best and are unlikely to stay on long in the organisation."[36]

According to Goddard, "Once the policy has been laid down, the process of delegation must come into play. If it does not, the central authority will quickly find that it is overwhelmed with detail; and the co-ordination of the efforts of the total working force will become impossible. If delegation is to become effective, however, careful selection and placement of staff for that purpose are necessary; and staff members must be vested with authority appropriate to the responsibility delegated."[37]

So, to provide quality patient care in any hospital, each nursing personnel in the Nursing Service Organisation should be given authority commensurate with responsibility.

IMPORTANCE OF DELEGATION IN WARD ADMINISTRATION

It is essential for efficient functioning. It helps to build interpersonal relation and a team spirit among the staff as each will be responsible for certain task and every one will have to depend on each other. It makes subordinates feel important and increase their level of interest and competence.

Principle of Delegation Applied to Nursing Services

1. There should be clear description of jobs to be delegated and the limit. Everyone should know which work is delegated to which person. .
2. Authority should be given with responsibility. But this has to be within limits. Important decision should not be taken by sister grade II at her own but she should consult sister grade I also.
3. Critical tasks should not be delegated.
4. Tasks for which sister grade II is not capable, should not be delegated
5. Worker should not be overburdened with task.
6. Administrative tasks should not be delegated to students.

What to Delegate?

1. Inventory keeping.
2. Medicine indenting, stocking and issuing.
3. Ward cleanliness.
4. Preparing diet list and diet distribution.
5. Maintenance of equipment.
6. Supervision of patient care.
7. Supervision of Class IV employees.

How to Delegate?

1. List all functions in the ward.
2. Divide functions into 3 categories:

(A) Have to be done by sister grade I only, e.g.

- Making duty roaster
- Holding group conference
- Filling A.C.R.
- Writing anecdote
- Planning and implementing ward policies

(B) *Can be carried out by sister grade II and other, i.e.*

- Patient care activity
  - o Health teachings
  - o Preparing equipments
  - o Medicine indent and maintain stock
  - o Maintenance of store
  - o Carrying out physician orders

(C) Responsibility of sister grade I but can be done by sister grade II without ending in administrative problem, i.e.

- D Patient care activities to sister grade II
- Cleanliness to safai sewak
- Diet list, Patient list, Ward clerk and Census to ward clerk
- Supervision of Class IV by ward clerk or sister grade II.

3. From 3rd category decide whom you want to delegate responsibility for each function.
4. Weigh each according to capability, aptitude and willingness to take the responsibility.
5. Have individual conference before delegating.
6. Have dear description of duties delegated.
7. Review performance.[38]

Co-ordination of Work

In any organisation, the parts have to work in co-ordination with each other in order to produce effective results. Proper co-ordination entails adjustments of the parts to each other and of the movement of individual parts in time so that each can make its maximum contribution to the achievement of the results.

In Nursing Service Administration of any hospital, there is a need for proper co-ordination of work in each ward or unit.

(i) Division of Managerial/Supervisory Functions

The managerial and supervisory functions are divided among the Sisters Grade I (Nursing Sister), i.e. one is responsible for the management of personnel, i.e. of Sister Grade II (Staff Nurses) such as making their duty rotation plans and assignment of duties. Other is responsible for equipment and supplies in the ward such as drugs, linen and other equipment. Whereas the other may be responsible for the sanitation of the ward. Though all of them take up each other's responsibility in the absence of other due to leave or night/evening shift.

(ii) Division of Patient Care Activities

Each Nursing Sister Grade II (Staff Nurse) is assigned work/duty on the basis of patient assignment or functional assignment. Whatever the bases, coordination of work is there so that it avoids duplication of work, waste of men, money and material and friction or jealousies.

Patient Assignment

Each Sister Grade II is responsible to provide comprehensive nursing care to patients assigned to her. All patients are assigned to one or the other Sister Grade II.

Functional Assignment

Each Nursing Sister Grade II is responsible to carryout one or two activities for all patients which contributes to the total patient care, e.g. one will distribute medicine and other injections, whereas the other will check vital signs and carry out state instructions and so on. So, by coordinating the activities of all nurses, total comprehensive care is provided to all patients in the unit.

Therefore, according to this principle, work has to be distributed among its members. In Nursing Services Organisation, the work is dearly distributed among all nursing personnel as per job responsibilities.

Job Description

The Nursing Service Department assigns job description for each category of Nursing personnel as follows:

- Chief Nursing Officer
- Statement of Responsibility

The job involves responsibility for planning, organising and implementing high standards of care in nursing, control over in service and clinical nursing education programme and in clinical nursing research projects.

Supervision Received

Nursing Service as an independent department, the Chief Nursing Officer is responsible to the Director of the institute/hospital.

Supervision Exercised

Supervision and guidance to the senior nursing staff to ensure maximum efficiency and productivity. Disciplinary measures at all levels of nursing staff.

DUTIES AND RESPONSIBILITIES

(i) Plans and estimates nursing man-power, material resources and budget for the Department of Nursing and collaborates with other department of the hospital to determine institutes needs.

(ii) Co-ordination and control of nursing staff and their activities towards achieving institutional aims.

(iii) Determines nursing policies to achieve reasonable and attainable standard of nursing care, preparation of nursing policy manual, nursing procedure manual and job description for each cadre of Nursing.

(iv) Recruitment of nursing staff from best possible sources. Assesses the availability of nursing personnel for recruitment in the community.

(v) Ensure adequate material resources for patient's optimum comfort, e.g. linen, basic necessities and food, etc.

(vi) Maintains reports, records and confidential files pertaining to nursing department.

(vii) Guides nursing supervisors in carrying out their functions of teaching and supervision.

(viii) Plans and organises clinical programmes of specialities for post-graduate nursing students.

(ix) Assesses the needs of in-service education programme for hospital staff.

(x) Co-ordinates, cooperates and collaborates with members of the multi-disciplinary team in formulation of policies and decision-making.

(xi) Establishes and maintains good interpersonal relations with professional and non-professional agencies in the community and participates in programmes in public relations.

(xii) Encourage a problem-solving attitude among the staff during her rounds and guides them in research.

(xiii) Participate in teaching and research.

(xiv) Evaluates activities of Nursing Service Department periodically.

Nursing Superintendent

General Nature and Purpose of the Job

The Nursing Superintendent is responsible for administration and supervision of nursing services and patient care.

Lines of Authority

She is directly responsible to the Nursing Service Administrator for the posting of nursing personnel, management of the patient care in the hospital and improvement of nursing services and patient care. She has indirect relationship with the Hospital Administrator/Medical Superintendent with whom she collaborates in the absence of Nursing Service Administrator. She is responsible for the Assistant Nursing Superintendent and other nursing personnel for performance of their duties.

(i) Assigns Nursing Personnel to the Ward/Deptt. in collaboration with Assistant Nursing Superintendent.
(ii) Manages the casual and earned leaves and arranges leave reserves.
(iii) She conducts ward rounds for implementing nursing service policies.
(iv) Maintains discipline of nursing staff and domestic staff of the nurses hostel.
(v) Manages the nurses accommodation and meals through the house keepers.
(vi) Investigates complaints and reports from the nursing personnel regarding the mess.
(vii) Develops and maintains office records pertinent to the administration of nursing services.
(viii) Writes confidential reports of nursing staff in collaboration with Nursing Sisters Grade-I/Ward Sister.
(ix) Notifies the nursing administrator regarding special emergencies.

Supervision

In the Supervisory capacity Nursing Superintendent is responsible for:

(i) Establishing efficient nursing services.
(ii) Upkeep of hospital environment and cleanliness through the sanitation department.
(iii) Promotion of good interpersonal relationship between all categories of staff.
(iv) Encouraging and supervising incidental teaching in order to maintain high standard of patient care.
(v) Encouraging the staff to maintain good health habits and keep health fit.
(vi) Supervise regular physical check ups and immunization programmes.
(vii) Ensuring proper care of the nursing personnel during illness.
(viii) Encouraging the nursing personnel to be active in professional association and educational programmes.

(ix) Keeping discipline and report matters pertaining action to the appropriate authority.

(x) Making surprise and regular rounds of the hospital wards and departments to ensure high standard of patient care through the day.

(xi) Encouraging the nursing personnel to maintain proper recording system regarding nursing treatment and care.

(xii) Evaluating with the nursing sisters the standard of care in the wards and departments.

1. Maintenance of records such as:
   (a) Attendance
   (b) Assignments of duties
   (c) Confidential records/reports
2. Correspondence
3. Leave and holidays
4. Issue of hospital certificates and transcripts
5. Shortage and condemnation.

Deputy Nursing Superintendent

Deputy Nursing Superintendent is responsible to the Chief Nursing Officer/Nursing Superintendent and assists her/him in the Nursing Service administration of the hospital—

- Officiates in the absence of Nursing Superintendent.
- Participates in the formulation of Nursing Services' philosophies, objectives and policies.
- Assists in the recruitment of Nursing Staff and Student's selection.
- Makes master duty roster of the Nursing Staff.
- Helps in allocating Nursing personnel to various Nursing Services Departments.
- Keeps records and reports of the Nursing Services.
- Assists in planning and organizing the new units in the hospital, e.g. LCU/CSD, etc.
- Maintains confidential reports and records of the Nursing staff.
- Takes regular hospital rounds.
- Supervises care given in various departments.
- Serves on several hospital committees, e.g. purchase committee, Class IV employee committee, etc.
- Interprets policies and procedures of the hospital care to subordinate staff and others.
- Acts as a Liaison Officer between the Nursing Superintendent and the nursing staff of the hospital.
- Receives night reports from the night supervisor.
- Maintains the attendance and leave register for nurses.
- Pays visit to the sick nurses in the nurse's hostel and nurse's home.

- Initiates condemnation of old and worn-out articles and procurement of new articles.
- Conducts regular physical verification of hospital stock.
- Attends to emergency calls in rotation concerning hospital or hostel problems.

Educational Functions

- Assists in planning and implementing staff development programmes.
- Ensures clinical experience facilities for student nurses in various clinical areas of the hospital.
- Guides and counsels' nursing staff.
- Arranges orientation programmes for new nursing staff.
- Maintains discipline among nursing personnel.
- Organises experience programmes for post-graduate students from different hospitals.

General Duties

- Escorts special visitors, Nursing Superintendent, Medical Superintendent for hospital rounds.
- Arranges and participates in professional and social functions of the staff and students.
- Maintains good public relations.
- Carries out the duties assigned to her by the Nursing Superintendent/CNO.

Nurse Educator

Nurse Educator is responsible to Chief Nursing Officer. She is independently responsible for in-service Education for Nursing staff and domestic staff.

Functions (Teaching)

(i) Responsible for organizing in-service education cell.
(ii) Responsible for planning and implementation of all teaching programmes for nursing staff.
(iii) She should make an arrangement for external lectures.
(iv) Organizing orientation programme for new staff and to conduct bedside clinical demonstration.
(v) Preparing and maintenance of teaching aids.
(vi) Participating in clinical teaching.
(vii) Supervision of all teaching programmes in clinical areas.
(ix) Sending and receiving staff for training/teaching courses.
(x) Evaluation of nursing staff performance from time to time.

Administration and Supervision

(i) Assist in Nursing Administration.
(ii) Supervision of training staff nurses in clinical field.
(iii) Helps in social activities relating to nursing department.
(iv) She is accountable for the maintenance of library.
(v) Counseling and guidance of nursing staff.
(vi) Helping nursing administration formulate nursing philosophy, policies and procedure manual.
(vii) Preparing for budgetary proposal for in-service education.
(viii) Participate in professional activities, e.g. staff meeting, staff education.
(ix) Carry out other duties assigned by nursing administration.

The Nurse Epidemiologist works under the immediate supervision of Nursing Administrator, in collaboration with the doctor in-charge of infection control from Microbiology Department.

(1) She is responsible for the infection control in the hospital.
(2) She is also responsible for health teaching to the patients and attendants in the wards, including Class IV employees.
(3) She assists nursing personnel to prevent cross-infection in the ward by various isolation techniques, such as barrier nursing, etc.

Function

(i) She will work as a liaison officer between all those concerned with infection controls.
(ii) She collects various records indicating incidence of infection and cross-infection in the hospital patients.
(iii) She organises periodic surveys of post-operative surgical infection through the theatre and ward.
(iv) She conducts bacteriological studies among the nursing personnel in areas such as operation theatre, labour room and neonatal nursery.
(v) She also conducts the bacteriological studies of the sterile equipments used in hospital.
(vi) She maintains accurate and complete records of various investigations and findings.
(vii) She recognizes infected patients promptly and advises Nursing Sister Grade-I/Ward Sister regarding the isolated organisms.
(viii) She will maintain records of infection among the members of nursing staff, particularly of infection prone nurses who can be source of infection to the patients and new born babies.

Supervision and Teaching

(i) In addition to her responsibilities regarding infection control she should take active part in the teaching good health habits to the patients and planned health teaching in the wards.
(ii) She motivates the patients and families through health teaching to prevent infection.
(iii) She introduces patient's attendant and ambulatory patients to the working of lavatories and bath room area.
(iv) She orients the patients regarding disposal of garbage.
(v) She organise the collection and supervises the proper disposal of soiled linen.

Assistant Nursing Superintendent

General Nature and Purpose of the Job

The Assistant Nursing Superintendent is responsible for supervisory administration of the nursing services.

Lines of Authority

She is directly responsible to the Nursing Service Administrator, for the supervision of the nursing services and the patient care in the hospital. She is responsible for apprising her of development and improvement of nursing services and patient care.

She has indirect relationship with the Hospital Administrator/ Medical Superintendent with whom she collaborates in the absence of Nursing Administrator.

She is responsible for the Nursing Sister Grade I and the Nursing Sister Grade II and other nursing personnel for performance of their duties.

Function

I. Administration

(i) Assigns nursing staff to ward and departments in collaboration with other nursing service administrators.
(ii) She conducts ward rounds to see seriously ill patients.
(iii) Maintains discipline of nursing staff and domestic staff attached to the ward/units and reports observations if any.
(iv) Investigates complaints and reports to the nursing service office.
(v) Writes confidential reports of nursing staff under the direction of Nursing Service Administrator.
(vi) Develops and maintains office records pertaining to the administration of her department.
(vii) Co-operates with nursing service administration in interpreting and implementing the administrative policies.

(viii) Communicates with patients and their relatives and friends during hospital rounds.
(ix) Notifies the nursing service administrator of any special emergencies in the ward.

2. Supervision

In a supervisory capacity Assistant Nursing Superintendent is responsible for:

(i) Establishing efficient admission and discharge policy in each ward.
(ii) Ensuring efficient nursing care and personal comfort.
(iii) Ensuring proper administration of drugs, treatment and diets.
(iv) Encouraging accurate observation, recording and prompt reporting by the nursing staff.
(v) Standardizing ward routines, e.g. handing and taking over charge, maintenance of intake/output chart; recording vital signs of seriously ill patients, etc.
(vi) Ensuring the smooth functioning of each department through efficient job allocation.
(vii) Ensuring efficient stock maintenance in each ward.
(viii) Maintenance of ward cleanliness.

3. Education

(i) Collaboration with clinical instructors/tutors to provide adequate facilities for clinical teaching programmes in various wards and departments.
(ii) Encourages Nursing Sisters Grade I/Ward Sisters to carry out incidental teaching wherever possible in order to maintain a high standard of nursing care to the patients.

4. General Responsibilities

(i) Attends and participates in staff meetings.
(ii) Attends meetings and participates in activities of professional organisations.
(iii) Carries out any other duties assigned by nursing and medical administrator from time to time.

Nursing Sister Grade I

The Nursing Sister Grade I/Ward Sister is a professional registered nurse who is responsible for the administration of nursing services of a single nursing unit/ward/department. She is accountable to the nursing service administration office for her functions.

Duties and Responsibilities in Relation to Nursing Team

(i) Assesses nursing needs of the patients by classifying patients and assigns patients to the Nursing Sister Grade-II/Staff Nurse recognizing the abilities and expertise of nursing personnel-available.
(ii) Assigns responsibilities and duties to the Class IV personnel.
(iii) Supervises and guides all nursing and non-nursing personnel.
(iv) Assesses nursing needs of individual patients and assists in preparing nursing care plans.
(v) Reads instructions of medical staff and assigns these to nursing personnel.
(vi) Interprets ward policies to nursing and non-nursing personnel.

In carrying out the above duties the Nursing Sister Grade-I/Ward Sister must know the following:

(i) Every individual patient's nursing problems and needs.
(ii) Each nurse's educational and professional background, experience and personality.
(iii) Hospital policies, rules, regulations and ward policies.

Main Functions

Nursing Sister Grade I/Ward Sister creates an environment for an efficient and adequate nursing care by:

(i) Maintaining good relationships with the patients, attendants, staff and others.
(ii) Co-operating with medical and other staff to meet total needs of the patients.
(iii) Ensuring comfortable, orderly and clean environment for the patients.
(iv) Providing and supervising the administration of medicines and treatments as ordered by the doctor.
(v) Co-ordinating the activities of the nursing and non-nursing personnel for optimum patient care.
(vi) Identifying nursing care problems and solving them with the staff.
(vii) Evaluating the quality and quantity of nursing care given and counselling personnel on the basis of the findings.
(viii) Utilizing all opportunities to enrich the clinical expertise for professional nurses.
(ix) Assisting in the teaching of staff and students and participating in the In-service Education Programme.
(x) Providing a planned orientation programme for all new personnel to the unit.

(xi) Carrying out administrative procedures in conformity with the policies of the hospital.

(xii) Keeping all nursing personnel and others informed of hospital policies and practices. .

(xiii) Evaluating staff nurses' (Nursing Sister Grade-II) performance and maintains evaluation records quarterly.

(xiv) Maintaining records of equipment and supplies according to hospital policies.

(xv) Writing reports as required and submit to the appropriate authorities.

(xvi) Providing adequate equipment, supplies and facilities to enable staff and students to carry out the patient care adequately.

(xvii) Maintaining economy in the use of supplies and equipment.

(xviii) Ascertaining proper use and upkeep of all equipment used in the ward.

Daily Responsibilities

(i) Report on duty at the time indicated and take roll call of nursing staff and Class IV employees.

(ii) Attend morning report and hold a short conference with staff and students to discuss problems and difficulties, if any, and make suggestions for improvements in nursing care and nursing service.

(iii) Check equipment and supplies and make certain that all is in readiness for the day's requirements.

(iv) Visit all critically ill patients and patients for surgery or special treatment. Classify patients indicating nursing needs.

(v) Check all patient's charts and records for accuracy and completeness.

(vi) Make assignments for staff nurses (Nursing Sister Grade-II), according to the patient's needs, according to classification of the patients. Critically ill patients should be assigned, considering the nursing abilities of the staff nurses (Nursing Sister Grade-II).

(vii) Notify Nursing Superintendent regarding problems and difficulties and make suggestions for improvements in nursing care and nursing service.

(viii) Check all new orders for medications and treatment and make certain that they have been carried out as ordered.

(ix) Check medicine and treatment lists and make certain that they are correct and upto date. Make any changes that are required.

(x) Accompany Nursing Superintendent on rounds and reports to her the condition of the patients, etc.

(xi) Accompany the doctors on rounds.

(xii) Assist in the care of critically ill patients and post-operatives several times during the day to ascertain their condition.

(xiii) Assist staff nurses (Nursing Sister Grade-II) and students in making out nursing care plans.
(xiv) Notify the doctor immediately of any change in the patient's condition.
(xv) Write reports as required and give report of the patients before going off duty to the evening nurses and the evening supervisors.
(xvi) Maintain records as required.
(xvii) Carry out clinical supervision and teaching as required.
(xviii) Assist staff nurses (Nursing Sister Grade-II) and students in planning for health teaching in the ward for patients and relatives.

Weekly Responsibilities

(i) Plan time schedules and post one week in advance.
(ii) Evaluate and check all ward equipment to see that it is in good working condition.
(iii) Check all supplies to see that there is sufficient to meet requirements.
(iv) Check inventories of all equipment to see whether there is any loss.
(v) Report breakages and losses according to hospital policies.
(vi) Attend conferences and in-Service Education Progarmme.
(vii) Conduct all staff nurses (Nursing Sister Grade) ID conference to discuss problems, changes or improvements.
(viii) Conduct weekly planned teaching programmes.
(ix) Carry out clinical teaching and supervision of incidental teaching.

Staff Nurse/Nursing Sister Grade II

A Staff Nurse/Nursing Sister Grade II works under the immediate supervision of the Nursing Sister Grade I/Ward Sister. She is responsible for the nursing care of the patients assigned to her and as a team leader she directs others in giving quality patient care:

(i) She knows the philosophy, purposes, policies and standard of the hospital and Nursing Department.
(ii) She communicates with patients' relatives and other hospital visitors and explains the nursing care needs of the patient.
(iii) She recognises signs and symptoms in patients and reports on the condition of her patients.
(iv) She maintains accurate and complete records of nursing care and observations of patients.
(v) She has a knowledge of patients at all times and provides nursing care according to the patient's needs.

(vi) She has a knowledge of patients at all times and provides nursing care according to the patients' needs.
(vii) She provides total nursing care for seriously ill patients and keeps the Nursing Sister Grade-II informed.
(viii) She assists the medical staff in ascertaining medical treatment.
(ix) She administers drugs herself and is personally responsible for keeping records of drug which she administers.
(x) She maintains contact with her patients through formal and informal visits.
(xi) She keeps the Nursing Sister Grade-II doctors informed of any change in the condition of the patient.
(xii) She participates along with the family in individualized nursing care.
(xiii) As a team leader she assumes responsibilities for the development and performance of the nursing care.
(xiv) She participates in pilot studies for improvement of nursing care within her assigned unit.
(xv) She takes an active part in staff meetings and education programmes.

2. Administrative

(i) She organises the admission of patients and their nursing care according to the policy laid down for her Unit/Ward.
(ii) She relieves the Nursing Sister Grade-I whenever she is required to do so.
(iii) She maintains record of patient's condition, medicines and treatment given and initials it immediately.
(iv) She maintains hygiene of the patients at all times.
(v) She carries out teaching and keeps her knowledge upto date.
(vi) She supervises and maintains environmental hygiene.
(vii) She maintains privacy and confidentiality in all aspects of nursing care.
(viii) She supervises and teaches the Class-IV workers in the ward or department.
(ix) She assists the Nursing Sister Grade-I in writing staff and student's reports.
(x) She participates in the checking of inventories equipment and requisitions of all supplies.
(xi) She is responsible for supervising the care of patients property/ valuables.
(xii) In her work she co-ordinates and cooperates with workers in other departments, e.g. pharmacy, X-ray and physiotherapy departments, etc.

3. Supervision and Teaching

In addition to responsibilities of teaching, a Nursing Sister Graden should take an active part in teaching good health habits to patients and their relatives by an orientation on admission and health teaching throughout the stay in the hospital:

(i) She manifest her interest in the spiritual welfare of all patients.
(ii) She guides nursing and other personnel in the unit to assure efficient performance for the welfare of the patient.
(iii) She motivates the patient and the family through health care teaching and continuing care which is directed towards the optimal level of health.[39]

Thus the role of the nurse in the hospital setting is of utmost importance. In the words of Shanks and Kennedy: "the fundamental goal of nursing profession is to provide patients with the best possible nursing care. Throughout the history of their profession, nurses have strived to attain this goal while confronted by vast technologic, economic and sociologic changes that have exerted a challenging impact on the nature of the health services provided. Nursing has responded to the demands imposed by these changes and will continue to respond in order to accomplish the goals of the profession. As health services increase, the need for nursing services increases and more and more persons become involved in providing these services."[40]

Job Satisfaction

A person joins an organisation in order to fulfil his own objectives or to satisfy his needs. These needs may be material needs, social needs or psychological needs. If his objectives reconcile with the objectives of the organisation in which he works, then he is likely to satisfy his needs and thereby derive satisfaction at his job. If the individual finds that his job satisfy his needs, then he will continue to stick to his job and he will do it whole-heartily.[41]

This dictum also applies to nursing profession. A person who joins nursing profession must reconcile with the objectives of the nursing profession, along with the gratification. of her personal needs in the profession. When a nurse finds that her job satisfies her personal needs, she will continue to stick to the job and she will do it whole-heartily and efficiently in order to enjoy maximum gratification of her needs. Social scientists and psychologists have given this factor the name of "Job Satisfaction." Thus, Job Satisfaction occupies a prominent place in Scientific Nursing-Service-Administration.

According to Blum, "Job satisfaction is the generalised .attitude resulting from many specific attitudes in three areas-specific job factors, individual adjustment and group relationship." He further adds, "It is an individual phenomenon and is measured by ascertaining certain attitudes.

These attitudes result from summation of many likes and dislikes in connection with the job.

So, job satisfaction is the attitudes people hold towards different aspects of their job. Positive attitudes towards the job being conceptually equivalent to job satisfaction and negative attitudes towards the job being equivalent to job dissatisfaction.

Bush gives a more elaborate definition of job satisfaction as:

"The perception that one's job fulfils or allows the fulfilment of one's important job values, providing and to the degree that those values are congruent with one's needs."[42]

Thus, job satisfaction is generated by an individual's perceptions of how well his job on the whole is congruent with his needs. Since no two human beings are alike, their needs also differ from each other. Therefore, they also differ in the gratification of their needs through their jobs, and attain an experience different levels of job satisfaction. Not only this, the same individual may experience different levels of job satisfaction at different times. Further, the same individual may derive different levels of job satisfaction on different types of jobs.

Job satisfaction of nurses is of great significance as they deal with the living organisms in distress pulsating with the feelings, emotions, sentiments, etc. and the attitudes of nurses towards them can be one of the important factors in ameliorating their sufferings and in attaining well-being. Hence, the role of the nurse in the health delivery system is of utmost importance and the gratification of her needs in and through her job acquires a position of prime importance. Rider has genuinely emphasized that: "Unless the no human needs are met in her work, she will be unable to satisfy the human needs of her patients."[43] An investigation was conducted by the author herself in a teaching hospital to study the perceived dimensions of job satisfaction among the registered staff nurses.

The results established that 54% staff nurses were satisfied whereas 43% were dissatisfied with their job. Only 3% staff nurses had indicated an attitude of indifference towards their job as depicted in diagram. The major factors about which staff nurses were not satisfied were as follows:

1. Allowances.
2. Policies governing promotions.
3. Rewards for outstanding performance.
4. Respect given by society.
5. Respect shown by Class IV employees.
6. Guidance given by seniors in the performance of duties.
7. Communication about major plans before implementation.
8. 12 hours night shift system of duties.
9. Supply of equipment in the ward.
10. Changing room facilities in the ward.
11. Dining place facilities in the ward.

12. Health facilities.
13. Leave facilities.
14. Guidance given in personal matters.
15. Non-nursing jobs.
16. Work load.
17. Role of professional organisations.
18. Opportunities for higher education.
19. Prescribed uniform.
20. Wearing of cap.
21. Policy of losses in the ward.[44]

If all these factors are improved, the nursing personnel will be satisfied internally as well as externally at their jobs. They will feel encouraged to come forward and to meet challenges in which high standards of performance will be maintained to yield best possible results in terms of achievement of goals, i.e. provision of quality patient care.

According to Ford: "Job satisfaction mayor may'not be tied to happiness. But we will know that, we are doing something right if we can change the conditions of the job so that employees will stay on the work productively."[45]

In many countries, the nursing profession is in a state of crisis, resulting in lack of interest among the young to take up nursing. Until society values caring work and women's work more highly and rewards them accordingly, measures taken to attract new recruits will not succeed; well-educated, motivated women will continue to seek careers in occupations that have a higher social standing and higher remuneration. The social consequences of this for the health and well-being of populations will be disastrous. In developing and developed countries alike we need excellent nursing services administration.

CONCLUSION AND RECOMMENDATIONS

Wrong/Bad ways of eating and bad/wrong ways of living are the root cause of all the diseases. Ayurveda teaches us the means and methods to have healthy way of eating as well as healthy way of living.

The world trend has changed and the world community wants to try the medicines based on natural medicinal plants. India is losing a huge amount, estimated about $10 billion yearly, by misuse of Ayurvedic products and raw materials. If Chinese system of medicine can get recognition in the developed countries, why not India. Therefore, India must realise the over-all health scenario in the world and must take effective and collective steps to improve the health care delivery system in the country and show the world community, the ways, to get a long and healthy and diseases free life. The author has recommended the following suggestions as under:

(1) India must declare health care a priority sector like other infrastructure sectors.
(2) There is an urgent need of the hour is to adopt the integrated approach, so that the essentials of these systems may be incorporated for better health care.
(3) The marginalisation of the ISM was effected by the allocation of resources between allopathic and other systems which are completely disproportionate. The total allocation was raised from 35 crore last year to Rs. 100 crore this year. The total allocation for the ministry,of health this year is 43'19 crore, and ISM gets a mere 2.5% of the whole. A clear reflection of marginalisation of the Indian systems of medicine in the public health care system. It should be at par with the Modern system of medicine.
(4) India must revive the old glory as well as upliftment of Indian System of Medicine in the country. For this, a well planned strategy and measures should be implemented to:
   - o Popularize the Indian System of Medicine.
   - o Give equal status to the medical officers, scientists, researchers and administrators of the Indian System of medicine.
   - o Standard the Indian drugs and manufacturers.
   - o Prevent the misuse of Ayurvedic products and raw materials at the earliest.
   - o Do Extensive research on the medicinal plants for modern purposes.
   - o Combat the new menace and challenge of western MNCs, which are taking patents based on Ayurvedic formulas.
(5) There should be an integration of potential of all the systems and should be under one umbrella.

In the health care delivery system of India, the Policy-makers, organizers, administrators and leaders should work in coordination with each other in order to produce effective results. Proper coordination entails adjustments of the systems to each other and of the movement of individual systems in time so that each can make its maximum contribution to the achievement for good health in 21st century.

Notes and References

1. Mehra, P., "The role of nursing personnel in the health delivery system", National Convention of Nurses, D.G.H.S., New Delhi, 1988, p. 9.
2. Immanuel, M.S., "Nursing in India—Health for All", *Health Action*, Vol. 3(9), p. 12, 1990.
3. Osler, Sir William, Acquanimitans and other addresses, Philadelphia, Blackistan Co., p. 163, 1925.

4. Brown, Esther Lucie, Nursing for the future, Russell sage, New York, p. 73, 1948.
5. Jaidev, Charaka Samhita I, Moti Lal Bansarsi Das, Delhi, p. 284, 1985.
6. Gupta, J.P., "Preface", National Convention of Nurses, D.G.H.S., New Delhi, p. 7, 1988.
7. Charaka Samhita, "Quoted in India Medical Review", p. 169, 1938..
8. Olivia, M. Sister, "Aims of Nursing Administration", Washington School of Nursing Educaiton, Catholic Uni., University of America, p. 3, 1947.
9. Charaka Samhita, *op. cit.*, p. 170
10. International Council of Nurses, special and committee report, presented to the ICN Board of Directors and Grand Council meeting at Frankfurt, p. 6 quoted in WHO TRS 347, p. 9, 1965.
11. International Council of Nurses, basic Principles of Nursing Care, TNAI, New Delhi, p. 15, 1969.
12. Kind, E.M., "A Conceptual Framework of Reference for Nursing", *Nursing Research*, Vol. 17(1), pp. 27-31, 1968.
13. Finer, H., Administration and Nursing Services, Mc-Graw Hill, New York, p. 15, 1959.
14. Goddard, H.A., Principles of Administration Applied to Nursing Service, WHO, Geneva, p. 21, 1958.
15. *Ibid.*, p. 30.
16. Gaus, J.M. *et al.*, The Frontiers of the Public Administration, University of Chicago Press, Chicago, pp. 66-67, 1936.
17. Gladden, E.N., The Essentials of Public Administration, Staples Press, London, p. IDS, 1953.
18. Dale, Yoder, Personnel Management and Industrial Relations, Prentice Hall, New Delhi, p. 281, 1956.
19. Schein, E.H., Organisational Psychology, Prentice Hall, New Delhi, p. 92, 1973.
20. Pfiffner, J.M. and Sherwood, F.P. Administrative Organisation, Prentice Hall, New Delhi, p. 30, 1968.
21. Etzioni, A., Modern Organisations, Prentice Hall, New Delhi, p. 3, 1965.
22. Dimock and Dimock, Public Administration, Rinehart, New York, p. 129, 1959.
23. Gladden, E.N., *op. cit.*, p. 105.
24. Bhandari, R.D., "Management of Change", *Hospital Administration, 26(384)*, pp. 235-45, 1989.
25. Simon, H.A., Administrative Behaviour, Macmillian Company, New York, p. 108, 1984.
26. Goddard, H.A., pp. 24-25, 1992.
27. White, L.D., Introduction to the Study of Public Adminitration, Macmillan, New York, p. 355, 1955.
28. Pfiffner,].M. and Presthus, R. Vance, Public Administration, Ronald Press, New York, p. 3, 1960.
29. Fayol, Henri, General and Industrial Mangement, Pitman, London, p. 24, 1949
30. Seckler-Hudson, C., Organization and Management—Theory and Practices, The American University Press, Washington, DC, p. 15, 1957.
31. Dimock and Dimock, *op. cit.*, p. 110.
32. Seckler-Hudson, C., *op. cit.*, p. 99.
33. White, L.D., *op. cit.*, p. 37
34. Avasthi, A. and Maheshwari, S., Public Administration, Lakshmi Narain Aggarwal, Agra, p. 59, 1978.
35. Hansten, R. and Washburn, M., "How to plan what to delegate", *American J.*
36. Joseph Raj, "Unseen Negligence", *Times of India*, p. 5, 29th March, 1994.
37. Goddard, H.A., *op. cit.*, p. 16.

38. Management Techniques: A Module for Nursing Sisters, Punjab Health Systems Corporation, pp. 12-13, 1998.
39. Ghai, Sandhya, Nursing Service Administration: A Case Study of Nehru Hospital, PGI (unpublished Ph.D. thesis submited to Panjab University, Chandigarh), 1998.
40. Shanks, Mary, D. and Kennel-Dorothy, A., "A Theory and Practice of Nursing Service Administration", McGraw-Hill, New York, p. 3, 1965.
41. Blum, M.L., "Industrial Psychology and its social foundations, Harper and Row, New York, p. 124, 1951.
42. Bush, J., "Job Satisfaction, powerlessness and locus of control", *Western J. NUTS. Res.*, 10(6), pp. 718-31, 1988.
43. Rider, "Human Needs and Nursing", *Public Health Nurse*, 42(7), p. 388, 1950.
44. Hands, S.R., "Perceived Dimensions of Job Satisfaction among registered staff nurses" (unpublished M.A. thesis submitted to Panjab University), 1980.
45. Ford, Robert N., 'Motivation through the work itself. American Management Association, New York, p. 199, 1969.

3

Classification of Nursing Personnel and Nature of Duties in Hospitals

The institution of nurses is the backbone of the organisation that provides health services to the community. Nursing is a vocation, implying dedicated service to suffering mankind and a missionary service to be rendered at any hour of the day and night as the need arises. It is a demanding and exacting profession. The ideal relations of the doctor, patient, nurse and the medicine are the four pillars upon which a cure must rest.

Definition of Nursing

A study carried out by the International Council of Nurses defined nursing as:

> "The nurse is a person who has completed a programme of basic nursing education and is qualified and authorised in her country to supply the most responsible service of nursing nature for the promotion of health, the prevention of illness and the care of the sick."[1]

Nursing in its broadest sense, may be defined as the provision of nursing care to individuals, families or communities in connection with the restoration or preservation of health, and comprising the nursing component or the organised health care and preventive services. Such care may be provided by personnel ranging from the nursing aide to the professional nurse and nurse-midwife. The National League for Nursing has adopted the following principles of nursing care:

Nursing care encompasses health promotion, the care and prevention of disability, and rehabilitation, and involves teaching, counselling and emotional support, as well as the care of the sick. Nursing care is an integral part of total health care and is planned and administered in combination with related medical education and welfare services. Nursing personnel respect the individuality, dignity and rights of every person regardless of race, colour, creed, national origin, social or economic status.[2]

The following is a statement taken from the Code of Ethics as Applied to Nursing published by the International Council of Nurses:

Nurses minister to the sick, assume responsibility for creating a physical, social and spiritual environment which will be conducive to recovery and stress the prevention of illness and promotion of health by teaching and example. They render health service to the individual, the family and the community and coordinate their services with members of other health professions.

The words and expectations appear to vary a great deal, and, as with many other professional groups, the nurses' role is a shifting one. A unique function of the nurse has been identified as to assist the individual, sick or well in the performance of those activities contributing to health or its recovery (or to peaceful death that he would perform unaided if he had the necessary strength will or knowledge). And to do this in such a way as to help him gain independence as rapidly as possible.[3]

From these definitions, we infer that nursing is—to nurse the patients or to serve the patients. It is the duty of the nurse to ensure the healing touch of sympathy for the patients. In view of these, Florence Nightingale felt a nurse should be chaste, sober, honest, truthful, trustworthy, punctual, quiet, cheerful and kind.

Categories of Nurses and their Education

There are a large number of categories of nursing personnel depending upon the duration and purpose of training and the level of general education. Let us discuss these categories briefly:

1. *Auxiliary Nurse Midwives*

This category of nurses are trained to function as multi-purpose workers in rural areas. Their functions are: care of the sick, home visits, treatment of minor ailments, maternal and child health care, family planning follow-up, nutritional education, etc. The entrance qualification for training to such category is Middle Standard and the age between 18-30 years. The duration of the training is two years and includes shorter and simpler courses in nursing and midwifery. Students are provided stipends and free accommodation.

2. *Lady Health Visitors' Course*

This is of one and a half year's duration. This is a modified Auxiliary Nurse-Midwives Course with more emphasis on maternal and child health. The minimum entrance qualification is matriculation.

3. General Nursing and Midwifery

Minimum education is matriculation with 45 per cent aggregate marks, having science subjects. Duration is 3 years. They are trained to function efficiently both in hospitals and in the community. It is also called "A" Grade Nursing Course.

4. B.Sc. Nursing Degree Course

This is a University Programme in General Nursing and Midwifery of 4 years' duration. Educational requirements are higher secondary or intermediate with science subjects. Degree programmes are conducted in colleges of nursing in our country at Delhi, Bombay, Bangalore, Chandigarh.

5. Post-Certificate B.Sc. Degree Course

This course is conducted for diploma-holders in seven colleges of nursing in India. Duration of this course is two years.

6. Masters or Doctorate in Nursing

Master is of 2 years' duration and is conducted at Delhi, Bangalore, Chandigarh and Bombay. Doctorate is a 3 year course.

7. Specialised Course

A large number of specialised courses are conducted for diploma-holders. They are:

(a) Ward Sister's Course for efficient management in the wards.
(b) Public Health Nursing is for better community health services.
(c) Tutor's Course
(d) Administration in Nursing
(e) Operation Theatre Training
(f) Pediatric Nursing
(g) Psychiatric Nursing
(h) Orthopedic Nursing

These are essential for efficient functioning of specialised departments.

8. Nurse Technician

This category includes Senior Dressers, Assistant Nurses and Community Nurses. More than one but fewer than three years of nursing education and training is required with a minimum of nine years of general education.

9. Nursing Aides

This category at present includes servants, messengers or other personnel actually performing certain nursing functions. Although aides must be literate, formal training is not generally required, since they are trained on the job to assist in patient care.

On examining critically, we find that it is illogical to classify all the personnel engaged in the assistance of health care as 'Nursing Personnel'. We must restrict the classification of nursing personnel to the nurses formally trained to do the job. We may give different names to the personnel helping the nurses. This would enhance the status of nursing personnel and would focus our attention on a definite category of personnel. The numerous categories of nurses diffuse functions and responsibilities. Dr. Gunaratne, the present Regional Director of the South-East Asia Regional Office of WHO observed that Sri Lanka had experienced some faculties because of the numerous categories of nursing personnel, including staff nurses (who underwent three years' training), emergency nurses (with only three to six months' training), assistant nurses, nursing aides and ward attendants. The Government intended to have only two categories of personnel staff nurse (a fully qualified nurse) and ward labourer (who would have nothing to do with patient care). The same is the problem in many countries. There is a need of rational classification of nursing personnel so that their duties may be clearly demarcated.[4]

In order to provide incentive and motivation to nursing personnel, five per cent of the seats in the proposed short-duration course of medical education may be reserved for the nursing personnel who fulfil the minimum qualifications and have set good standards of service. This would also attract good candidates to this profession.

Let us explain the duties of Important Nursing Personal.

Staff Nurse

Job Summary

Staff Nurse is a first-level professional nurse who provides direct patient care to one patient or a group of patients assigned to her/him during duty shift. She/he Assists in ward management and supervision. She/he is directly responsible to ward supervisor.

Direct Patient Care

- Admits and discharges the patient.
- Maintains personal hygiene and comforts of the patient.
- Attends to the nutritional needs of the patient, prepares invalid's diet and feeds helpless patients.
- Maintains clean and safe environment for the patients.
- Implements and maintains ward policies and routines.
- Co-ordinates patient care with various health team members.
- Follow doctor's rounds.
- Performs technical tasks, e.g., administration of medication, assisting doctors in various medical procedures, preparing

articles and the patient for medical or nursing procedures, recording vital sings, tube feeding, giving enema, bowel wash, dressing, stomach wash, eye and ear-care, collection and sending of specimens, pre- and post-operative care, Assists in administration of transfusion. Perineal care, breast care, baby care, etc.

- Helps doctors in diagnosis and treatment.
- Maintains intake and output chart.
- Observes change in patient's condition and records, takes necessary action and reports to the concerned authority.
- Imparts health education to the patient and his/her family.
- Accompanies very ill-patients sent to other departments or transferred to other institutions.

Ward Management

- Hands over and takes over the patient and ward equipment and supply.
- Keeps the ward neat and tidy.
- Maintains safety of the ward equipments.
- Prepares and checks ward supplies.
- Assists Ward Supervisor/Sister in ward management and officiates in her/his absence. Assists in taking inventories.
- Maintains ward record as assigned to her/him by the sister incharge.

Nursing Sister/Supervisor

Job Summary

Nursing Supervisor is accountable for the nursing care management of a ward or a unit assigned to her/him. She is responsible to the Nursing Superintendent/Assistant Nursing Superintendent for her ward management. She takes full charge of the ward and assigns work for various categories of nursing and non-nursing personnel working with her. She is responsible for safety and comfort of the patients in her ward. In a teaching hospital she is expected to ensure good learning fields.

Direct Patient Care

- Ensures proper admission, discharge of her patients.
- Plans nursing care and makes patients' assignment as per their nursing needs.
- Assists in the direct care of the patient as and when required.
- She/he sees that total health needs of her/his patients are met.
- Ensures safety, comfort and good personal hygiene of her/his patient.

- Assist in planning and administration of therapeutic diet to her patient.
- Sees that helpless patients are regularly fed as per direction.
- Sees that proper observation records of the patients are made and necessary information imparted to the concerned authorities.
- Takes nursing rounds with staff and students.
- Makes rounds with doctors. Assists him in diagnosis and treatment of the patients.
- Implements doctors' instructions concerning patient treatment.
- Assists patient and his/her relative to adjust in the hospital and its routine.
- Co-ordinates patient care with other departments.

Supervision and Administration

- Ensures safe and clean environment for the ward.
- Makes duty and work assignments.
- Indents Ward store keeps necessary records.
- Does regular inventory checking of her/his ward.
- Makes list for condemnation of articles and submits it to all concerned.
- Assists in making ward requirements.
- Establishes and reinforces ward standards prescribed in the procedures and manuals of the ward and the hospital and policies that are in force.
- Acts as liaison officer between ward staff and hospital administration.
- Maintains good public relations in her/his ward.
- Sees that ward statistics are regularly submitted.
- Maintains discipline among the ward workers, e.g., Staff Nurses, students and domestic staff.
- Deals appropriately with any adverse situation that has occurred in the ward and reports to the concerned authorities.
- Reports about any medico-legal cases in the ward.
- Writes and submits confidential reports of the staff.
- Sees that students get desired learning experience in the ward.

Educational Function

- Organises orientation programmes for new staff.

INDIAN NURSING YEAR BOOK: 1983

- Organises formal and informal ward teaching, conducts bedside clinics and demonstrations.

- Conducts ward conferences/meetings.
- Gives incidental teaching to patients, relatives, Staff Nurses, students and the domestic staff.
- Guides in formulation of Nursing care studies, and Nursing care plans, etc.
- Evaluates the students' performance and submits reports to the school authorities.
- Helps in medical and nursing research.
- Encourages staff development programme in her/his ward.

Assistant Nursing Superintendent

Job Summary

She/he is responsible for developing and supervising Nursing Services of a department of a floor consisting of two or more wards or units managed by the ward supervisors. These Units may be In-patient wards, Out-patient Departments/Clinics, Operation Theatres, Obstetric units, central supply departments, etc. She/he is responsible to the Nursing Superintendent and Deputy Nursing Superintendent.

Patient Care and Ward Management

- Organises and plans nursing care activities of the department or floor according to hospital policies and service needs.
- Plans staffing pattern and the other necessary requirements of her/his department.
- Compiles and submits nursing statistics to the concerned authorities.
- Conducts and attends to departmental and intra-departmental meetings/conferences from time to time. Makes regular rounds of her/his department.
- Sees to the safety and general cleanliness of the department.
- Look into general comforts of the patient and his/her relatives.
- Receives report from the night Superintendent of her/his department.
- Evaluates nature and quantum of care required in each unit/ward.
- Makes rotation plan for the Nursing staff under her/his jurisdiction.
- Plans ward management with the ward/unit supervisor of each ward/unit.
- Reinforces the principle of good ward management in each ward.
- Helps ward/unit supervisors to procure their ward unit supplies.

- Supervises the proper use and care of the equipments and supplies in the department.
- Acts as a Public Relations Officer of the unit and deals with problems faced by the ward supervisor, if any, especially with the Class IV employees and patient's attendants.
- Keeps the Nursing Superintendent/Deputy Nursing Superintendent's office informed of the needs of the nursing units/wards under her/him and of any special problem/ problems.

Educational Functions

- Arranges classes and clinical training of nursing students in the department, related to the specialty experience.
- Implements the teaching programme and clinical experience of the students with the help of doctors and Ward Sisters.
- Does counselling guidance of staff and students.
- Arranges and conducts staff development programmes of her/ his department.
- Assists in planning for and participation in the training of auxiliary personnel.
- Writes the confidential reports of her/his ward/unit supervisors.

General

- Escorts the Nursing Superintendent/Deputy Nursing Superintendent and special visitors in the department.
- Participates in various professional activities, e.g. staff education, staff meetings, etc.
- Acts as a liaison officer between the Nursing Department and higher hospital authorities.
- Carries out any other duties delegated by the Nursing Superintendent/Deputy Nursing Superintendent.

Deputy Nursing Superintendent

Job Summary

Responsible to the Nursing Superintendent as assistant to her/him in the Nursing Service administration of the Hospital. She/he is independent incharge of Nursing Service Department of a less than 400-bedded hospital.

Nursing Service

- Officiates in the absence of Nursing Superintendent.
- Participates in the formulation of Nursing Services, philosophies, objectives and policies.

- Assists in the recruitment of Nursing Staff and Students' selection
- Makes master duty roster of the Nursing Staff.
- Helps in allocating Nursing personnel to various Nursing Services Departments.
- Keeps records and reports of the Nursing Services.
- Assists in planning and organizing the new units in the hospital, e.g. I.C.U., C.S.D., etc.
- Maintains confidential report and records of the Nursing staff.
- Takes regular hospital rounds.
- Supervises care given in various departments.
- Serves on several hospital committees, e.g., purchase committee, Class IV employees committee, etc.
- Interprets the policies and procedures of the hospital care to subordinate staff and others.
- Acts as a liaison officer between the Nursing Superintendent and the Nursing staff of the hospital.
- Receives night reports from the night Supervisor. Maintains the attendance and leave register for nurses.
- Assist in the supervision of Nurses' Home, Nurses' Hostel.
- Conducts regular physical verification of hospital stock.
- Initiates condemnation of old worn-out articles and procurement of new articles.
- Attends to emergency calls in rotation concerning hospital or hostel problems.

Educational Functions

- Assists in planning and implementing of staff development programmes.
- Ensures clinical experience facilities for student nurses in various clinical areas of he hospital.
- Guides and counsels Nursing staff.
- Arranges orientation programmes for new Nursing staff.
- Maintains discipline among nursing personnel.
- Organises experience programmes for post-graduate students from different hospitals.

General Duties

- Escorts special visitors, Nursing Superintendent, Medical Superintendent for hospital rounds.
- Arranges and participates in professional and social functions of the staff public relations.
- Maintains good public relations.
- Carries out other duties assigned to her by the Nursing Superintendent.

Nursing Superintendent

Job Summary

Nursing Superintendent is responsible to the Medical Superintendent, in a hospital having 400 or above bed strength. She is accountable for the safe and efficient running of the various Nursing departments in the hospital. She is assisted in carrying out her duties, by the Deputy Nursing Superintendent/Assistant Nursing Superintendent, Ward Supervisors and Clerical, linen room and domestic staff.

Nursing Service

- Participates in the formulation of the philosophy of the hospital in general and those specific to the nursing service.
- Determines goals, aims, objectives and policies of the Nursing Services.
- Implements hospital policies and rules through various Nursing Units.
- Decides and recommends personnel and material requirement for running various Nursing Service departments of the hospital.
- Interviews and recruits Nursing staff.
- Assists in student selection and recruitment of other auxiliary staff whose duties are related to Nursing.
- Ensures the safe and efficient care rendered in the various Nursing departments of the hospital.
- Makes regular hospital rounds in hospitals and wards.
- Checks if standard of care is maintained and patients are nursed in clean, orderly and safe environment.
- Takes hospital rounds with Medical Superintendent.
- Selects and secures proper equipment needed for the hospital or nursing home.
- Looks after the welfare of the patients, their relatives and the Nursing Staff.
- Prepares budgets for the Nursing Services Departments.
- Functions as a member of the condemnation board for linen and other hospital equipments.
- Prepares duty roster, plans staff leave, and disburses salaries.
- Gives counselling and guidance to the subordinate staff.
- Maintains discipline among Nurses and other auxiliary staff.
- Enforces implementation of the hospital rules, regulations and policies.
- Participates in the hospital and intra-Hospital meetings/ conferences.
- Investigates complaints and takes necessary steps.
- Evaluates confidential staff reports and recommends for promotion or higher studies.

- Plans staff development programmes and arranges for in-service education and orientation programmes, etc.
- Inspects hospital kitchen and dietary services of the hospital.
- Arranges students' clinical experience and Council examinations.
- Initiates and participates in Nursing Research.
- General and Office Duties.
- Attends to the general correspondence.
- Maintains necessary records concerning the Nursing Staff, students, confidential reports and health records, etc.
- Submits annual reports of the Nursing Service departments to Medical Superintendent, Indian Nursing Council and Nurses' Registration Council.
- Participates in professional and community activities.

SCHOOLS OF NURSING

Clinical Instruction

- Supervision and teaching of students in the Clinical Public health field.
- Planning and supervision of Clinical teaching schedule including assignment of patients.
- Supervision and guidance of patient care activities carried out by students.
- Assisting in evaluating students' progress.
- Maintaining records related to Clinical experience and teaching.
- Guidance of students.
- Helping students with extra-curricular activities.
- Assisting in conduct of practical examinations.
- Any other duty assigned.

Tutor

- Teaching Nursing subjects.
- Supervision of students in clinical field.
- Arrangement for external lectures.
- Assists in planning and implementation of specific courses.
- Participation in clinical teaching.
- Participation in the School's Committee work.
- Conducting tests (theory and practical).
- Helping students with extra-curricular activities.
- Guidance and counselling of students.
- Maintenance of class-room equipment, supplies and teaching aids.
- Evaluating students' assignments.

- Preparing teaching material under guidance of senior teachers.
- Any other duty assigned.

Senior Tutor

- Responsible for planning and implementation of teaching programmes.
- Teaching subjects in the curriculum.
- Over-all supervision of Clinical teaching programme of subject in hospital/Public Health field.
- Assisting in the administration of the School of Nursing.
- Supervision and guidance of junior teaching staff including in-service education of teacher.
- Supervision of students' health, welfare and security.
- Assisting in the selection of students and admission.
- Assisting in examination, tests (sessionals and terminals).
- Supervision of living conditions of students in the hostel.
- Preparation of reports on students' progress.
- Assisting in maintenance of School records.
- Participation in student guidance activities.
- Guiding students' extra-curricular programmes.
- Assisting the Principal Tutor in the general administration of the school.
- Assisting the Principal Tutor in the procurement of School supplies and equipments.
- Assisting in the Library.
- Planning, implementation and evaluation of specific courses.
- Officiating as Principal Tutor in her/his absence.

Principal Tutor

- General administration of a School of Nursing.
- Administration and overall supervision of teaching programmes.
- Supervision and guidance of teaching staff including organization of in-service education of staff.
- Responsibility for organizing work-load of staff including teaching assignments.
- Supervision of students' welfare, health and security.
- Guidance and counselling of students.
- Administrative arrangements for students' clinical experience and teaching in hospital and Public Health field.
- Recruitment of students and staff.
- Responsibility for conduct of examinations.
- Supervision of living conditions of students in hostel.
- Maintenance of permanent School records.

- Preparation of reports (School reports, progress reports).
- Review and revision of policies, rules, regulations, philosophy of the School.
- Performing Public Relations duties for the School.
- Procurement of School equipments, supplies, stationery.
- Preparation of budgetary proposals
- Supervision of hostel and office staff.
- Participation in the School's committee work.
- Participation in professional activities.
- Supervision of library services.
- Planning for development of the school.

PUBLIC HEALTH COMMUNITY NURSING ORGANIZATION

Auxiliary Nurse-Midwife/Female Health Worker

Under the Multipurpose Workers' scheme, a Health Worker (Female) is expected to cover a population of 5,000. At present, however, she covers a population of 10,000, of which about 4,000 are in her intensive area and the remaining are in the twilight area. In the intensive area, she is responsible for all the activities listed. She carries out the following functions:

Assisting in conducting MCH and Family Planning Clinics; surveying the area and maintaining contact with the local Dais; supervising the work of local Dais, especially in conducting delivery cases, and assisting in the training of minor ailments, antenatal care, intra-natal care, post-natal care: Family Planning follow-up, Nutrition education; maintaining records of daily work; assisting in the registration of deaths and births and births and other vital events occurring in her area, assisting in the immunization programmes; associated with the school health programme; providing Primary Medical care, treatment of minor ailments; first-aid in emergencies and referring of cases; any other duties assigned to her by LHN/PHN/Medical Officers.

Male Health Workers

Under the Multipurpose Workers' scheme, a health worker (male) is expected to cover a population of 5,000 wherein he is to carry out the responsibilities assigned to him. He will have different sets of responsibilities of MCH, Family Planning, immunization and nutrition in the intensive and twilight area of the Health Worker (female).

- Making a visit to each family once a month.
- To identify and notify communicable diseases like Malaria, T.B., etc.
- Educate public about identification, prevention and control of diseases.
- To maintain contact with and educate people about

environmental sanitation. To carry out immunization and Family Planning Programmes.

- To carry out nutrition programmes and identifying cases of malnutrition and helping in their treatment.
- To record vital events and maintain records and statistics. To provide treatment for minor ailments and emergencies.

Lady Health Visitor

Lady Health Visitors are directly responsible for the preventive, promotive, curative and rehabilitative health care carried out in the health centres, maternity homes, hospitals and in the community. Each Health Visitor is responsible for the care of 40,000 populations in the community. She is responsible to the Medical Officer incharge of the center. She independently runs the family planning and maternity centres, maternity home, maternity section of the P.H.C. and Anganwaries in I.C.D.S. projects.

Area of Work

Clinics, fields, maternity homes and hospitals, family planning camps, Emergency duties in flood and epidemic area.

Clinic

Organises ante-natal and post-natal clinics, well baby and family planning clinics; runs full-time clinic with the help of ANMs, Dais, Family Planning social workers, etc. Principal motivator for achieving net Family Planning targets; independently runs 20-bedded or more maternity home; assists doctors in the insertion of I.U.D. and other emergencies; responsible for error of audit, condemnation, etc.

Field Duties

Making regular home visits; arranging educational programmes, raising total health care planning and implementing community health education programmes; arranging seminars, group meetings, etc.

Public Health Nurse (Junior)

Assists senior PHN in carrying out her responsibilities.

Public Health Nurse (Sr)

- Provides health care (preventive, promotive, and curative/rehabilitative) to all individuals, families and community in any field that she is appointed.
- Trains, supervises and guides the health workers in the delivery of health care services to the community.
- Plans health and family welfare programmes along with Health Workers.
- Carries out supervisory home visits in the area covered by the health workers.

- Coordinates the work of male and female health workers and other personnel
- Arranges educational programmes for the community.
- Assists in conducting medical examination of the school children. Reports any anomaly to the concerned specialist.
- Does follow-up and maintains records of the school health care programmes.

Public Health Nurse Supervisor

- Public Health Nurse is responsible to Chief Public Health Nurse/Medical Officer for the provision, supervision and improvement of community health care within the assigned area. She carries out preventive, promotive, curative and rehabilitative care.
- Assists in determining the philosophy and objectives of the community health programme.
- Gives leadership in planning total health care to all individual; families and community in any field that she is appointed.
- Assists in the development of standards of health care in assigned area in harmony with the accepted philosophy, objectives, aims and health policies.
- Assist in the preparation of a budget for the Community Health department and administers the approved budget for the department.
- Major responsibility in guidance and supervision PHN/LHV/ANM/students who are under her care.
- Organizes educational programmes for the Community members including school children, mother and other interested groups in her area.
- Ensures that the workers under her maintain proper records and achieve their targets of work.

Chief/District Public Health Nurse

Provide health services to the Community according to the policies of the department in the area of preventive, promotive, curative and rehabilitative care.

Determines the philosophy and objectives of the Community Health Department of the assigned area; gives leadership in organising and implementing the various health schemes; provides effective supervision and guidance to the members of the health team (community workers); plans, implements and evaluates training programmes at the P.H.C. for various categories of health team; recommends appointments, transfers and promotions of her staff; effectively discharges the responsibilities as administrator and manager of P.H.C.; carries work in the P.H.C. area; contributes to research planned by other health services; Plans and implements community education programmes.

UNION MINISTRY OF HEALTH AND FAMILY WELFARE

Nursing Officer

- Assists Nursing Advisor in all matter of Nursing.
- Relieving Nursing Advisor as and when required.
- International Assistance—UNICEF equipment and supplies and vehicles for all training institutions of Nurses/ANMs.
- Organising and conducting Refresher Courses on an all-India basis, e.g., Nursing Superintendents, Tutors, Principals, Public Health Clinical areas.
- Representing on Committees, give advice and teaching as and when required specially in the area of Public Health Nursing.

Deputy Nursing Advisor (Department of Family Welfare)

Training of various categories of Nursing personnel in Family Planning on an all-India; periodical assessment of the needs of Nursing personnel working in the Family Planning in terms of quantity and quality advising State Government on ways and means of meeting the situation; advising the Government of India in term of policy-making as regards Nursing training. Any other responsibilities assigned.

Nursing Advisor (D.G.H.S.)

- Nursing Advisor being the Head of the Nursing Services in the country is responsible for advising the Government of Indian on all matters concerning Nursing Service, Nursing Education and specialization in Nursing, etc.
- She/he guides, supervises, and co-ordinates Nursing Service and Nursing Education in the States.
- She/he plans total Nursing manpower requirements of the country in the area of Nursing Service, Nursing Education and Continuing Education, etc., in co-operation and co-ordination with State Government units and voluntary agencies.
- Responsible for developing the national and international projects concerning Nursing in India.
- She is a programme officer for Nursing Section in the office of the D.G.H.S., which involves components of all the National Health programmes.
- Maintains liaison with all professional bodies concerned with improving the standard of Nursing Service and Nursing education in the country.

Changing Concept to Meet Present Needs

There has been a change today in the concept of nursing care. In the words of the WHO Expert Committee on nursing, "Minor modifications of existing nursing systems will be inadequate to meet new situations and demands in a rapidly changing society nursing must break with some of its traditions as well as alter existing stereo-types.[5]

The current trend is to involve the nurse in the planning, implementation and evaluation of health programmes rather than simply expecting from her a subservient role in patient care. This requires a great change in the contents and methodology of nursing education. The present nursing education does not encourage research. The nursing journals contain articles of descriptive nature. There is a need to encourage research among the post-graduate nursing students and the faculty members to prepare them for senior positions in the health care delivery system. In a report of an international seminar on Research in Nursing. Brotherston has summarised the position thus:

Whereas the ability and opportunity to carry out research must be limited to a minority in any profession, an urgent and understanding sense of the need for research should be part of the mental equipment of every member of any profession worthy of the name.

He further adds that there is a need for the profession to cultivate research-mindedness which he defines as readiness to look analytically at the events or working methods, a willingness to encourage scientific study or experimentation and an ability to accept the proven conclusions and act accordingly.[6] Research is a fundamental function of a profession which is necessary to ensure its growth and progress. The professional competence of nursing personnel also greatly depends on the availability of research reports based on basic as well as applied researches. A recent book on Essentials of Nursing Research by Notter says that "Research is serious business. It should not be entered into lightly, but neither should it be feared." Nursing research in India still remains neglected.

In order to keep the nursing service up-to-date it is necessary to organise programmes of in-service education and training for all nursing personnel as a means of improving the quality of patient care. The contents of these programmes may be carefully scrutinized. At present, wherever such programmes are being carried out, they are few and lack in seriousness and purpose.

The literature available for the study and research in nursing services and administration is in the context of the developed world and is written by the writers and their professional associations from the developed world. This situation needs to be improved by rejuvenating the nursing professional associations to inculcate professional standards among their members and produce stimulating literature in the context of the needs of their countries. Dr. Chitt (Thailand) while speaking in the Regional Committee meeting of the WHO suggested that steps should be taken to stimulate the establishment and development of professional nursing associations. The essential part to be played by them in the overall growth of the profession has not been fully appreciated even by the nurses themselves.[7] Besides, the nursing associations can help in building professional standards for the professional growth of their members. According to Gardner:

Standards are contagious. They spread throughout an organisation, a group, or a society. If an organisation or group cherishes high standards, the behaviour of the individual who enters it is inevitably influenced.[8]

The future of the nursing profession is in the hands of its members who must strive for creativity, academic excellence and the pursuit of a lofty standard in their professional activities.

CRITICAL APPRAISAL OF NURSING EDUCATION

The quality of nursing education needs immediate change so that qualitative nursing care can be assured. The following facts and suggestions can be taken into consideration to improve the situation:

1. Classification of Nurses Need Review

There should be two categories of nursing personnel—Graduate Nurse and an Auxiliary Nurse/Midwife. The nursing aides may not be included while classifying or defining nursing services.

2. Strict and Higher Entrance Qualifications to Attract Better Quality of Nurses to the Profession

The entrance qualifications should be higher secondary with science. At present, there is no admission policy, i.e., a fixed criteria for admission to nursing schools. It was learnt from direct interviews of some nurses that "merit is no criteria to get admission in a nursing school. Those who have political and other pressures get admitted leaving the best available candidates." It is suggested that nursing schools and colleges should declare their admission policy to ensure fairness, impartiality and proper selection. This would go a long way in improving the nursing profession.

3. Continuous and Well Planned Nursing Education

All nursing education should be continuous and not terminal. Besides, the in-service training programmes may be arranged to keep them abreast of the latest development. The nursing leaders do not appreciate the need for higher education among nurses as they think that nurses are to carry out only routine and mechanical duties which as already mentioned in the earlier part of this chapter is quite short-sighted and wrong. A nursing superintendent of a big hospital informed the present author that the nurses did not need higher education as they were responsible only for elementary activities like bed-making, spongebath noting the temperature, pulse-rate, respiration, etc. The doctors in a hospital hold the same view about the status of nurses. Mrs Narinder Nagpal, Secretary, Trained Nurses Association of India. in her article 'Noble Profession in Neglect' in *The Tribune* (Nov. 15, 1979) had rightly mentioned: "The nursing profession is treated as an auxiliary to the medical profession. We have been telling the medical men that they should leave the nursing profession to the nurses. But, so far we have not met with success." This is the reason why most of the nursing superintendents and hospital authorities are not in favour of deputing their nursing personnel for higher education. Some nurses even seem to feel that they are not allowed to improve their qualifications so that they may not become more qualified than the existing nursing leaders thereby posing a professional threat. It is strange to find that most of the nurses have improved their general qualifications through correspondence courses or by appearing in examinations in a private capacity. Many of them have completed the university degree courses while some of them have passed M.A. examinations from first rate universities. It is suggested that correspondence courses in B.Sc. Nursing may be instituted by some universities to ensure professional growth of nurses otherwise they would be misutilising their energy for improving general qualifications.

4. Status of Nursing Institutions should be Autonomous and not under Medical Personnel

Nursing schools and colleges should be independent institutions. There may be arrangement for formal and informal coordination between the hospital and the nursing institutions. This would save the exploitation of nursing student—perhaps relieve them from excessive clinical work and thus neglects of their studies. Miss Simone Liegois, Secretary, International Committee of Catholic Nurses, New Delhi, has rightly mentioned that the shortage of nurses led to the use of student nurses for services much to the detriment of theoretical instructions. This problem needed to be studied in order to raise the quality of basic training. Besides, nursing schools should adopt some hospitals to enlighten and develop the existing nursing personnel with the latest developments in the field of nursing education and administration. The nursing personnel in the hospital should be encouraged to study in the library so that they keep themselves aware of the latest developments.

5. Developing Quality Nursing Faculty

The nursing teachers of right quality and caliber should be prepared. Some research degree may be instituted. This would encourage research among the nursing educators. Their conditions of service must be the same as of Lecturers in a college. Besides, the time devoted by them in the nursing institutions is about 9 hours which is too much. This leaves no time for research and library reading. They must be encouraged to do independent work by reducing their duty hours. Most of the nurse educators interviewed by the writers were unaware of the system of health care prevailing in the country. They were only equipped in the paper they were teaching. It is suggested that an independent paper on "Health Care Administration" may be started to inform them of all the developments in this sector from the international to the local levels. Whenever a new post-graduate course in a particular medical speciality is started for doctors—

a course for nurses and other workers should also be started simultaneously to prepare a team and provide effective services to the patients. The school and college subjects may include 'Nursing' as one of the papers which can create interest among the students to pursue this profession.[9]

6. Status of Nursing Faculty is too Low: Need of Upgradation

The dearth of nurses especially really well qualified and the unsatisfactory standards of education are because of the poor status of nursing as a career. Besides, the teachers of nursing institutions are not at par with their counterparts in schools and colleges. Professor P.K. Devi has suggested that: "In order to improve the image of nursing, the profession has to consider three aspects. First, the independent way in which nursing benefits humanity by taking crucial decisions at critical times where timely action by nurse-in-charge has led to saving of life, e.g., early diagnosis of fatal complications like pulmonary embolism, collapse, hyperpyrexia, etc. Secondly, administrators must recognise the place of nursing in the medical team and nurses must prepare themselves to take their due place and accept this challenge. Thirdly, economic rewards must be commensurate with the nature of their responsibilities. Employment conditions must not be laid down unilaterally, nursing personnel must have a voice in determining how best and efficiently their services can be utilised.[10]

7. Need of Introducing Administration as a Component of Curriculum

There is a need of introducing principles of management and administration of health care in the curriculum of B.Sc. and M.Sc. Nursing. At present, the principles of administration are taught without making them understand their application in the provision of health care. It is suggested that an independent paper on 'Health Care Administration' may be started at B.Sc. and M.Sc. levels.

8. Need of Expansion of Nursing Institutions

There is a need to open more colleges/schools for imparting nursing education. The delegates at the Third All India Nursing Education Conference held at Chandigarh from 14 to 16 November 1979, strongly demanded a sizable increase in the number of seats in nursing colleges to tackle the growing need for nursing personnel in the country. The conference also urged that the nursing education curricula may be improved so that nurses are able to manage minor ailments on their own.

Indian Nursing Council

We may mention here briefly the role of the Nursing Council. It is a statutory body constituted under the Indian Nursing Council Act, 1947. The Council is responsible for regulation and maintenance of a uniform standard of training for nurses, midwives, auxiliary-nurse-midwives and health visitors. The Council prescribes syllabus and regulations for various nursing courses. In every meeting, the council discusses the issues pertaining to education and training of nursing personnel. There is a need of developing Nursing profession at par with other medical personnel. For this Nursing Council of India should make earnest efforts.

Nursing Associations

Besides there are Nursing Associations at the union level and in all the states. These Associations are engaged in routine activities and are not taking active steps to improve the status of the profession. They should publish material based on research in their journals which can influence policy-makers to look into the demands of the Nursing Profession.

Notes and References

1. International Council of Nurses (1965) Special and Committee reports presented to the IGN Board of Directors and Grand Council meetings in Frankfurt, June 1965, p. 6.
2. National League for Nursing, What People can Expect of Modern Nursing Service, New York, 1959.
3. Henderson, Virginia (1969), Basic Principles of Nursing Care, Geneva, International Council of Nurses, p. 4.
4. WHO, SEA/RC/19/2, p. 96.
5. WHO, Technical Report Series, 1966, No. 347, p. 7.
6. Brotherston, J.H., Research Mindedness and the Health Profession, quoted in International Council of Nurses, Learning to Investigate Nursing Problems, London, 1960, p. 24.
7. WHO, SEA/RC/21/2, p. 111.
8. Gardner, John W., Excellence, New York, 1961, Harper and Brothers, p. 74.
9. WHO, SEA/RC/21/2, p. 111.
10. The First All-India Nursing Education Conference, Chandigarh, April 19-24, 1971, Proceedings of the Conference, p. 26, (Address of Prof. P.K. Devi, P.G.I., Chandigarh). Applied to Nursing published by the International Council of Nurses:

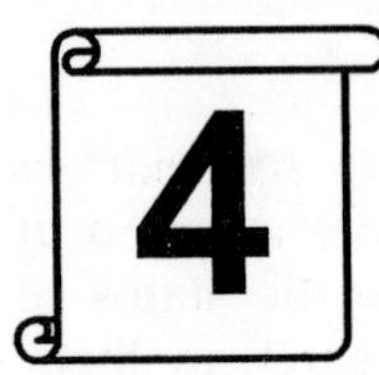

Planning Nursing Organisation and Administration in a Hospital

In a hospital, Nursing Organisation is the most important ingredient of hospital administration. After the formulation of the plan, the organisation is designed to implement the plan. According to Mooney, "Organisation is the form of every human association for the attainment of a common purpose."[1]

And this is what Dimock and Dimock have to say of organisation. "Organisation is the systematic bringing together of inter-dependent parts to form a unified whole through which authority, coordination and control may be exercised to achieve a given purpose . . . Organisation is both structure and human relations."[2]

Herbert A. Simon has concluded,

". . . Organisation affects the people who work for it in five different ways:

(i) The organisation divides work among its members; by giving each employee a particular task, it limits and concentrates his attention on that task.
(ii) The organisation establishes standard practices: by working out detailed procedures, it relieves employees of the need to determine such procedures, each time they use crossways;
(iii) The organisation transmits authoritative decisions by despatching such decisions downward, upward and crossways;
(iv) The organisation provides a communication system; and
(v) The organisation trains and indoctrinates its members by providing for the internalization of influence relating to knowledge, skills and loyalties; training enables employees to make decisions as the organisation would like them to be made."[3]

It would, therefore, be of utmost significance to stress that organisation is not merely a structure; in fact, it embraces a structure as well as the human beings who man and run it in order to realise the pre-conceived objectives. Organisation can be formal and informal. According to Simon formal organisation means, "a planned system of cooperative effort in which each participant has a recognised role to play and duties and tasks to perform. The key to the whole process is effective cooperation among the persons engaged in the operation."[4]

But the actual working of any organisation is not according to the formal plan. The informal relationship of the persons working in the organisation may be different from the formal expected relationship. It is better to encourage informal relationships among nursing organisations to and the community promote decent patient care.

Keith Davis has enumerated the following five practical benefits which can be derived from informal organisations which may be kept in mind by the Nursing Superintendent and other hospital administrators.

1. It blends with the formal organisation to make a workable system for getting the work done.
2. It lightens the workload of the formal manager and fills in some of the gaps in his abilities.
3. It gives suggestion and stability to work groups.
4. It is a very useful channel of communication in the organisation.
5. Its presence encourages the manager to plan and act more carefully than he would otherwise.[5]

Likert has called this general principle, the principle of 'supporting relationships', in which decision-making, leadership, motivation, communication and control move together. He states, "the leadership and other processes of the organisation must be such as to assume a maximum probability that in all interactions and all relationships with the organisation each member will, in the light of his background, values, and expectations, view the experience as supportive and one which builds and maintains his sense of personal worth and importance.[6]

Thus, the Nursing Superintendent and other top nursing personnel should strive as far as possible to create the atmosphere of an informal organisation which would develop the genuine feeling of goodwill and mutual trust among the nursing personnel. It may not be understood that the Nursing Superintendent should not follow the formal plan. The idea is to supplement the good elements of formal organisation with informal organisation to get the best out of the employees.

There are many aspects or problems which must be taken care of while planning an organisation. Let us discuss some of them which are important:

(i) Authority and responsibility—Development of team nursing.

(ii) Delegation and decentralisation.
(iii) Public relations.
(iv) Communication.
(v) Coordination within the nursing unit and coordination with the entire hospital system.
(vi) Supervision and control.
(vii) Personnel management.

AUTHORITY AND RESPONSIBILITY

Authority is the right or power of a person to command other people, to do things and to get work done from them. This authority in a hospital organisation relating to nursing services is exercised by the Nursing Superintendent subject to the overall control of the Medical Superintendent/ Director. It requires complete understanding of the decisions by the Nursing Superintendent and communicating them to the subordinates for implementation responsibility means a charge for which one is responsible or accountable. Since it would not do just to hold a person responsible for performing a task without first giving him/her the authority necessary to get the job done, responsibility should always be coupled with commensurate authority. If a Nursing Superintendent and her team is to perform efficiently, she should know what her job is and with how much authority she has to perform it. This parity is not mathematical but rather co-extensive, because both relate to the same assignments. According to Ernest Dale, Authority should be equal to responsibility. That is, if a man is responsible for the results of a given operation, he should be given enough authority to take the action necessary to ensure success.[7]

The trend today is to make use of authority in collaboration with colleagues-developing team work. Team nursing is a plan of nursing care which makes possible utilisation of all levels of personnel to provide optimum patient care. The nurse should be a team member. This means that the nurse is to be totally integrated into the function of the team. It means involvement of all nursing personnel in the planning and implementation of patient care. It implies "expert planning and assigning of the duties to be performed by all those concerned with the care of the patient, so that nursing will be improved and the entire staff will function smoothly, efficiently and happily."[8]

The team leader must ensure effective communication to ensure effective participation. We can represent the merits of team work with the help of the diagram. Thus, the fuller staff participation is important both as a means of tapping the practical and intellectual resources of all the nursing personnel for the benefit of the organisation and as a way of making work in the organisation more meaningful for each nurse.

Such participation though theoretically available in one form or the other is practically non-existent. Most of the nurses interviewed revealed that the nursing leaders allow superficial participation which serves as an eyewash indicating the presence of distrust in the mind of the nursing leaders. The consequences of this can be represented with the help of the Schematic Chart.

CHART 4.1

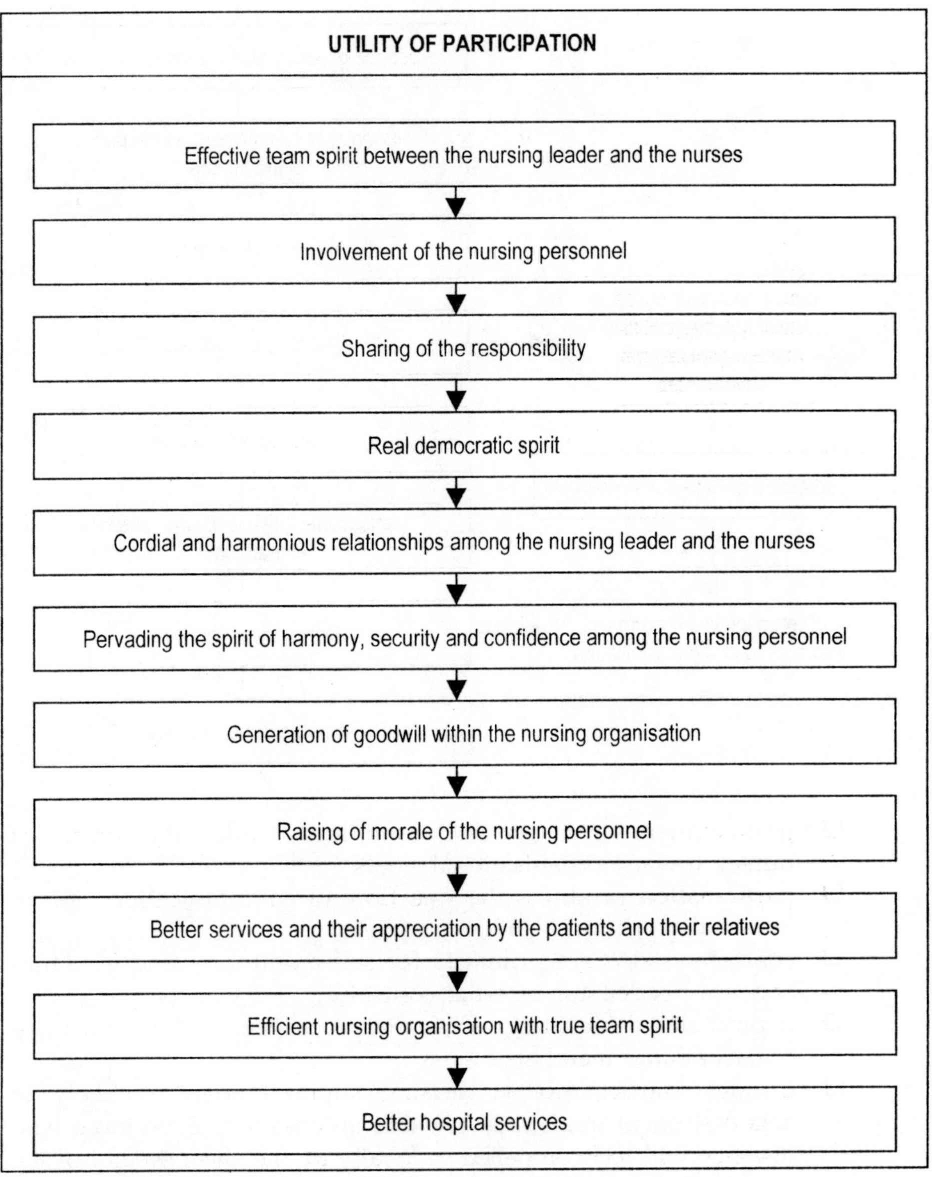

The following advantage would result from the participative management:

CHART 4.2

Implications of Lack of Participation

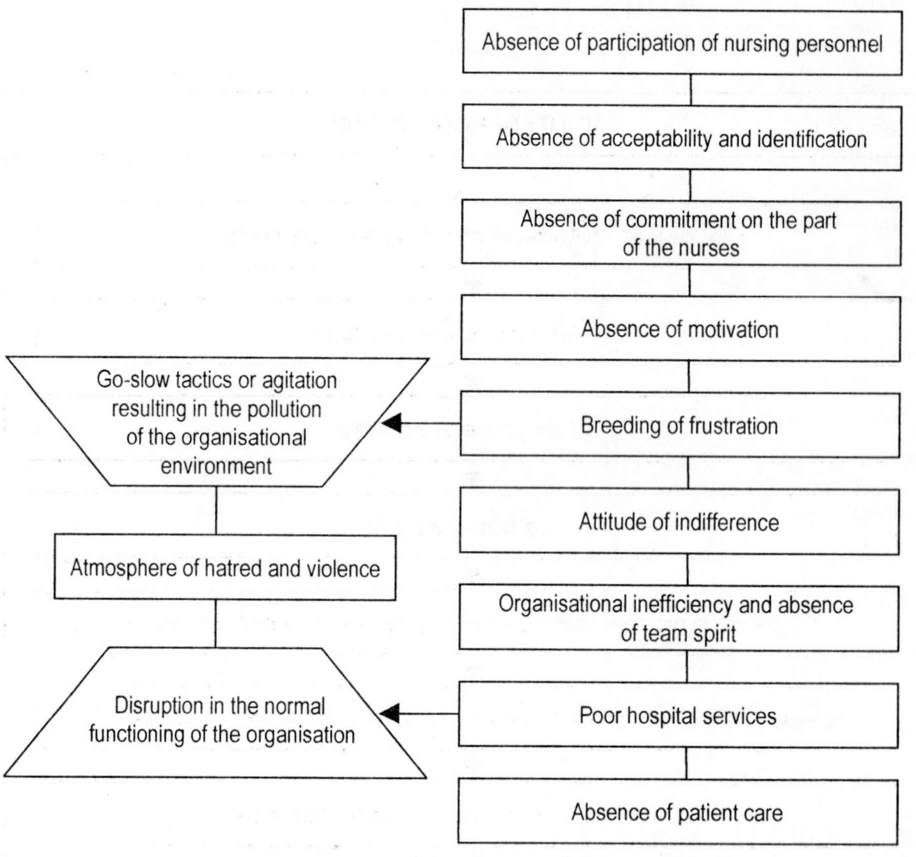

- participation yields personal commitment and involvement of nurses toward organisational goals;
- participation produces the free flow of communications for an informal work force and atmosphere;
- control systems are primarily for self-monitoring and guidance and not needed for external control;
- it produces a high degree of mutual respect and trust among organisational members;
- through participation a nursing superintendent is likely to obtain stronger motivation towards an objective. Even those who disagree will feel compelled to loyalty by the sheer weight of the group opinion; and
- a high degree of confidence is shown in subordinates which facilitates interpersonal processes.

Therefore, we should encourage nurses participation in the promotion of patient care. An employee's participation would build his morale and ultimately his efficiency. An ILO document mentions that the individual worker "is not just a cog in the very big wheel, but that his personal effort is essential for the achievement of the overall production plan."[9]

The research theory in social organisational psychology has also suggested that participation in group decision-making enhances satisfaction among members and removes tensions. Micheal R. Cooper and Micheal T. Wood have shown that satisfaction is effected by the participation. Satisfaction was greater where participation was complete than where it was partial.[10]

There is a need to practise 'Management by Objectives' to ensure fruitful participation. Management by objectives shifts the focus to goals, to the purpose of the activity rather than the activity itself. It is a process whereby the superior and subordinate personnel of an organisation jointly identify its common goals and ensure performance. The Nursing Superintendent must encourage such concepts to develop among nurses. The Nursing Superintendent/Nursing leaders should check the nursing organisation in the context of the essentials of a good organisation to ensure parity between authority and responsibility—

(a) Clear definition of objectives.
(b) Systematic grouping of related activities.
(c) Maximum delegation of authority.
(d) Minimum layering.
(e) Clear demarcation of line and staff functions.
(f) Unity of command.
(g) Correct span of control.
(h) Proper conditions of work.
(i) Provision for easier communication.

For a Nursing Superintendent it is one thing to have the legal right to command, and quite another to have effective direction over the nursing personnel. The former is a matter of formal power. The latter is largely a matter of appeal and influence. It requires, first of all evidence of interest, intelligence, and energy. Unless there is single-mindedness that will enable the Nursing Superintendent to generate and sustain a general concern for the fufilment of the goals of his/her programme he/she cannot hope to assert the authority that signifies the true leadership.

These qualities—interest, intelligence, and energy—are fundamental to strength of personality. But they must also be in balance. Unless the individual's traits are so combined that they enable one to win and hold the devotion of other colleagues, one will have little chance of meeting the demands made on him or her. The nursing personnel must be able to feel that they know the Nursing Superintendent and can trust her because she is the leader of their team. More specially, an executive must have that quality about his or her personality which enables him or her, without sacrificing integrity of purpose, to lubricate human relationships.

Let us understand the psychological reasons for participative management with the help of extracts from the scholars of organisational psychology. This would help the Nursing Superintendent and hospital authorities to manage their personnel efficiently.

McGregor categorised the traditional motivational assumptions as theory X, a string of self-consistent notions about human nature.

Firstly, the theory X assumes that the ordinary man is selfish, lazy, and stimulated by only economic rewards. Secondly, the average man is not interested in work unless goaded by the superior. Thirdly, the individual and organisational goals are contradictory and tend to clash against each other. Fourthly, the average man is devoid of self-discipline and self-control. Finally, he tends to submit himself to the control and direction of others and avoids responsibility.

McGregor, however, points out that man's motivation is far too complex and varied to be explained away wholly by the aforementioned assumptions. In line with other thinkers of social psychology school, McGregor describes his alternative model of motivation as theory Y. The assumptions of theory Y may be stated as:

1. The average man is not really against doing work.
2. The ordinary man can show self-control and self-direction, depending upon the involvement in the work he is doing.
3. The average man craves self-actualisation and it is the responsibility of the management to provide genuine conditions for satisfying his creative abilities and yearnings.
4. The ordinary man, under suitable conditions, would willingly shoulder responsibility.
5. The average man is capable of making significant contributions to the solution of many administrative problems but his potentialities are not fully utilised.

McGregor's assumptions in theory Y roughly correspond to what Maslow and Argyris have stated about human motivation. The running theme of all these thinkers has been to show that adequate attention has not been paid, so far, to the actual potentialities, creativity and responsible behaviour with which the ordinary man is endowed. That way, McGregor has successfully discarded the assumptions of classical school of thoughts. Douglas McGregor has rightly given his preference for theory Y which helps in true organisational building and development. He states:

> "Theory X leads naturally to an emphasis on the tactics of control to procedures and techniques for telling people what to do, for determining whether they are doing it, and for administering rewards and punishments. Since an underlying assumption is that people

must be made to do what is necessary for the success of the enterprise, attention is naturally directed to the techniques of direction and control. Theory Y, on the other hand, leads to a preoccupation with the nature of relationships, with creating an environment which will encourage commitment to organisational objectives and which will provide opportunities for the maximum exercise of initiative, ingenuity, and self-direction in achieving them."[11]

Elton Mayo and his colleagues who pioneered the 'Human Relations' school also recognised and emphasised the use of techniques as given in theory Y. They outlined the following principles, which may be followed by the Nursing Superintendent and other top personnel of the hospital to develop and maintain sound organisational health:

(i) The need for recognition of the 'human' element and the well-being and motivation of the working teams.
(ii) Good supervision is exercised with proper understanding of the subordinates.
(iii) It is important to have proper communication and consultation between the managers and the workers. This creates a sense of participation and involvement among the employees. There should be means of keeping the management informed of what the employees are thinking, fearing, hoping and equally of keeping the employees informed of what the management is thinking or proposing to do.
(iv) The Hawthorne experiments showed that economic incentive is far less powerful than the personal or social incentives.
(v) The flow of work and arrangements of operations should give full play to the informal organisation of the workers.

In Argyris' view an organisation following these principles would be able to achieve efficiency as well as keep its employees satisfied. He says:

"Every individual has 'psychological energy' to expend. Exerting that energy in a way that helps him fulfil his own social and egoistic needs is what motivates an individual. Therefore, provided a hospital is structured in such a way that an individual is able to meet these self-fulfilment needs, the psychological energy will be used in the Hospital's interests. If the reverse is the case the psychological energy can easily be used to thwart the hospital's aims."[12]

This would promote dynamism. To quote Howard P. Smith:

"Dynamism in an organization cannot be declared by fiat, nor can it be generated by the artificial insemination of imposed systems, procedures, and job demands. The enthusiasm people express about their jobs, about each other, and about their organization is a priceless corollary of effective management. Without it, the whole management effort can easily become a kind of drudgery, never moving beyond a mechanical process with little sense of personal involvement. A spirit of dynamism in the organization, a sense of personal involvement in the organization's affairs, is particularly necessary as the setting for meaningful appraisal and development because of the high personal relevance of this activity. Good leadership is the real determinant of such a spirit."

Thus we can say that the Nursing Superintendent must encourage participative management among nursing personnel to raise their morale. Such a situation will be conducive to the growth and development of nursing personnel and they, in turn, would do their best to provide decent patient care. In such a situation, the energy and initiative among the nursing personnel would be self-generating. Besides, all their latent potential energy would be changed into kinetic energy which can be utilised for the promotion of health among the persons visiting the hospitals.

DELEGATION AND DECENTRALISATION

The decentralisation and delegation can lighten the burden of the Nursing Superintendent and enable her to devote attention to important aspects of planning, policy-making and coordination. She should clearly make use of delegation and decentralisation through Sisters and staff Nurses to achieve the objective of best patient care. According to Fayol, "Everything that goes to increase the importance of subordinate's role is decentralisation. Everything which goes to reduce it is centralisation."[12]

Let us first understand the meaning of delegation and decentralisation and their utility.

Delegation is a process whereby a superior divides his total work assignment between himself and subordinates or operative personnel in order to achieve both operative and management specialisation. It is the entrustment of responsibility and authority to others and the creation of accountability for performance. It is to be clearly understood that delegation is not a process of abdication. The person who delegates does not divorce himself from the responsibility and authority which he entrusts.

There are three aspects of delegation: "the entrustment of work of responsibility to another for performance, the entrustment of powers and rights, or authority to be exercised; and the creation of an obligation, or accountability, on the part of the person accepting the delegation to perform in terms of the standards established."[13]

Speedy and realistic decision-making is one of the essentials of efficient administration. In a big and complex organisation like the hospital, the number of decisions to be taken from time to time is so large and the points at which decisions are to be implemented are so many that it becomes necessary to distribute decision-making powers among a number of organs, rather than concentrate in one organ. This is expected to prevent the emergence of bottlenecks which bedevil highly centralised power structures. Thus, one of the important problems of organisation is to reconcile the administrator's desire for centralised control for the sake of uniformity and certainty of decisions and actions, with the people's view that administration should be so organised as to deal with the needs of the different segments of the society in an effective manner.[14]

Effective decision-making can be facilitated by decentralisation and delegation of powers. The word decentralisation is derived from Latin.[15] In modern times, it has been so widely .and differently used that, as Norman D. Palmer says, it has become less precise.[16]

Decentralisation is a twin process of deconcentration and devolution. In deconcentration, a superior officer, in order to make his department function effectively and efficiently, delegates to his sub-ordinate field officials the power to act in his name without transferring to them the authority he enjoys.[17] Devolution, which also implies dispersal of authority, is a process wherein power is transferred from one organ of government to another by means of a piece of legislation or constitution. A certain sphere of jurisdiction, either functional or territorial, is set apart for a legally-constituted body which while administering its authority, enjoys "some power of self-determination."[18]

Besides, proper delegation of authority promotes effective control over operations, due to a clear definition of responsibility and action at each level. When decisions are no longer to be referred up the line, the delay in execution is minimised.[19]

Such delegation can prove to be of considerable value. It can lighten the burden of the Nursing Superintendent and enable her to devote her attention to more important things. The Sisters/Staff Nurses under her may feel more responsible and act more effectively if they are entrusted with responsibility and authority.

The importance of delegation was also stressed by Goddard: "Delegation of responsibility and authority is an important aspect" of successful administration to place the responsibility for decision at the lowest possible organisational level in order to attain decision as speedily as possible. No administrator can do in detail all the work he is administering, for by definition an administrator manages the work of others. Therefore, the principle of delegation of responsibility should be followed to the utmost extent consistent with efficiency and coordination of policy. The responsibility and authority of individuals should be clearly defined in writing, and the authority placed in each position must correspond to the responsibility which the position carries.[20]

PUBLIC RELATIONS

Public relations is the establishment of a climate of understanding. It means interpreting the programme of an organisation to the public and *vice-versa*. According to J.L. McCany:

> "Public relations in government is the composite of all the primary and secondary contacts between the bureaucracy and the citizens and all the interaction of influences and attitudes established in these contacts."

According to Harwood:

> "Public relations may be defined as those aspects of our personal and corporate behaviour which have a social rather than private and personal significance."[21]

The purpose of public relations is not only to supply information, but also to encourage an understanding and cooperation between the citizens and the public servants. This is very important in a hospital situation as the patients and their relatives are demoralised and psychologically insecure. It is the duty of every member of the nursing personnel to maintain public relations in the hospital at various stages of contact with the patients and the visitors.

At present, we find a great deal of alienation between the patients and nursing personnel. A large number of patients who were contacted in various hospitals were of the view that the attitudes and behaviour of the nursing personnel were negative and they lacked sympathy and courtesy. Some even went on to say that their tone was biting and insulting. This has undermined the legitimacy, effectiveness and credibility of the hospital system in our country. We need to promote harmony and mutual trust among the patients and hospital authorities. The objectives of public relations should be to increase prestige and goodwill and to protect the life of the organisation by safeguarding it against unwarranted attacks as well as to remove the genuine complaints and grievances of the people. This would be possible only if all the employees of the hospital, especially the nursing personnel, make it a point to remove the misunderstandings prevailing in the minds of the people about the nature and scope of hospital services.

To improve understanding between the citizens and the hospital personnel, public relations need to be developed in an effective manner to create favourable community opinion towards the hospital services. This would create confidence in the minds of the people towards the competence, fairness, honesty, impartiality and sincerity of the hospital personnel. The following do's and don't may always be kept in mind for better public relations:

1. The patient is never interruption to work: the patient is our work. Everything else can wait!
2. Greet every patient with a friendly smile. Patients are people and they like friendly contact. They usually return it.
3. Call patients by name. Make a game of learning patients' names, and see how many you can remember.
4. Teach your staff members that for patients, all staff members are as important as the doctor.
5. Never argue with a patient. The patient is always right (in his or her own eyes). Be a good listener, agree with them where you can, and do what you can to make them happy.
6. Never say, "I don't know." If you don't known the answer to a patient's question, say, "That is a good question. Let me see if can find out for you."
7. Remember that the patient pays your salary: treat him like your boss!
8. Choose positive words when speaking to a patient. This is a valuable habit that will help you become an effective communicator.
9. Brighten every patient's day, and you'll soon discover that your own life is happier and brighter.
10. Always go the extra mile, do just a little more than the patient expects you to do. For example, make it a habit to phone the patient after discharge from the hospital, to ensure he is doing well. Exceeding patient expectations is the best way to keep your patients happy and keep them as your patients for life

COMMUNICATION

Communication is central to the exercise of authority in an organisation. In the words of Ordway Tead:

> "Communication is the touching of mind by mind, of person with person whether it be one man, to a thousand. It can include conversation, interview, dialogue, visual techniques carefully used."[22]

This is of great significance in case of a nursing situation since any wrong communication or mis-understanding can be responsible for the death of the patient. There is a need to issue orders, instructions and prescriptions to be implemented clearly, simply and understandably. The Nursing Superintendents should not think that their job ends after conveying the commands to the subordinates. He or she should encourage effective participation from the nursing personnel to ensure proper understanding.

Most of the nurses complain that the Nursing Superintendent issues orders as these are received from hospital authorities above her. She does not take pains to understand the implications resulting in confusion. It is her duty to clarify the details of the orders before passing these on for implementation. Nursing Superintendent and Sisters may keep the following facts in mind to achieve effective communication:

(a) Clarity of Thoughts

The first *sine qua non* of good communication is that the idea to be transmitted must be absolutely clear in the mind of the communicator. It must spring from a 'clear' bead. It should be understood by the nursing personnel so that it may be fully appreciated and acted upon.

(b) Attach Importance to Action rather than Words

In all communication, actions are more significant than words. Example is better than precept. A Nursing Superintendent or Sister who is not punctual cannot succeed in enforcing the time-rules on the subordinates.

(c) Participation

In this connection the essential is that both the parties (communicator and the recipient) should participate in the communication. It is the only way to make the communication effective.

(d) Transmission

In this connection the communicator must plan carefully what to communicate, to whom to communicate and how to communicate. How can the Nursing Superintendent/Sister communicate with the workers when they themselves do not know or cannot understand all the facts about the new plans? Further, delegation of authority without responsibility breaks down the spirit of communication.

(e) Keep the System Always Alive

The system of communication should be kept open and alive all the year round. It is only by honest attempts that good communicative relations can be developed.

(f) Cordial Employer-Employee Relations

Effective communication requires good employer-employee relations which enables mutual appreciation of different viewpoints. According to Terry, eight factors are essential to making communication effective:

(a) Inform yourself fully.
(b) Establish a mutual trust in others.
(c) Find a common ground of experience.
(d) Use mutually known words.
(e) Have regard for context.
(f) Secure and hold the receiver's attention.

(g) Employ examples and visual aids.
(h) Practice delaying relations.

According to Millet, seven factors make communication effective, viz., it should be clear, consistent with the expectation of the recipient, adequate, timely, uniform, flexible and acceptable.

To quote Goddard:

> "Efficient communications are essential to all aspects of effective administration. Staff must be adequately and currently informed about plans, methods, schedules, problems, events and progress. It is necessary that instructions, knowledge, and information be passed on for practical application to all concerned, and that they be so clearly presented as to make misinterpretation or misunderstanding impossible. Proper and adequate communication is not just in one direction; it requires a two-way passage. Administrators must be certain that they know and understand the problems of workers for whom they are responsible. Communication must flow from the bottom upwards, as well as from the top down."[23]

Because of the lack of proper communication and resultant misunderstandings, we observe a lot of conflict among the nursing personnel and between the nursing personnel and other staff working in the hospital. This causes a lot of inter-personal rivalries and jealousies. Such conflict may not be treated as an evil. According to Mary Parker Follett, it is possible "to conceive conflict as not necessarily a wasteful outbreak of incompatibilities, but a normal process by which socially valuable differences register themselves for the enrichment of all concerned."[24]

According to her, there are three ways of dealing with conflict. She says, "By domination only one side gets what it wants; by compromise neither side gets what it wants; by integration we find a way by which both sides may get what they want."[25]

She favours integration through uncovering the conflict and bringing the whole thing into the open. The Nursing Superintendent and hospital authorities should encourage methods to remove conflicts in a positive manner.

COORDINATION

In the nursing organisation, different nurses perform different duties because of the adoption of specialisation and division of work achieve maximum results. This is possible only if all the nurses work to achieve the common purpose—welfare of the patient. This can be achieved by devising a proper system of coordination according to J.C. Gharlesworth.

"Coordination is the integration of the several parts into an orderly whole to achieve the purpose of the undertaking."[26]

It is the centripetal force in administration. It is the duty of the Nursing Superintendent to ensure this coordination among the different wards in the hospital and among the nursing personnel in the same ward through effective communication and sharing responsibility. Besides, the Nursing Superintendent has also to coordinate in the hospital authorities. This is very important as she has to slan her activities only in consonance with the total needs of the hospital. She has to liaison with the different departments, e.g., Stores, Central supply, Pharmacy, Dispensary, Registration, Laboratories, etc., to ensure smooth functioning.

Where the central purpose of the organisation is known, understood and considered to be worthy by the workers, it binds them together as a coherent group and unifies their separate efforts into common endeavour to realise the goal. A stimulating leadership Nursing Superintendent/Nursing Sisters can create enthusiasm among the nurses for the common cause and spur them to overcome difficulties.

Ideally, coordination should be achieved through voluntary cooperation of the members of an enterprise. Each member should be ready and willing to adopt his work to secure unified action. Coordination can be secured by:

(a) instilling dominant objectives among the members of the group;
(b) developing generally accepted professional standards and norms making it easy for nurses to work with one another enthusiastically;
(c) promoting informal contacts to supplement formal communication;
(d) encouraging Nursing Sisters to maintain close contact with nurses working under them; and
(e) using group methods for informal exchange views.

SUPERVISION AND CONTROL

Planning communication steps in the process of directions. Like every other aspect of organisation, supervision is also becoming very complicated and complex. The responsibilities of a supervisor has increased and of a good supervisor it is expected that he should have the qualities of head and heart. There is an old saying, "that which is not inspected is not done." Hence inspection, overseeing and supervision, arise in response to needs inherent in the functioning of an organisation.

Supervision is a compound word and its two parts are 'super' and 'vision' which means overseeing. In a hierarchical organisation no one can claim to work without proper supervision. Generally, each officer is given certain powers and responsibilities and is supposed to be responsible to the officer above him for proper execution of the decisions and use of delegated powers. Moreover, for proper functioning of an organisation it is very essential that there should be proper coordination and link among different parts and organs of an organisation. It is also to be ensured that departments of an organisation do exactly the same work which is expected of them. In common parlance, by supervision we mean direction accompanied by authority. In a broad sense we mean superintendence and overseeing. Margaret Williamson has defined supervision as "a process by which workers are helped by a designated staff member to learn according to their needs, to make the best use of their knowledge and skills and to improve their abilities so that they do their jobs more effectively and with increasing satisfaction to themselves and the agency."

The purpose of supervision and control is to ensure that the purpose of the organisation is being fulfilled. In nursing organisations, the supervision and control is still on the old philosophy, i.e., to find faults and award punishments. The purpose of supervision is not only to inspect and inquire but to encourage and inspire, and thus achieve team work. To quote Pfiffner:

The supervisor on the lower levels secures cooperation and production by de-emphasizing his own ego, stimulating group participation, and encouraging the maximum satisfaction of individual egoes that is consistent with coordination.[27]

The supervisor should have training in human relations, public relations and human dynamics. Supervision and control should ensure higher efficiency through clarification and encouragement by the supervisors. John D. Millett rightly observes:

Supervision is more than a process, it is a spirit which animates the relationship between levels of organisation and which induces maximum administrative accomplishment or when unsuccessful, generates administrative paralysis. Effective management is concerned to realise the first and to avoid the second.[28]

According to Newman and Summer, "The aim of control is to assure that the results of operations conform as closely as possible to established goals."[29] Henry Fayol says that "Control consists in verifying whether everything occurs in conformity with the plans adopted, the instructions issued and principles established. It has to its objects to point out weaknesses and errors in order to rectify them and prevent recurrence."[30]

Nigro has identified the following aspects of the supervisor's job:

(i) To satisfy the employees' desire for recognition.
(ii) To keep them informed.
(iii) To allow subordinates to make as many independent decisions as possible.
(iv) To avoid invading the specialist's bailiwick.
(v) To keep the door open for conference and consultations with subordinates.

(vi) To accept the probability of being unpopular with at least a few subordinates.
(vii) To avoid over-optimism.
(viii) To assure the proper interpretation and execution of orders.
(ix) To abolish useless regulations.
(x) To recognise that assistants will sometimes be more intelligent than oneself.
(xi) To make no promises that cannot be fulfilled.
(xii) To expect loyalty and give it too.
(xiii) To avoid discrimination even in favour of a friend.
(xiv) To resist undue pressure and fight for the interests of subordinates.

According to Chester Bernard, subordinates obey authoritarian command only when: (1) they understand what the order is and what purpose to achieve through their collective effort; (2) they feel in their cognition that the command is consistent with the organisational purpose and obeying that they are trying to be moral beings respecting a commitment; (3) they realise and understand that the command is the authority as issued and is compatible with their personal interests. If they see some gains or their personal interests are served in obeying the command, they generally accept it; and (4) they know that they are qualified, competent and capable of complying with the orders. In other words, the nature of the command is such that they are mentally and physically fit to execute it.

The Nursing Superintendent and other nursing leaders must understand the implication of the true meaning of supervision and control. If properly understood, supervision and control would ensure good healthy cooperation among the nursing personnel. Such a situation would be beneficial and rewarding both to the supervisors and employees working under them. The Nursing Superintendent should see that the supervision and control should promote better understanding and cooperation rather than conflict, jealousies, heart-burning, enmity, which are detrimental to the smooth functioning of an organisation, through her role as a friend, guide and philosopher.

PERSONNEL MANAGEMENT

Management of nursing personnel—recruitment, training, promotion, conditions of service, etc.—is an area which holds the key to the success of health care administration especially the hospital services. Bacon, philosopher and administrator, has rightly said: It is vain for princes to take counsel concerning matters if they take no counsel likewise concerning persons; for all matters are as dead images; and the life of the execution of the affairs lies in the good choice of person.

Therefore, the first and foremost task is to pay attention to the administration of personnel in nursing organisations if we expect the effective performance of such organisations.

Several steps, however, need to be taken if the health systems are to succeed in their avowed attempt to attract, retain and utilise the best talents available in the country. This includes healthy internal environment, competitive wage structure, potentialities of rapid growth and advancement and opportunities to create change/challenge and work for the promotion of decent health care.

Inspite of the inherent merits of attending to personnel management, nursing manpower planning has not received due attention in the hospital management in spite of the expansion and diversification of hospital services. The image of the hospital services depends to a great extent upon the requisite skills, aptitudes, integrity and organising capacity of the personnel working in the hospitals. In order to optimise the performance of the nursing personnel as a component of health care administration, we have to harness, coordinate and channelise their capacities and energies in meaningful and fruitful ways.

It is very difficult to deal with all aspects of nursing personnel management as it is a subject by itself. We may mention here briefly one of the serious challenges facing the performance of nursing organisations, i.e., unsatisfactory terms of employment. The importance of pay or compensation is very great for every employee. The standard of living and the social prestige of an employee depends to a great extent on the pay he draws. A man chooses his carrer on the basis of pay which he expects to receive. Rightly does Mason Haire remark, "Pay in one form or another is certainly one of the mainsprings of motivation in our society."[31]

The tempo of challenging and arduous tasks to be undertaken by the nursing personnel can only be accelerated in case they have the right number of employees, with the right level of talent and skills, in the right job, at the right time, performing the right activities and to achieve the right objectives. But the health care systems cannot attract such talented and motivated nursing personnel unless they are able to provide good conditions of service and good status.

Because of the poor conditions of service, it is very difficult to attract better qualified people to take up the nursing profession. Besides, their avenues of promotion are very limited. A staff nurse can be promoted to a Ward Sister and it is very difficult to be promoted beyond that as the positions are very limited. The status of Nursing Superintendent in a hospital is very low which affects the morale of the nursing personnel. In many hospitals, it is the medical Superintendents who are all in all. The Nursing Superintendents are mere decorative pieces. They have no authority. Even the Nurses duty rosters are made by the Medical Superintendents. This leads to a deterioration in the quality of Nursing care. It is suggested that the status of Nursing Superintendent should be raised to the level of Medical Superintendent and more avenues of promotion may be made available to Nursing Sisters. It has been the feeling of most of the nursing personnel interviewed by the writer that, "inadequate salary structure, poor service conditions, want of scope for career development, long duty hours, are the general features of employment causing frustration and low morale."

Thus, an adequate and sound salary structure together with healthy working conditions is the *sine qua non* for the organisational efficiency and effectiveness. Otherwise, as the Administrative Reforms Commission aptly observes, the lack of those conditions has been:

> "one of the major factors for strikes, agitations, inter-service tensions and rivalries, indifferent attitude to work, poor performance, frustration and low morale of the employees."[32]

In other words, the aim of health care systems should be to create and maintain such conditions whereby an employee feels like giving his best, gets satisfaction out of his job and is suitably rewarded. Besides the conditions of service, the personnel management may look after the following aspects of nursing personnel:

(a) to treat the nurses as key personnel and as partners along with the other members of health care and medical team;
(b) to help the nursing personnel reach self-actualisation and thereby help release their creative energy for the promotion of health;
(c) to create facilities for continuous growth, development and training of nursing personnel to make them fit for higher jobs;
(d) to ensure adequate working arrangements and maximum participation in management and decision-making of the health system by nursing personnel;
(e) to provide institutional safeguards for redressal of their grievance esp. to bring their emoluments at par with other professionals and improve their working conditions;
(f) setting good professional standards by senior nursing personnel;
(g) development of unity, energy, initiative and loyally among nursing personnel;
(h) to promote their creativity, insight and loyalty; and
(i) to improve the nurse-patient ratio from 1:12 to 1:3.

Notes and References

1. Mooney, J.D., Principles of Organisation, p. 1.
2. Dimock and Dimack, Public Administration, p. 104.
3. Simon, H.S., Administrative Behavior: Study of the decision-making process in administrative organization (2nd Ed.), New York, Macmillan, 1960.
4. Simon, H., Public Administration, p. 5.

5. Keith Davis, Human Behaviour at Work, 4th Edition, New Your, McGraw Hill, 1972, pp. 257-59.
6. Rensis Likert, The Human Organisation, New York, McGraw-Hill Book Co., 1967, p. 103.
7. Ernest Dale, Management—Theory and Practice, 1973, Tokyo, McGraw-Hill, p. 149.
8. Elizabeth Jones and Joan Grube Ellsworth, "An Experiment in team assignment," *The American Journal of Nursing*, 49, 146 (March), p. 34.
9. ILO, International Labour Conference, 33rd Session, Provisional Records, p. 34.
10. Micheal, Cooper R., and Micheal, Wood T., "Member participation and commitment in group decision-making on influence satisfaction and decision riskness", *Journal of Applied Psychology*, Vol. 59, No. 2, April 1974.
11. Douglas McGregor, *op. cit.*, p. 132.
12. Fayol, Henri, General and International Management, London, Pitman, 1956, p. 26.
13. Lyndall Urwick, The Element of Administration, New York, 1953, pp. 41-42.
14. James, Charlesworth C., Government Administration, New York, 1951, p. 207.
15. Arthur, Machmohan W., Delegation and Autonomy, New Delhi, 1961, p. 15.
16. Norman, Palmer D., "Experiments in Democratic Decentralisation in South Asia", *The Indian Political Science Review*, Delhi University, Vol. I, Oct. 1966-March 1967, Nos. 1 and 2, p. 49.
17. White, L.D. (Ed.), Encyclopaedia of the Social Science, The Macmillan Company, 1951, Vol. 5, p. 43.
18. *Ibid.*, p. 18.
19. *Ibid.*, p. 16.
20. Goddard, H.A., Principles of Administration Applied to Nursing Service, World Health Organisation, Geneva, 1958, p. 85.
21. Harwood, Childs L., An Introduction to Public Opinions, *op. cit.*, p. 2.
22. Ordway Tead, The Art of Administration, New York, McGraw-Hill. 1951, p. 45.
23. Goddard, H.A., Principles of Administration Applied to Nursing Service, World Health Organisation, Geneva, 1958, p. 85.
24. Mary Parker Follet, Creative Experience, New York, Longman's, 1924, pp. 101-02.
25. *Ibid.*, p. 300.
26. J.C. Charlesworth, Government Administration, N.Y, Harper and Brothers, 1951.
27. Pfiffner John M., The Supervision of Personnel, Human Relations in the Management of Men, N.Y., Prentice-Hall, 1951, p. 215.
28. Millett, John, D., *op. cit.*, p. 122.
29. Newman and Summer, The Process of Management, p. 561.
30. Henri Fayol, General and Industrial Management, p. 107.
31. Mason Haire, *et al.*, "Psychological Research in Pay: An overview" in *Personnel Administration*, Paul Pigos and Charles A. Myers, New York, 1969, p. 491.
32. ARC, Report of the Study Team on Promotion Policies, Conduct Rules, Discipline and Morale, Vols. I and II, Delhi, 1967, p. 72.

Decision-making in Nursing Profession in Hospital Services

Nothing is more difficult and therefore
More precious than to be able to decide

—*Napoleon*

Since nursing services have to deal with emergency situations, therefore, there is a need of prompt decision-making about patient care, inventory, facilities, etc. Nurses must be trained to take rational and prompt decisions, since their decision would affect the lives of patients

Webster's dictionary defines decision-making as "the art of determining in one's own mind upon an opinion or course of action." Decision-making has to be done by Nurses every moment since they are involved with the lives of people. Shull and his associates define the decision-making process as ". . . A conscious and human process, involving both individual and social phenomena, based upon factual and value premises, and which includes a choice of one behavioural activity from among one or more alternatives with the intention of moving toward some desired state of affairs."[1] According to Ishwar Dayal, "Decision is the commitment of the decision-maker to act, thereby committing the personnel, material and financial resources of the organization towards the action objectives."[2] Emory and Niland view a decision as only one step in an intellectual process of differentiating among relevant alternatives. It is . . . The point of selection and commitment . . . The decision-maker chooses the preferred purpose the most reasonable task statement, or the best course of action."[3] According to Hodge and Johnson, "Decision-making is to solve any obstacle (problem) that stands between decision-maker and the accomplishment of the organization." According to Donald J. Clough: "The decision-making process involves a problem to be solved, a number of conflicting objectives to be reconciled, a number of possible alternative courses of action from which the 'best' has to be chosen and some way of measuring the value or pay off of alternative courses of action."[4]

According to Kreitner: "Decision-making is a process of identifying and choosing alternative course of action in a manner appropriate to the demand of the situation. The act of choosing implies that alternative courses of action must be weighed and weeded out." According to Manley H. Jones: "Broadly, decision-making involves making organization committed to adoption of a specific course of action and use of resources in a particular manner."

New problems demand new solutions and the Nursing Executives which come out from the routine are highly prized. This requires creativity in the sphere of decision-making. Newsman has indicated five distinct stages which can help the Nursing Executive in this process.[5]

1. *Saturation*: to be familiar with the problems.
2. *Deliberation*: to consider alternative solutions and to rearrange them.
3. *Incubation*: to let the sub-conscious mind work on the problem.
4. *Illustration*: to get new ideas and sensing that it may work.
5. *Accommodation*: to work out the new ideas so that it is a practical solution to the problem.

Hicks[6] gives the following types of creativity in sound decision-making:

1. *Innovative*: Creativity to think total new ideas.
2. *Synthesis*: Creativity to absorb, combine and use ideas from different sources and making it new.
3. *Extension*: Creativity to use old and new ideas.
4. *Duplicaiton*: Creativity to use the other's successful ideas.

According to W. Brooke Groves, "Decision-making is the selection from two or more reasonable possibilities of a course that will, at the time and under circumstances, provide the most suitable solution of the problem at hand.[7]

Nursing personnel must understand as to how decision-making is done about persons, materials, and other activities. This will help them in optimising patient care. In a hospital, nurses are not encouraged to take independent decisions, as there is a supremacy of Director and Medical Superintendent who are from Medical background. There is a need of decentralisation of decision-making to nurses. This would save the time of the medical superintendent and result in better decision-making. As seen from the Chart 5.1, Nurses must take decision on the basis of wide variables.

CHART 5.1

Problem-solving

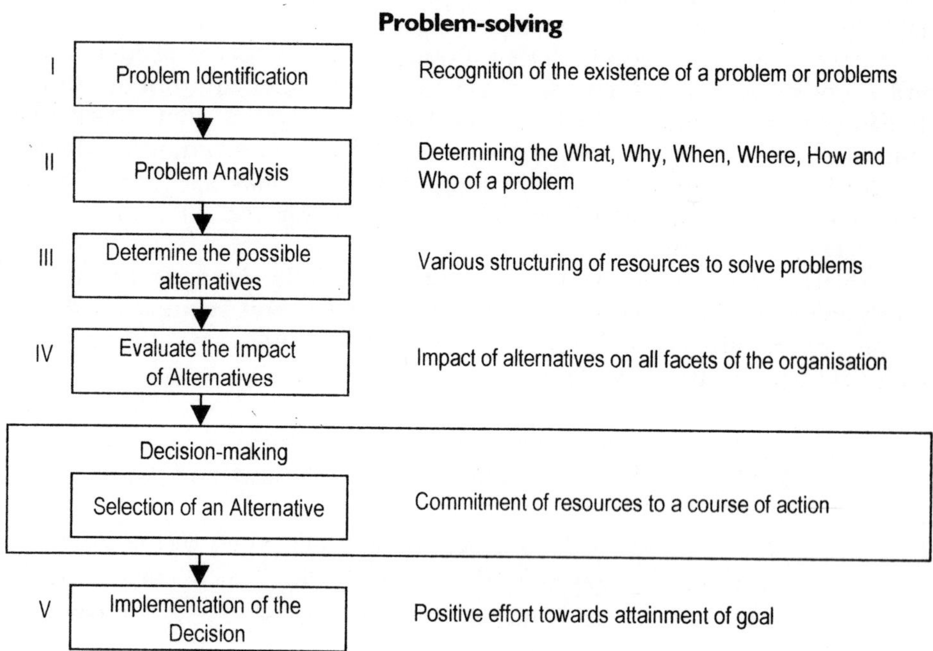

STEPS IN DECISION-MAKING

For nursing personnel, they must engage in five distinct steps as shown in the Chart 5.1. These steps, however, are quite elusive and difficult for the nursing personnel to follow in attempting to reach a wise decision. Most of us take a decision on the basis of emotion or hunch, rather than logic. Therefore, it is necessary for the top level nursing personnel and the middle level nursing personnel working in a health organisation or hospital to take decisions on the basis of the steps outlined below. Let us analyse these steps in detail.

I. Problem Identification

Diagnosing the problems is an essential step for nurses to make rational decision-making. The ability of a nurse to identify problems can be compared to that of a medical doctor diagnosing human problems. Sometimes, decision-maker is led astray by identifying the symptoms as causes and when he subsequently treats the symptoms, he fails to eliminate the cause of the problem. Therefore, it is necessary that the problem is recognized and identified and not simply the symptoms. In this step, the decision-maker must separate the relevant from the irrelevant; the material from the immaterial, the important from the unimportant. In this step, clear thinking and open mindedness should prevail. Once the real problem has been identified and thus stated by the nursing personnel the chances of solving it to a large extent increases. The old proverb that 'a problem defined is a problem half solved' is more than true in this situation.

There are no definite steps in regard to problem identification. Handerson and Soujanen have indicated four main steps for the problem identification. In some situations, all of these may not be required. These are:

(a) determine expectation through present standards of performance,
(b) record actual performance by observation and measurement,
(c) observe differences between expected performance and actual performance; and
(d) identify the problem as to who, how and why of the observed differences.[8] Nurses remain too busy in routing activities, that they hardly find time to take rational decisions which can help the patients and hospitals to achieve decent patient care. Nurses in wards, OPD, Emergency wards, operation theaters want to be dependent on doctors for taking decisions. They should be bold enough to questions the legitimacy of the decision of the doctor. They must be active and smart to take decisions.

2. Problem Analysis

Problem analysis is the next step in successful problem-solving. Henderson and Suojanen have suggested four steps to help problem analysis:[9]

(a) Classify the problem—separate symptoms from problems; describe the causes and nature of the problem. If it is too large—sub-divide it.
(b) Search for and gather data, combine additional information with that what is known and determine relationships.
(c) Analyse data—determine if the data is useful in isolating and describing the problem.
(d) Evaluate data—relate data to symptoms and causes for initial development of solutions.

Nurses must develop analytical ability to analyse the problems from all angles. Nurses must analyse the problem from all angles as the situation would differ from case to case.

3. Determine Possible Alternatives

This is a difficult step in decision-making. The nursing personnel should keep in mind all logical solutions to the problems and not only those which tend to shape up her preconceived or pet solutions. The emphasis should be to minimize the impact of previous solutions to the problem. There is nothing wrong to take into consideration the previous solutions; but the thing to be avoided, however, is relying on these previous solutions as the only source of ideas. In trying to generate new alternatives, it is useful to list all and even the most remote alternatives, one can think of, write on a piece of paper. Alternative solutions are in fact our only tools to mobilize and to train the imagination.

Decisions made without considering alternatives may have unfortunate consequences. Drucker makes this point succinctly in the following passage. Whenever one has to judge, one must have alternatives among which one can choose. A judgement in which one can only say 'yes' or 'no' is no judgement at all. Only, if there are alternatives one can hope to get insight into what is truly at stake . . . A decision without an alternative is a desperate gambler's throw, no matter, how carefully thought it might be. If one has thought through alternatives during the decision-making process, one has something to fall back on, something that has already been thought that has been studied, that is understood. Without such an alternative, one is likely to flounder dismally when reality proves a decision to be inoperative.[10]

4. Evaluate the Impact of each Alternative

The nursing personnel now takes into account each alternative solution to the problem and weighs it in terms of the parameters within which the decision must be made. In fact, the Nurse is forecasting here the impact of a certain alternative, if it is implemented. If the decision is of national importance, then the view of public advisory committee, pressure groups and interest groups are also obtained. In brief, we can list four steps for determining possible alternatives, and examining their impact.

(a) *Identify resources*—list everything available to assist in solving the problem.
(b) *Develop alternative solutions*—develop various resources leading to problem solutions.
(c) *Test each alternative*—analyse for:
Suitability—will it solve the problem; partially, permanently or temporarily.
Feasibility—will it work? How much will it cost? Can we afford it?
Acceptability—is it acceptable to those involved and responsible?
(d) List benefits, cost and risks associated with each alternative. Each alternative and improvement, its benefits and cost of action be weighed. What are the odds and successes of each alternative?

Druker has rightly said that the right decisions grow out of the clash and conflict of divergent opinions and out of the serious consideration of competing alternatives.

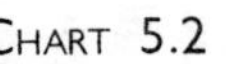

CHART 5.2

The Inter-Disciplinary Framework of Decision-making

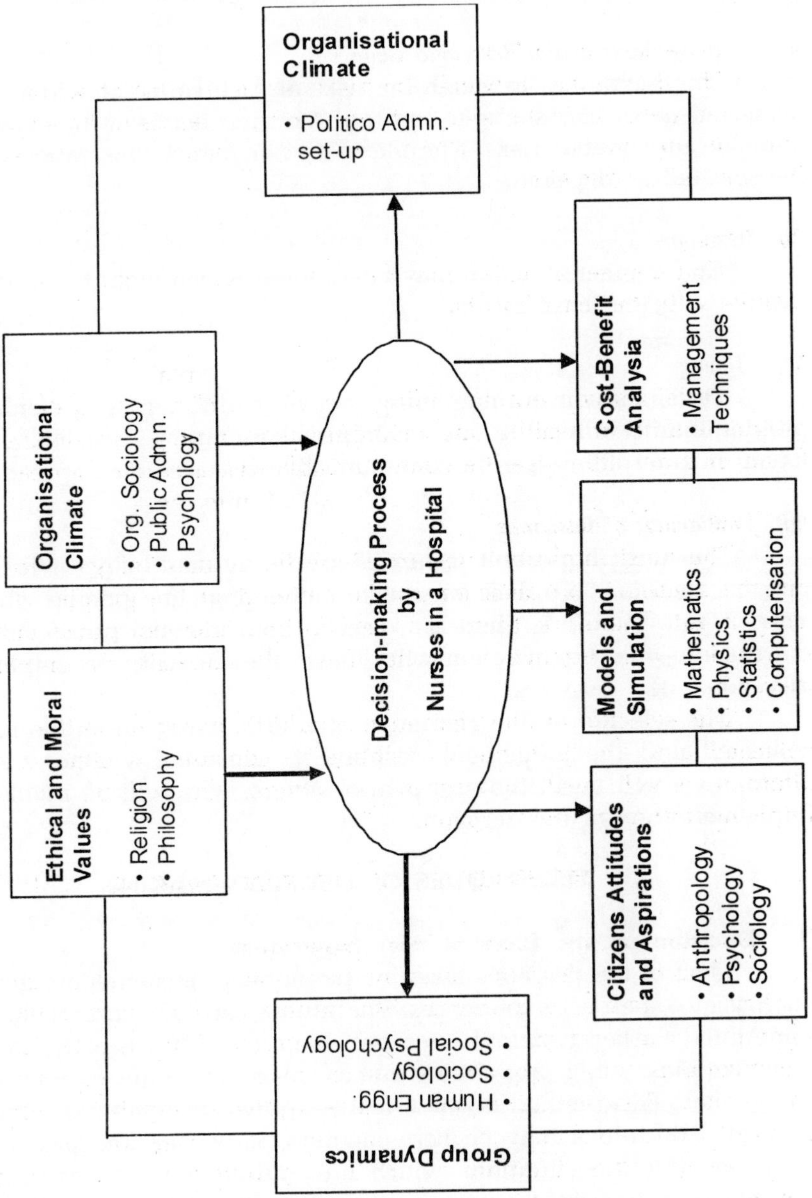

Ethical and Moral Values
- Religion
- Philosophy

Organisational Climate
- Org. Sociology
- Public Admn.
- Psychology

Group Dynamics
- Human Engg.
- Sociology
- Social Psychology

Decision-making Process by Nurses in a Hospital

Organisational Climate
- Politico Admn. set-up

Citizens Attitudes and Aspirations
- Anthropology
- Psychology
- Sociology

Models and Simulation
- Mathematics
- Physics
- Statistics
- Computerisation

Cost-Benefit Analysia
- Management Techniques

5. Selection of an Alternative

This is the final stage of the decision-making. All the alternatives except the one chosen are cut-off. There are four important criteria for picking the best solution:

(a) Management of the Risks and Gains

The Nurse has to weigh the risks of each course of action against the expected gains. He/she is to find out the ratio between the expected gains and the anticipated risks. The alternative in which this ratio is high may be selected as decision.

(b) Economy

That course of action may be adopted which would give the greatest results with the least efforts.

(c) Timing

Decisions concerning timing are very difficult to systematise. In a predominantly unhealthy and malnourished country, decisions have to be taken in time otherwise the communicable diseases may spread.

(d) Availability of Resources

The most important resources are the human beings who will carry out the decision. No decision can be better than the people who have to carry it out. Therefore, there is a need to find talented nurses either inside or outside the organization who have the capacity to implement the decision.

The selection of the alternative should be based upon the information collected and the judgement desirable to consider whether the selected alternatives will meet the approval of others, who will be involved in the implementation of the decision.

TECHNIQUES OF DECISION-MAKING

1. Decision on the Basis of Past Experience

Most of the decisions taken by the nursing personnel are generally on the basis of the past experiences. The nurses can take care of the mistakes committed earlier perceptibly or imperceptibly. That is why, most of the organizations, while appointing nurses insist on some experience in the line earlier. This method is good, if it is applied to repetitive activities and changed conditions may be kept in mind. However, the past experience may not suit the situations which are entirely new, or there has been complete change in the organizational ecology. To quote Koontz and O'Donnell: "If experience is carefully analyzed rather than blindly followed and if, the fundamental reasons for success or failure are distilled from it can be useful as a basis for decision analysis. A successful programme, a well managed hospital, a profitable health promotion, or any other decision that turns out well may furnish useful data for such distillation. Just as no scientist hesitates to build upon the research of others and would be foolish indeed to duplicate it, a nurse can learn much from others. We may keep the following facts in mind to make this technique as a valuable guide to national decision-making:

(i) An effective record of the past experiences must be kept so that it can be retrieved whenever needed.
(ii) Past experiences must be anlysed in today's and future environment.
(iii) Past experience must be analysed critically to ensure their utility in the future.

2. Experimentation

It is better to do experimentation wherever possible, before taking a final decision. In most of the Hospitals, we try the impact of the particular decision through a pilot project. After examining the impact of this pilot project; it is either extended to the entire area/field or stopped.

The difficulties with this techniques are that it would require a lot of money, material and personnel resources to test the efficacy of a decision. It may also take a very long time before we ascertain the impact of that decision. As there would always be a time between the experimentation with the decisions and the ultimate decision, there is a possibility of the future changes as future may not duplicate the present. Nurses have to take decision whether to sterilize the needles for infection or use disposable needles.

3. Quantitative Techniques

In the words of Emory and Niland, "the contribution of quantitative techniques to decision-making is largely in the appraisal step—the analysis of decision possibilities. Quantitative techniques are unable to suggest hypotheses or to define problems or to suggest alternatives. These abilities remain in the domain of personality, experience and creativity. But, once alternatives have been defined, these techniques can be powerful tools for making quick and accurate appraisals.

We must always keep in mind that quantitative techniques are only an aid to management to better decision-making. These are no substitute for better decisions. We concentrate here on some of the techniques, which can improve rational decision-making. We can classify these techniques as follows:

(a) Those techniques which can help the nurses in taking decisions under certainty or deterministic situations, e.g cost benefit analysis, marginal analysis, net work analysis, etc.
(b) Those techniques which can help the management taking decisions under risk, but the decision-maker knows the

probability of each risk. Here we can use techniques like Operational Research.

(c) Those techniques which can help the management in taking decisions under uncertainties. Here we can make use of the utility theory or preference theory and decision trees.

INFORMATION TECHNOLOGY AND DECISION-MAKING

In these high tech times, marked by a revolution in informatics and electronics, an effective nursing administrator has to be a knowledge worker in the service sector, which is knowledge or 'information industry'. In such an industry, we receive information, process information and produce information as an output of decision-making. The time has come where there is hardly any scope of arbitrary and 'ego-based' decision-making. The behaviour of subordinates will be controlled not perhaps through the code of conduct rules but through better knowledge and information on the part of the boss. Hence, the information skill of the decision-maker in getting information, in storing information and using information is going to be the crux and future decision scenario.

Role of Information in Decision-making

- Information plays a significant role in identifying and defining the problem.
- It helps in developing tentative solutions and selecting a suitable one.
- Availability of required information encourages the Nurses for using quantitative techniques in decision-making which give better results.
- Adequate and relevant information on the problem situation may further help in reducing uncertainty and complexity associated with the problem.
- Availability of information may also encourage factual decision-making and ensure higher degree of objectivity and precision.

In the new Millennium, nursing administrators should be trained and encouraged to take patient (and community) friendly decisions, so that they can see the benefits of better health care percolating to them. A culture of not taking prompt and judicious decisions has been afflicting the hospitals and nursing administrators, causing great harm to the people. Things are changing fast, so should be the decisions. Nursing administrators responsible for slowing decisions should be held guilty and punished to set examples. The environment of apathy and indifference should be curbed, rather, the environment of activism should be encouraged, so that concerned persons can take timely decisions. It has been rightly said that a stitch in time saves the nine. We suggest the following for good and timely decisions by nurses:

(a) Nurses should be involved in the decision-making of hospital activities to promote management by objectives.
(b) Nurses should exert pressure to be an essential part of hospital functioning.
(c) Refresher Courses may be arranged for nurses to promote art and science of decision-making.
(d) Nurses should be encouraged to be creative.
(e) One of the top positions in a big hospital should be given to a senior nurse.

Notes and References

1. Fremont A. Shull, Jr. Andre, L. Delbecq. and L.L. Cummings: Organizational Decision-making (New York: McGraw Hill, 1970), p. 31.
2. Ishwar Dayal, "Organisation for Public Policy in Government", Paper presented to the Indian Institute of Public Administration, Annual Conference, New Delhi, 30, 10-73.
3. C. William Emory and Powell Niland: Making Management Decision, Boston: Houghton Miffin, 1968, p. 12.
4. Clough, Donald, J.: Concepts in Management Science, Prentice Hall of India, New Delhi, 1963, p. 51.
5. Newmann William, H. and Others: The Process of Mangaement (Englewood Cliffs, N.J., Printice Hall, 1967), pp. 338-45.
6. Hicks, Herbert G.: "The Management of Organizations" (New York, McGraw Hill, 1967), pp. 1698-1771.
7. W. Brooke Groves: Public Administration in a Democratic Society, Boston, 1950, p. 434.
8. Richer, I., Henderson and Waino W. Soujanen: The Operating Manager, New Delhi, 1975, p. 150.
9. *Ibid.*, p. 151.
10. Peter F. Drucker: The Effective Executive, (New York: Harper and Row, 1967), pp. 147-50.

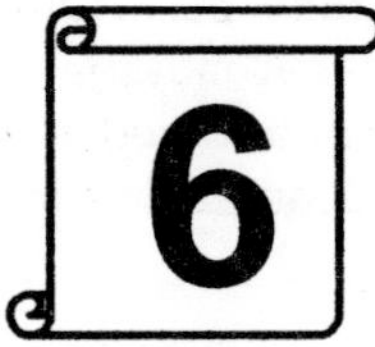

Nursing Leadership in Hospital Excellence

Nursing Leadership is the process to direct and co-ordinate activities of Nurses in a hospital towards the achievement of decent health services, honestly and efficiently.

SIGNIFICANCE

The quality of the health institutions run by Government would be dependent to a great extent upon the quality of the health personnel engaged in their operation. Personnel move the machinery. To quote Mrs. Indira Gandhi: "If Government has to do more for the people. its employees must play a more dynamic and more creative role as the instrument for implementing government policies and programmes."[1] The progress of development would also depend upon the personnel in an organisation. Among the three components required for developmental tasks—men, money and material (M3), it is more the men (or the human element) than any other factor which determines the quantity and quality of the performance and output. After all, even the contribution of money and material to performance depends substantially upon their manipulation by the men in an organisation. Walter R. Sharp has aptly remarked: "Good administration is a composite of effective organisation, adequate material facilities and qualified personnel—Even poorly devised machinery may be made to work if it is manned with well trained, intelligent, imaginative and devoted staff. On the other hand, the best planned organisation may produce unsatisfactory results if it is operated by medicore or disgruntled people."[2]

Personnel constitute an integral part of the organisation. It is with their requisite skills, aptitude, integrity and organising capacity that they can build the image of their organisations as effective institutions in the nation-building process.

Dr. Rajendra Prasad said at the concluding session of the Constituent Assembly:

Whatever the Constitution mayor may not provide, the welfare of the country will depend upon the way in which the country is administered. That will depend upon the men who administer it . . . it requires men of strong character, men of vision, men who will not, sacrifice the interests of the country at large, for the sake of smaller groups, and areas and who rise above the prejudices which are born of these differences.[3]

There is a general tendency in the organisations to lay emphasis on materials and financial management to the utter neglect of the personnel. What are the consequences? It is observed that the process of development takes longer, sometimes even fails. Why? The main reason for this is that we are not attending to the administration of personnel earnestly and forget that they are the real agents of development and ultimately the beneficiaries of the process of development. Persons, properly selected and given the job of their choice, produce excellent results otherwise they are a liability on the organisation.

A leader is a person who plans, organizes, makes decisions and influences people. Leaders have a positive attitude towards people and towards their work. Leaders are always helpful; they expect their efforts to lead to success. A number of factors are involved in the ability to lead, including the following:

(a) Insight into Nursing behaviour.

(b) Ability to plan, organize and direct efforts of other Nursing Personnel.

(c) Decision-making ability on a practical and realistic basis.

(d) Ability to co-ordinate the efforts of other Nursing Personnel.

(e) Keep the environment of work place stimulating.

As the profession moves forward into this new millennium, the need for strong nursing leaders at all levels and in all areas of the profession has been greater. Strong leaders are needed in hospital, professional organizations, in community organizations and in educational. Strong visionary leaders are needed in educational institutions to guide the faculty who will prepare the Nurse of the future. The earlier literature in this century frequently identified leadership as a managerial function. In health care, until recently, strong management skills have received more emphasis on leadership. Fedoruk and Pin come (2000) state, "If Nurses are to assume leadership positions in the health care system of the 21st century, nurse leaders will have to let go of traditional practices and behaviours." Marquis and Huston (2000): "A job does not make a person a leader. Only a person's behaviour determines if he or she occupies a leadership position."

Transformational leaders:

- Identify themselves clearly as agents of change who want to make a difference:
- Are courageous, but take prudent risks;
- Believe in people and work toward empowerment of the individual;
- Are able to describe their values and demonstrate them in their behaviors;
- Are life-long learners;
- Have the ability to cope well with complexity, ambiguity, uncertainly; and
- Are visionaries who can translate dreams and images to others (Wylie, 1994).

Conclusion

The effective Nurse leader must be able to understand the fast paced change of the health care system, management and leadership, and be able to have a clear vision of the preferred future and Nursing, role in this future. The many changes in the health care system include a shift from hospital care to community and home care: an increased emphasis on health promotion and prevention of illness; a better-informed and more involved consumer. Who take a more active role in decisions affecting their care; changes in demographics with an increase in the elderly; and increasingly more complex technology.

According to Warren Bennis and Bert Nanus, managers do things right, leaders do the right things. The success or failure of Nursing organisation depends, to a great extent, upon the administrative capability and motivation of its top Nursing leadership. Administrative capability is an important means of converting or processing programme inputs into outputs such as goods and services. "What makes the leadership variable so crucial in the implementation process is its dynamic, not passive, quality, i.e., its capability to act and react on these critical inputs. It is this administrative and transferring quality of Nursing leadership that could significantly determine the administrative capability of implementing organisation."[1] Dr. Rashmi Diwan in her article, "Self-Development, must for Transformational Nursing Leadership" feels that Transformational leadership would call for drastic changes in the behaviour of self before it could be applied to the organisation. Good managers can be transformed into successful leaders but through real world leadership training.[4]

Professor Yadu Kul Bhushan pinpoints the importance of leadership. He says that henceforth, people and organisations will get "Cash for Kash" where Kash stands for Knowledge, Attitudes, Skills and Habits. HRD focus will increase as Nursing Organisations realise that they are as good as their people. If the people do not measure up, empowerment can backfire.[5]

Peter Drucker defined it as the lifting of man's visions to higher sights, the raising of man's performance to higher standard, the building of man's personality beyond its normal limitations. According to Chester I. Bernard, "It refers to the quality of the behaviour of the individual whereby they guide people on their activities in organised efforts."

The dictionary meaning of the word Leadership is "to lead" shows that the term is used in two different senses: (a) to excel, to be in advance, to be prominent; (b) to guide others, to be head of an organisation, to hold command.

Poonam Mittal and K.B. Akhilesh in their article, "Team Building: Quovadis" define leadership in broader context. To quote them, "Leadership at the individual level and institution building at the organisational level are important determinants of effective team building. Sufficient emphasis thus needs to be laid on the organisational and group building processes for effective movement of micro-identity orientation towards macro-identity orientations. This would essentially aim at issues of designing: (a) institutional spaces, activities and mechanisms which are not related to task but to community processes affiliation management, and learning from collective experiences; and (b) leadership processes and lateral relationships and relatedness."[6]

Leaders may keep in mind that the team members prefer involvement, good team-work, guidance from superiors, two-way communication, good inter-personal relationships, and freedom at work as important factors for success.

People, who are being led, must feel the touch of leadership. To quote Sally Brinkee and Paul Nakai, "Effective leadership is instantly recognizable by those who are touched by it. When a person acts with common sense, grace and intelligence, the people being led feel calm, certain and confident. This fosters humour, faith in the chosen direction, a willingness to pitch in and a sense that the hard work no longer seems difficult."[7]

For developing such leadership, he should possess the following:

(a) Stand on a foundation of values.
(b) Use values to shape your organisation or department and the direction it is headed.
(c) *Remember*: Values outlive goals, choose them well and live the values.

OBJECTIVES

The health personnel are appointed in a health system to achieve its goals. The primary objective of personnel administration, therefore, is to ensure the effective utilization of human resources in the achievement of organisational goals. The personnel administration departments should design and establish an organisational structure and an effective working relationship among all the members of an organisation by division of organisational tasks into jobs, defining clearly the responsibility and authority for each job and its relation with other jobs/personnel in the organisation. The personnel administration must create a soothing environment for the personnel to secure their integration so that they may feel a sense of involvement, commitment and loyalty to the organisation. Such an atmosphere would automatically discard the frictional situations leading to personal jealousies and rivalries, prejudices and idiosyncrasies, personality conflicts, cliques and factions, favouritism and nepotism.

Health personnel administration implies proper planning for work, selection, placement and training of employees so selected, and distribution and assignment of work among them. It includes the supervision, conduct and discipline, motivation, communication and welfare, grievance settlement, terms of employment, etc. It also deals with all other auxiliary functions starting from recruitment and ending with retirement. Personnel administration functions are comprehensive and cover the entire work career of the employees *vis-a-vis* the organisation. This function is universal and is useful for all organisations whether government, industry, hospital or universities.

All the functions performed by the health services must be oriented to rebuild their country, transform its health system, instil in people an ambition for higher standards of life and arouse in them the will and determination to work for such standards. The ambition of the greatest man of our times, Mahatma Gandhi, was to wipe out every tear from every eye. The work of the health service will not be complete until this noble objective is achieved, i.e. decent health care to all. In a broader sense, the Government through its health system should ensure happiness to the people (as given in sruti).

"All human beings may enjoy happiness and bliss. All should be free from troubles. All should promote the welfare of others. No one should suffer from any visible cause which can be prevented by human efforts."

Thus, it is of great importance for state and district level health functionaries, to manage health personnel efficiently to optimize the health services for the benefit of the people and the nation. Management can help them in the following ways:

(a) Detection

Detection is to find out or discover something, e.g. what is happening or what is wrong. We can include such techniques here as input-output analysis, attitude survey, production study, activity sampling, critical path examination, break-even analysis, etc.

(b) Evaluation

Evaluation is a measure or estimate of the value of an item. We can include such techniques here as job evaluation, work measurement, work estimation, performance appraisal, cost benefit analysis, etc.

(c) Improvement

Improvement is better performance, and includes such techniques as management by objectives, method study, value analysis, etc.

(d) Optimisation

To optimise performance, we can use such techniques as linear programming, operations research, etc.

(e) Specification

To specify a desired value or situation or action, we can use such techniques as strategic planning, office and plan layout, designing, etc.

(f) Control

Here we can include such techniques as cost control, credit control, labour control, budget control, etc.

(g) Communication

To communicate information, we can use techniques such as visual aids, suggestion schemes, report writing, communication theory, information theory, management information, etc.

(h) Demonstration

To demonstrate something would include such techniques as programmed learning, job instruction, management development and training, etc.

We are in a hurry; we wish to achieve most; we cannot afford the luxury of wasting our resources for experimentation. What is, therefore, needed is a proper identification of opportunities, setting out of priority areas and accordingly, continually devising technology and techniques appropriate to set-up our value system and to our environment. Let us strive to usher systems/technologies/techniques that are compatible. The call is, therefore, to stress on the know why rather than just on the 'know-how' of techniques and technology. This can materialise only when we bear in mind the following motto.

The Right Technique/Technology.
At the Right Place.
At the Right Time.
At the Right Cost.
With the Right Methods/Means.

There is a real need to reform the current personnel policies in government, semi-government, private, co-operative organisations through intellectual and idealistic approach. The day-to-day personnel administration is the responsibility of the personnel department, but, the major policy decisions in the form of rules or regulations would require the approval of the chief executive. Most of the personnel in an organisation agree that the personnel administration is passing through a crisis caused by the antiquated procedures backed by unwillingness and incapacity to introduce the desired reforms.

QUALITIES OF LEADERSHIP

The attributes that are required in Nursing leadership may be briefly summarized as: technical competence, missionary zeal, the capacity to motivate others, the ability to get along with people, cultural adaptability, the capacity to organise and manage, the capacity to inspire confidence in others, patience and dignity.

Besides, a Nursing leader must believe in the ideals of the organisation, be willing to accept hardships and be prepared to work in a spirit of service. His ambition and enthusiasm should not be dampened by local conditions which may not provide him with the necessary facilities.

EROPA has emphasized the following qualities:

First, there are certain specialised fields of knowledge and skill which are programme-relevant, such as substantive knowledge of engineering in infrastructure programme. Second, managerial expertise and skills are paramount in effective implementation, coordinating and scheduling work, planning and allocating resources, and so on. Third, modern administrative, leaders need human relations' ability to deal with a major resource in organisational life. Motivating people to perform beyond normal requirements to instill a strong sense of programme-commitment and integrity and to incite programme personnel to unfetter the suffocating bonds of anachronistic administrative values, traditions and practices are additional requisite skills. Finally, there are certain 'political' skills required to sustain, support and co-operation from the volatile public (legislators and ministers), mass media, clientele, local, political notables, etc.[6]

Stogdill classified in 1948 a leader's qualities as follows:

1. Capacity (Intelligence, alterness, verbal facility, original judgement).
2. Achievement (scholarship, knowledge, athletic accomplishments).
3. Responsibility (dependability, initiative, persistence, aggressiveness, self-confidence, desire to excel).
4. Participation (activity, sociability, cooperation, adaptability humour).
5. Status (socio-economic position, popularity).
6. Situation (mental level, status, skill needs and interests of followers, objectives to be achieved, etc.).

In lesson from the Top: the search for America's Best Business leaders, Neff and Citrin analysed 50 top-performing companies and identified six common characteristics which are relevant for Nursing Leadership:[7]

1. Focus on strategy;
2. Lead by example;
3. Build a great team;
4. Inspires employees to greatness;
5. Create a flexible organization; and
6. Arrange management and compensation to support these aims.

Leadership depends upon strength of character.

Mr. Justice A.M. Ahmadi, Chief Justice of India, delivered the Convocation Address at the thirty-ninth special convocation of Sardar Patel University. He said, "In the final analysis, what really matters is one's character and not the outward signs of achievement. It requires character to face the unending tests that life constantly puts one through; when faced with a crisis, it is only a person possessed of true character who is able to keep his head steady whilst others around are losing theirs."[8]

Samuel Smiles says in Self Help:

"Character is the noblest possession of an individual. It exercises a greater power than wealth and secure all the honour without the jealousies of fame.

Men of character are not only the conscience of society but in every well governed state they are its best motive power. The strength, the industry and civilization of nations all depend upon individual character. Mind without heart, intelligence without conduct, cleverness without goodness, are powers in their way, but they may be powers only for mischief. We may be instructed or amused by them. But it is sometimes as difficult to admire them as it would be to admire the dexterity of a pickpocket or the horsemanship of a highway man."

To quote Linda Klebe Trevisu and others:

Moral Person + Moral Manager = A reputation for Ethical Leadership.

Being an ethical leader requires developing a reputation for ethical leadership. Ethical leadership pays dividends in employee pride commitment and loyalty—all particularly important in a full employment economy in which good Organisations strive to find and help the best people.[9]

Leaders are responsible for the organisation's moral climate, which in effect, reflects the moral development of the leader as well as the followers. The leader's moral development is a result of character formation through the practice of virtue in private as well as public life. The moral development of followers can be facilitated by the leader through the use of morally appropriate influence strategies and tactics which are motivated and guided by moral intent. Ethical leadership therefore, manifests itself in three dimensions: The leader's motives, the leader's influence strategies and the leader's character formation. They endeavour to cultivate virtues and abstain from vices in order to build up their own inner strength.[10]

In brief we can say that:

A leader is a person who plans, organizes, makes decisions and influences his staff. Leaders are self-confident, and possess a positive attitude towards their work.

Leadership traits mostly include:

- Intelligence
- Emotional stability
- Energy and enthusiasm
- Accommodation and adaptability
- Human Engineering
- Co-existence with subordinates
- Objectivity
- Willingness to make personal sacrifices to assist subordinates
- Develops team spirit.

NEED OF COMMITMENT AND EMPATHY

Quality Nursing needs team work and mutual understanding. Personnel must work in a team to achieve quality. S.J. Maricodoss mentions two ingredients of team work commitment and empathy. To quote him:

Commitment is a deep and profound value of emotional intelligence. It means aligning oneself with the goals of a group or organisation. It is applying oneself completely for a cause. People possessing this competence readily make sacrifice to meet larger organisational goals. Hence more than the individual interests, the group's mission or interest takes priority. It is very deep to the extent of sacrificing oneself. It also involves taking sides or taking stance. Emotionally balanced and committed people don't yield to any pressure or threat, instead they courageously proceed whatever may be the consequences.

Emotionally balanced people are generally empathetic and not sympathetic. Sympathy perpetuates oppression and makes people dependent. Sympathy is a form of judgement. We should therefore avoid being sympathetic towards others. Empathy means understanding the issue or concern that lie behind another's feeling. It is an ability to look at things from other's point of view or to read another's emotions or to put oneself into other's shoes and think from their angle. Avoiding pretension, it enables sensing and responding to a person's unspoken concern or feelings. It can be called the foundation skill for all the social competencies. Empathetic listening is a tremendous deposit in the Emotional Bank Account. Empathy includes understanding others, service orientation, developing others, leveraging diversity and political awareness.[11]

Azim Premji in his article, "Leader for the Knowledge Era" rightly suggests that leaders must build star performers and teams. They must not only attract the best of minds to join the organisation but create a strong sense of ownership in them. Ownership is not just offering stock options. It has more to do with an emotional engagement and integration with the organisation.

Ward sister is the manager of ward. She is responsible for ensuring efficient working of the ward. In district hospital there may not be enough ward sisters, so she has to look after several wards.

Qualities of Ward Sister to be an Efficient Leader

1. Integrity and sincerity.
2. Intelligence.
3. Clarity of vision and able to change vision into reality. She must be able to visualize what improvement can be made in the ward and how she can achieve that.
4. Will power to take difficult decisions or dicisiveness.
5. Shrewd, Independent of men and matters.
6. Flexibility of mind and resourcefulness.
7. Fellow Felling.
8. Progressive and enthusiastic enough to improve the performance of organization.
9. Source of inspiration for subordinates. Motivate others to provide high quality of work and bring out best in other.
10. Ability and willingness to take extra responsibility and committed to work.
11. Emotionally mature and has higher level of competence.
12. Technically competent, teaching ability.
13. *Appraisal*: Able to evaluate her subordinates as well as self-appraisal.
14. *Communication skill*: Patience in explaining her view point to public and know their reaction. Able to maintain positive relationship with public.
15. Possess listening skill, i.e. learn to listen and listen to learn.
16. Role model for her subordinates.
17. Have managerial and supervisory ability.
18. Ready for unforeseen situation and to be a scapegoat.

What a Nurse Leader has to Do

Primary Functions

1. To do supervision, co-ordination and control.
2. To plan and organize functioning in ward for quality patient care.
3. To coordinate with other department for smooth functioning of ward and to provide quality patient care.

4. To evaluate for work done and take action on feedback.
5. Act as counselor to staff, patients and relatives and direct them.
6. Act as clinic specialist in difficult situation when her staff Nurse find it difficult to do.
7. She acts as role model for her subordinates.
8. She takes interest in search.

Secondary Function

1. She attends patiently and sincerely to personal needs of Nurses.
2. She is a father figure for group.
3. She divides their sorrow and multiply their joys.
4. Arrange for social gathering in the group.
5. She be a symbol of group and group has faith in her.
6. She is the star figure among Nurses.

Nursing Leaders must be the persons with vision, initiative and desire to achieve the operational goals with dedication and perseverance. In the words of Jawaharlal Nehru, "No administrator, I suppose, or anyone else for the matter of that, can really do first class work without a sense of function, without some measures of a crusading spirit. I am doing this, I have to achieve this, as a part of great movement in a big cause. That gives a sense of function, not the sense of individual's narrow approach of doing a job in an office for a salary or wage, something connected with your life's outlook or anything, perhaps being interested, as people inevitably are, one's personal preferment in that particular work.[12]

The greatest efficiency and productivity will flow from the efforts of those who find satisfaction in their work and conditions of service, who sense an awareness of usefulness of their functions, who feel encouraged to move ahead and to meet new challenges, who perceive their working environment as one in which high standards of performance are maintained and rewarded and not one in which indolence and incompetence can be ignored or even protected and rewarded. Motivation can do miracles, as a motivated worker can achieve more than an expert with no motivation. Leaders must, therefore, devote considerable time and effort in planning for, and achieving, high levels of motivation and morale. In such a situation, we would achieve goal congruence, i.e., identity between the individual goals and the organisational goals.

Living together is a beginning.
Keeping together is progress.
Working together is success.

Norman Vincent Peale has advised the leaders to be highly charged. To quote him: Think excitement, talk excitement, act out excitement, and you are bound to become an excited person. Life will take on a new zest, deeper interest, and greater meaning.

LIMITATIONS

The performance of the personnel functions by the personnel department is limited in practice because of the following drawbacks:

(a) Inadequate understanding and appreciation of the basic and the essential problems of personnel management;
(b) No future personnel planning resulting in the absence of timely corrective measures;
(c) Lack of control and supervision over the personnel especially of the field personnel;
(d) Lack of effective decentralisation to substantive departments resulting in delays and confusion;
(e) Absence of effective participation of the employees resulting in a gulf between the management and the staff;
(f) Lack of a manual setting out all the rules and regulations clearly and fully in a single document;
(g) Lack of effective communication between the staff and management; and
(h) Lack of personnel standards of performance which should be realistic, appropriate and flexible. Besides, these should be stated with sufficient clarity to allow measurement of achievements and rationale in the sense that it is based on acceptable criteria related to performance and to the degree of responsibility.

Therefore, there is a need to design properly structured personnel departments or personnel agencies staffed by competent personnel.

NOTES AND REFERENCES

1. Gabriel V. Legisias, College of Public Administration, University of Philippines, 'Administrative Capability as a Neglected Dimension in the Implementation of Development Programmes and Projects', Seventh General Assembly and Conference of EROPA on Implementation of the Problem of Achieving Results, October 24-31, 1973, Vol. III, pp. 3-14.
2. Rashmi Diwan, Self-Development Must For Transformational Leadership, in *Indian Management,* Vol. 39, No. 9, Sept. 2000.
3. Y.K. Bhushan, *Ibid.*
4. Poonam Mittal and K.B. Abhishek, Team Building, Quovadis in ASCI, *Journal of Management,* Vol. 23, No. 1, Sept. 1993.
5. Sally Brinkee and Paul Nakai, Leadership From Within, *Journal of Human Values,* Vol. 6, No. 1, January-June, 2000.
6. ERORA: Summary Report of the Seventh General Assembly and Conference on 'Implementation: the Problem of Achieving Results', Vol. II, pp. 1-8.
7. Thomas J. Neffand, James F. Citrin, Lessons from the Top, The Search For America's Best Business Leaders, New York, Doubleday, 1999.
8. *University News,* AIU, New Delhi, Feb. 17, 1997, p. 8.

9. Linda Klele Trivino, *et al.* Moral Person and Manager: How Executives Develop a Reputation for Ethical Leadership" in *California Management and Review,* Vol. 42, No. 4, Summer, 2000.

10. R.N. Kanungo and M. Mendonce, Ethical Leadership in Three Dimensions in *Journal of Human Values,* IIM, Calcutta, Vol. 4, No. 2, July-Dec., 1998, pp. 136-37.

11. Robert H. Rosen, Learning to lead, in Frances Hassellein *et al.,* 'The Peter Drucker Foundation', 1997, p. 302.

12. Jawaharlal Nehru and Public Administration, *IJPA,* New Delhi, 1975, p. 88.

7

Nurse-Patient Relationship in Hospitals: Nurture and Nourishment

The nurture and nourishment of every human being starts, right at birth and is required throughout life. The role of a nurse may be assumed by different individuals at different times, e.g. nobody is a better 'nurse' than one's own mother, in most situations and stages of life. The concept of a professional nurse came much later. In the earlier ages religious orders took to nursing out of compassion or charity. Even now many medical and surgical relief camps are held by temples, churches and gurdwaras, where the devotees perform selfless nursing service for the care of the patients with dedication and earnestness. Many consider such 'nursing service' as the greatest Dharma, as ordained by God. The Sisters of Mercy order, which still exists today, was set-up in the 1830s by the Roman Catholic Church in Dublin. It became known throughout the world for its work in caring for the sick and elderly. In the 1800s, the famous prison reformer Elizabeth Fry set-up the Institute of Nursing Sisters, which offered training in how to care for the sick. Nursing emerged as a profession in the late 19th century. Before this time, nursing did not require any training, was badly paid and did not have a respectable reputation. Florence Nightingale was instrumental in bringing about this change. In 1860, Nightingale set-up the first nurse's training school at St. Thomas's Hospital; this became the foundation of most nursing programmes within the world.

Now, nursing as a profession is practiced throughout the world and is in no way less important than medical profession, in giving succor and rehabilitation to the sick, elderly and disabled. Nursing-service is a devoted profession in the service of mankind, which provides curative, preventive and promotive health services to individuals and community irrespective of cast, creed, religion and gender. Nursing has a great role in national health programme. A nurse is an assistant to a doctor, but has an independent

CHART 7.1

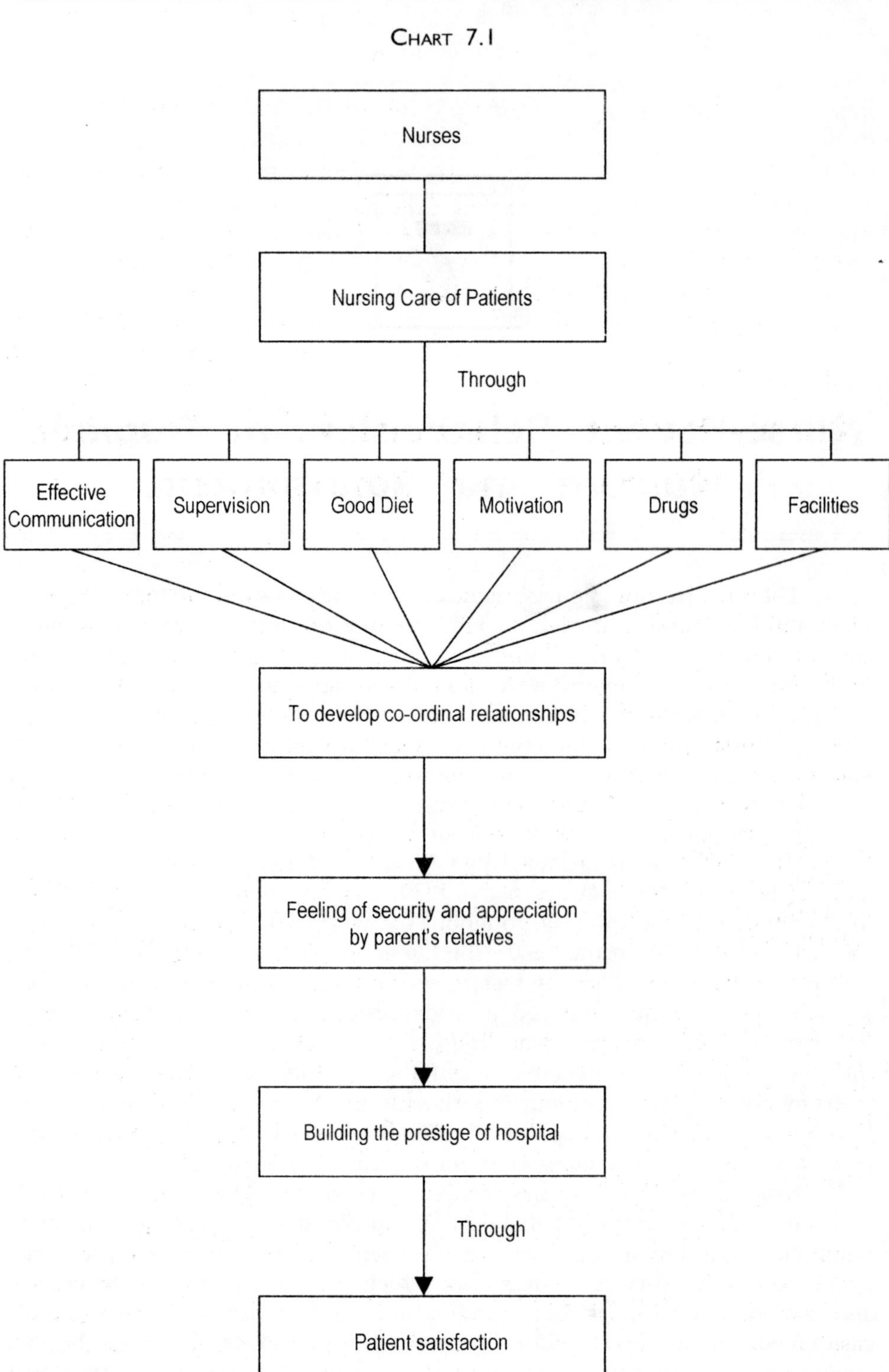
Nurses
Nursing Care of Patients
Through
Effective Communication
Supervision
Good Diet
Motivation
Drugs
Facilities
To develop co-ordinal relationships
Feeling of security and appreciation by parent's relatives
Building the prestige of hospital
Through
Patient satisfaction

part to play in several areas, where a doctor need not be present. They do work as complimentary to the physician in caring the sick, but her relationship with the patient is continuous and involves both the state of illness as well as state of well being. This service is based on knowledge of nursing, skill, affection and cleanliness. Charka defined the 4 attributes of a good nurse: (i) the manner in which drugs are prepared and administered, (ii) cleverness, (iii) devotedness, (iv) purity of mind. Besides the above a good nurse must be intelligent, healthy, possess good manners and even temper, sympathetic at heart and with deft hands. She must have habits of obedience, cleanliness, a sense of proportion and accuracy of statement.

Since the nurse has continuous contact with the patient, she understands the problems of a patient better and has opportunity to redress his complaints better. In fact it is the nurse, who is at the centre-stage of patient care, all others come and go; either reporting to her or enquiring from her.

I. HUMAN ASPECT OF NURSING CARE: NURSING STUDENTS MUST LEARN IT

Florence Nightingale (known as the 'Lady with the Lamp') believed that a nurse's work was never ceasing. She would have taken considerable interest in the nurse-patient relationship in today's fragile health care delivery system, if she were alive today. The relationship must culminate in a connectedness beyond a physical presence. Nightingale had dedicated herself to one purpose, i.e. care of the sick. The nurse, must be an extension of the person who is in the bed or on the stretcher. Nursing students must always have a true understanding of that situation and Nightingale's style of human touch, along with good communications skill and acknowledging the respect and dignity in patients. Nursing students are advised to treat patients as they would like to be treated themselves. No body wants himself to be treated only as a patient, he is a full-fledged human being. So treat him like one. Even in a jail, the prisoner is not happy to be pronounced as No. 1084—he has a name and his entity extends beyond, his numerical identity. In a hospital, his expectations and rights demand that he is addressed as Mr./Mrs./Miss ___________ and not pronounced as bed No. 1, 2, 3, etc. He has to be treated with respect, compassion and care, which he is entitled to and he also deserves as a part of patient care.

For teachers of nursing it's a world dedicated to students and consequently to their future patients. "I don't want the patient to get lost in the health care delivery system," says C. Polifroni, a professor of nursing in US. So each nurse or nursing student has to exercise her skill to put in her best in providing the personal and social dignity to the human being admitted under her care, besides the professional assistance.

2. RESPONSIBILITIES OF A NURSE

The nurse acts as team leader to the staff within the span of her control, by organizing and monitoring their work either in OPD, Ward or Operation Theatre. She has several responsibilities at hand.

(A) Clinical

She provides professional leadership, direction and motivation by giving support, advice and guidance to the nursing team within the span of her control. She ensures the patients are nursed in a safe environment according to their need. Some of the responsibilities are:

(i) Responsible for the quality nursing care.
(ii) Exercises professional judgment in assessing short-term priorities.
(iii) Responsible for the safe administration of drugs (and keeping a record of them).
(iv) Responsible for ensuring that all policies are adhered.
(v) Ensures that the agreed policies and procedures are implemented.

(B) Managerial

She is responsible for the supervision and development of staff within her span of duty and provision of all supplies viz.,

(i) Medicines, instruments, equipment and laundry.
(ii) The safe operation and repair of equipment.
(iii) The Staff adheres to and are fully acquainted with the unit's health and safety policy.
(iv) To seek advice and discuss problems on all matters with the superiors and physicians/surgeons.
(v) To be assessed on their own performance as Nurse, through the appraisal system.
(vi) Be responsible for communications between theatre and other departments and disciplines, and liaison with the medical staff.

(C) Education

Responsible for the teaching and training of all members of the team and nursing students with a learning environment. They ensure that the staffs within their area of responsibility are prepared and participate in continuous learning:

(i) In their role as teacher—nurse will keep uptodate with the new trends by attending review discussions on nursing, medicine and education, and by reading literature.
(ii) They will encourage junior staff to progress in their careers and to take responsibility.

(iii) They should assess their staff and discuss their progress with them.

(iv) Assistance in any research projects within their area of responsibility.

(D) Integrated Day Care Unit

Criteria	*Essential*	*Desirable*
Skills/Abilities	Good written and verbal communication skills; able to work within a multiple disciplinary team, able to work effectively under stress; facilitation of the clinical learning environment; clinical skills required to assess, plan, evaluate and monitor nursing care; supervise and support the nursing team; contribute to the performance management and development staff.	
Education	Staff nurse/sister. Evidence of appropriate skills development.	Teaching qualification/ course
Experience	3 year post-basic experience in the relevant speciality; previous experience with managing own caseload and junior staff; ability to prioritize workload effectively.	
Other Requirements	Have a working knowledge of current research and ability to implement and develop nursing practice understanding of budget and resource management.	
Knowledge	Flexibility, ability to undertake shift patterns, continues to develop clinically and managerially.	
Skills/Abilities	Good written and verbal communication skills; able to work within a multiple disciplinary team, able to work effectively under stress; facilitation of the clinical learning environment; clinical skills required to assess, plan, evaluate and monitor nursing care; supervise and support the nursing team; contribute to the performance management and development staff.	
Education	Staff nurse/sister. Evidence of appropriate skills development.	Teaching qualification/ course

(E) Theatre Nurse

She is a key manager for maintaining supplies of usable, linen, instruments, their maintenance and repair, etc. She is also the leader of different type of assistants to the surgeons. See details in the chapter on theatre nurse.

3. NURSE-PATIENT RELATIONSHIP

This relationship is based on mutual trust, mutual-respect, good communication, safe and affectionate care, total dedication and nurse-patient partnership to ameliorate the lot of the later. For good patient care, neither the nurse can arrogate herself due to her knowledge or status as a care giver, nor the patient, due to his status as a money provider. See Appendix about the aspects of restoration of sanctity of patient and nurse-doctor team relationships.

3.1 Good Patient Care

The study of nurse-patient relationship is of paramount importance, in the context of good patient care. It is to be realized that in this set-up both the participants are under a degree of stress. The nurse has to use her professional knowledge and skill, observing a degree of discipline and ethics to improve the patient's lot, who in turn looks upon her as a person of knowledge and science and who is pictured as kind, friendly thoughtful and affectionate person, committed to do everything possible for patient's care. In this task she may be constrained by her ability, time, communication, money, attitude, hospital systems, hospital environment, etc.

It would be desirable to keep the nurse free from hunger, wants, exploitation and extraneous stresses, if the health care delivery is to be saved and made more useful. This entails giving her the conditions of confidence and comfort, so that she is neither affected by ego, nor enters into unhealthy competition with other employees to muster more and more money. If she is assured of decent status and adequate salary, her performance will improve and thus patient care will also improve.

3.2 Physical and Social Factors

Man's social and physical environment determines susceptibility to disease-conditions. His lifestyle, the work he does, the place in which he lives, recreation or lobbies which he pursues, may all increase the likelihood of his contracting a disease. The patient may be more concerned with primary symptoms of pain than the underlying disease, the doctor and nurse may be more concerned about the diagnosis and treatment of illness and its cause, than to produce an immediate comfort. This may lead to conflict. It is the nurse, whose role is important not only to keep them cool, but also provide valid professional service.

Similarly, a well read layman's effort at self-diagnosis and self-medication are dangerous to the patients' health and welfare. The role of a nurse as a source of health education is again important in such situation.

3.3 What brings a Patient to the Nurse

It need not be the serious disease always, it could be morbid episodes of life, illness conditions, disabilities, disorders, psychological stress, symptoms, non-diseases as well as their attempted cures. Whatever may be the complaint, it indicates disturbance in smooth pattern of existence or a change in his/her external or internal environment. Hence, while diagnosing and treating diseases, it is often important to study illness behaviour, i.e., the way in which given symptoms may be differentially perceived, evaluated and acted upon by different kinds of persons.

The meeting between a nurse-doctor team and patient can be turned into a positive, congenial and curative relationship, with the support and co-operation provided by the nurse. Patients do not always find it easy to reveal their worst anxieties or betray their real notions without encouragement and certainly not outside the framework of relationship based on mutual confidence and respect. Understanding the patients' symptoms will require a peep into his work environment, his relation with the employees and the associates at work, his sexual life, his social inter-relations and his friends. This all may not be possible for the doctor to elicit, but a nurse may explore important and relevant points in his personal life and present them to doctor.

Whether the patient's basic complaint is physical or emotional, the work of a nurse starts with imaginative listening so that the patient feels that his condition is being taken seriously. It should be possible to strike a happy mean between a cold impersonal attitude adopted for the sake of objectivity and an over-identification with the patient, resulting in personal/emotional involvement.

3.4 The Relationships

It is the nurse-patient relationship where the lay and professional perspective and priorities most intimately meet, accommodate each other or may clash. Beside patients, nurses too vary widely in their responses to illness situations. However, the nurse being member of a professional group, her actions are defined and confined by the law, ethics, time, space, inter-professional relations and organization of medical practice. Any contact between a patient and doctor-nurse team is usually as a result of conscious choice on the part of the patient. Such a contact on the part of the patient may represent a desire as much for emotional support as for physical diagnosis or medication. The patient's assessment of the professional's performance will be based upon his view of such things as the interest taken by nurse (or doctor) in him, the amount of information given to him, the willingness to show concern, her commitment to the welfare of the patient. A busy doctor may fail to come up to the expectation of his patient, but intervention of the nurse may bring cheer to him.

3.4.1 The Interaction

The relationship of a patient with nurse-doctor team is that of expert-layman and it is the physician's expertise which is ultimate resource in his interaction with others. This relationship varies from complete passivity on the part of the patient, to the patient's consent to accept the advice and follow it. The interaction is expected to follow the model of guidance-co-operation; the physician's team initiating more of the interaction than the patient. A patient is expected to do what he is told by the experts. It may extend to mutual participation where patients are able or are required to take care of themselves, e.g. in diabetes. In other model of interaction the patient guides and the doctor cooperates, i.e. the patient is active and the doctor is passive. In fee-for-service situation, it may be certainly a case that the patient guides and the doctor co-operates. A nurse may act as an advocate for patient as well as doctor and also safeguard the interests of both parties.

3.4.2 Privileged Access

The nurse often deals with human beings in a manner, which outside the context of the professional relationship would be criminal, immoral, scandalous or ridiculous. As part of her basic task, it is frequently necessary that the patient's body be exposed and touched, that it should be mutilated in some way or that it's bio-chemical functioning should be interfered with. While such activities become part of the professionals take-for-granted perspective, it is clearly a source of conflict, tension and upset for patients, who must readjust their usual concept of appropriate behaviour in relation to their body. To see a person naked when this is not usual and to touch and manipulate their body is a privileged access. Some acts of the doctors or nurse's such as vaginal or rectal examination, may not be permitted to any other person not even a sexual partner. The patient's usual concept of the inviolability of his body is temporarily shelved in this relationship.

3.4.3 The Prescription

It is not surprising that practitioners frequently choose to treat rather than to wait, when they think that the patient expects to be treated. Prescriptions are seen as rewards at the end of nearly all consultations. Often the time honoured methods to send the patient away after consultation, e.g. sliding one's chair back, rising to one's feet, holding the door open, fail to work, only a prescription succeeds. But the doctor must weigh the risk of doing something against the risk of delaying or deciding not to do anything. The doctor may develop a vested interest in the perpetuation of this system of doing something, since he will earn after each prescription given or medicines dispensed. This will reduce the chances of real patients getting due attention. Should the reward for declaring a person perfectly fit or free of disease be also not available? A nurse can educate a patient, about the perils of unnecessary medication.

3.4.4 Non-Diseases and Non-Medical Problems

Non-disease is defined as a diagnostic label which is established after a person has been incorrectly diagnosed as ill or suspected of having a disease and then after subsequent examination and tests is ruled not to have it. Such false positives are non-diseases. The cause may be mimickery normal variation or a laboratory error. It would seem that having a non-disease is hardly serious and involves nothing more than a certain amount of worry and time wasted on one or more visits to clinic. The non-diseases highlight the importance of a variety of emotional and psycho-social problems and the tendency on the part of some doctors to define them as non-medical problems. But the doctor is too close to his patients and the community to shirk in this manner. It is natural that such problems be presented to the doctor, whether he sees them as a part of his task or not. In such non-disease situations, the importance of health education by a nurse is all the more.

3.4.5 Informed Consent

The controversy about the informed consent has been there in connection with clinical research or with non-therapeutic research, such as drug trials where the benefit is not for the particular patient (volunteers) but for patients in general at sometimes in the future. In such case the nurse has to seek consent of the subjects after giving an adequate information about the facts and outcome of the drug trial, etc. This step is very important in saving one's skin later.

3.5 Ethics

Till recently, the concept of ethics was simple one, since it did not have to deal with knotty problems like euthanasia, abortion, forensic medicine, iatrogenic diseases, ethics in context of drug industry, public service, registration, hospital services, nursing home as a business venture, specialization to promote professionalism, an association safeguarding their own interests in the community. This was irrelevant in the practice of nursing in the earlier times. The ethics are as important for a nurse as far doctor to earnestly help the patient.

3.6 Community Nurse

A doctor-nurse team is responsible for good deal of primary medical care, notwithstanding the stiff competition offered to him by quacks of different hues. The area of primary care and preventive care can better be dealt by a nurse with due training and supervision. A nurse with her training and experience can understand the patient's symptom better and present her case to the doctor. Though there are several posts of Lady Health Visitors (LHV) and ANMs, they need to be given the work of real and active community nurses for liaison with community and their education.

3.6.1 Minor Ailments

Once the doctor and the patient is aware of the vast field of untreated minor emotional or psychiatric illness, it will be possible to offer considerable help by ventilation of problem. When a patient of common cold presents to the doctor, it is necessary to ask what is the reason of his visit, rather than ridiculing the patient. May be the patient has something more to unburden, which he needs to settle by discussion and advice. A nurse can be a good middle-person/shock absorber to help the patient.

3.6.2 The Neurotic

A patient with minor Stress or nervousness will be unwilling to visit a psychiatrist even if referred. Also the psychiatric services will be over-burdened if patients start coming for psychiatric help in all neurotic problems. More so, a psychiatrist is not the best person to treat minor aberrations in behaviour. Best to attend such a case is one's own family doctor, who knows the person and his environment. It would be prudent to assume that there is none in this world who does not have any neurotic trait.

It will be useful to attach a nurse (who may act as psychiatric social workers/medical social worker) as assistant to doctor in practice as well as those working in hospitals, to reduce their workload and to provide psychotherapy based on situations and difficulties. Such a nurse can attempt to manipulate the patient's environment after studying his social difficulties, as well as his organic and emotional problems. It will take several visits for the patient, before he accepts the ailment to be of emotional origin. This management will provide an effective assessment of the patient's non-medical problems and would prove less expensive, time-saving and acceptable. A nurse can ably perform the job of a social medical worker.

3.7 The Government Nurse: Private Nurse

In our set-up, most of hospitals, dispensaries, and the so-called health centres are managed and financed by the Central Government/State Government/Municipalities, etc. The salary of the staff, including that of the nurses is paid from the public funds. The patients have generally not to pay any fee to get consultation and other services. Now certain States have come out with user's charges for investigations, surgery, patient care, etc.

3.7.1 Impersonal Attitude

Since it is not a fee for service situation, the nurses tend to be impersonal to the extent of being apathetic. The human beings in distress are treated like subjects or even objects. With the result, the ailing citizens tend to get a feeling of non-attendance, neglect and indifference, even if the treatment administered is timely, correct and adequate. Though, it is the citizen, who is the master of all—since he votes the Government in/out—it is he who is neglected most. He is not given any information. No one treats him as a person and his social, personal and emotional needs are overlooked. A nurse can fill this gap by explaining and giving a feeling of attendance.

3.7.2 Indifference to Job

The Government nurse often refuses to develop any relationship with the OPD/Ward patients and tend to just mark her time. Some of them attend to only VIPs, who can bestow favours in one way or the other, others do it for a consideration. Some doctors and staff report only on the day of visit of the boss, while others tend to limit it to the salary day. Many of them continue to run their business outside, even during the stipulated hours of the hospitals. A minority of them who work earnestly and with devotion, are called worldly unwise, eccentric or even foolish. Nurses observe such misadventures and can't remain unaffected. In this process, the patient care is wholly or partially sacrificed. When the reluctance to look-after even the seriously ill is visible, where is the scope for preventive health, community education or to look into the promotional or rehabilitation aspects? Let the nurse get rid of this indifference and develop rapport with patient and his family.

3.7.3 Patient is a Person

In any case, if a human being falls ill, he does not cease to be a person and hence he has to be treated as human, keeping in view this fact. The hospital doctor or nurse cannot arrogate to herself to maltreat these unfortunate persons who happened to seek help and support from the hospital. Hospital is a public institution which thrives on public funds and which is designed to serve the public, and the hospital staff is there to be sub-servient to the public. If the practicing doctors and nurses undertake to provide the front line medical and health care and the hospitals are used only for serious and referred cases and the two segments of health team work in unison, the coverage of population and the quality of health care will improve.

3.8 Sixth Sense

Examination of a patient involves the employment of the five senses of the doctor and nurse team. There is a sixth sense to provide information about the patient: the emotional experience evoked by the attitude and hearing of the patient. This experience is generally excluded while making a diagnosis. It is proper to some extent that this exclusion of feelings should be encouraged. It would be improper for the surgeon to be prevented from performing his technically essential but emotionally brutal function by the intrusion of his emotional feelings during an operation. All doctors spend much of their time in a physical environment of deformity, pus and excreta, and an emotional environment of pain, unhappiness and anxiety. Barriers against the evocation of disgust by the physical and emotional environment are necessary to enable him to tend the patient. People are made into cases and feelings which may sway or prejudice judgement are suppressed to obtain objectivity. When objective findings are equivocal or inconclusive, however, the feelings evoked by the patient in the doctor may be the vital data for the doctor's diagnosis and assessment of therapy. A nurse can be asked to shake the emotional aspects of the patient.

Of all the emotions that can be evoked in the doctor or nurse is the one least likely to be reported by the patient is depression. A depressed person does not express himself readily, but easily produces a feeling of depression in the people with whom he is in contact. If depression is not talked about, it is because this is integral to the nature of the emotion. A feeling which may be almost as difficult to talk about is sexuality. A good nurse assistant can help a lot to the patient as well as doctor. She can assume the role of a psycho-social analyst as well as an advocate and emotional support for the patient, while sparing the valuable time of the physician. The doctor can objectively and freely concentrate on examination and interventions, while nurse records the history of emotional symptoms and knotty complaints. The role of a nurse is important here. Nurse will alleviate the anxiety of the patient by her sweet words and style.

We may consider the situation when a woman presents complaining of a lump in her breast. The 'bad' nurse will refer her immediately to a surgeon. If suspected diagnosis is malignant tumor, she must send her to a surgeon. The 'good' nurse will examine her and she will get her treated medically and take the responsibility of managing her, or coping with her emotional reaction.

3.9 Sympathy

The feelings and expression of sympathy is an integral part of the approach to a patient. But sympathy, however genuine and heartfelt, is far from being therapeutic. Sympathy is an emotional response to be used under conscious intellectual control. It may act as a barrier to effective communication between nurse and patient, and secondly, it may be used by the patient for his own ends; the doctor may be maneuvered into actions which may serve only to foster the patient's neurosis and be the reverse of therapeutic. Sympathy part may best be left to the nurse.

Tears are a time honoured weapon in the armory of a patient, especially females, sometimes used in doctor's chamber to enlist sympathy. Most commonly this is done to avoid discussing unpleasant issues. In many circumstances, they can be a very convenient refuge but they are then a barrier to further communication, diagnosis and effective treatment. The doctor's response may be: 'if you are crying I know you are miserable. If you can talk I will then know why. When we know why we may be able to find out some way of relieving it.' Excessive sympathy, when evoked, may be used for purposes which would be contrary to the doctor's judgment The doctor need not be a puppet into serving the patient's ends. Experiences with such patients leads the doctors withdrawing their sympathy from professional relationships. Undue and unnecessary sympathy can lead to clouding of clinical judgment and misuse of doctor's precious time. However, nurse may assume this part of the role.

3.10 Communication

Ideal relation involves a state of communication, in which the nurse and the patient can converse with mutual confidence. It demands her interest, consideration, empathy, friendly objectivity, understanding and the patient's full faith and co-operation. If she clumsily alarms her patient while explaining the treatment or the patient gets frightened, it is a failure in communication. The good nurse can step in. The doctor may fail to understand the idiom, dialect, phraseology or use of words. The patient will either take such a doctor as stupid, in-attentive or uninterested or a snob. Often the patient does not understand what the doctor or nurse wants to know and in turn the doctor gets impatient and starts shouting in a loud voice. But a doctor who shouts, ridicules or shows indifference would forfeit patient's respect. The nurse has to keep him cool and has to extract the information as to what the patient really means.

3.11 Hospital Visitors

All hospital visitors require proper attention, viz. the attendants looking after the patient, his relations, children and courtesy-callers. Where one set of visitors comes and goes after leaving behind their 'get well soon' wishes, the other set has to keep hanging around the hospitals, to look for the patient.

The contact of the visitors and hospital-staff is at several points and starts right from the moment it is decided to seek hospital advice or admission. Generally, the first contact is with the enquiry/reception. This, if well-managed can help a lot to mitigate the subsequent sufferings of attendants and patients and can facilitate a great deal, the dispensing of medical care and the associated services, e.g., registration, OPD service, fee deposit, laboratory services and admission if required. Generally, the failure of hospital administration and its staff starts from here and gets accentuated as the patient proceeds further in various queues. More often the attitude of the reception staff is impersonal, indifferent, inadequate, curt to impolite. The visitor to this counter is more often dealt away by putting off, rather than by offering him any help. The same culture is perpetuated further, as he moves to get his card made, approaches the lift or awaits in the OPD at the mercy of the peon or a self-styled social worker. A Registration Nurse can be a great help for the patients and their attendants.

In the OPD, where he is waiting anxiously to get attention of one of the doctors or a doctor of his choice, he is pushed around. His turn to see the doctor becomes a 'mirage', with politicians, VIPs, bureaucrats, hospital staff and others who matter not showing only respect for the queue, or the human beings in distress, huddled there.

The waiting in the congested and polluted environment, involving standing for hours, uncertainty of the 'turn' for the patient, with hospital noise, cries, smells and infections all round, prove to be a real rest of nerves and physique, for the attendants. Getting a hospital bed/room is a measure of one's tactfulness, resourcefulness and manipulation. After passing through the rigmarole of formalities, the serious patient with his worried attendants arrive in the ward, where the nurses receive him with a shower of "get out attendants, do not crowd here, allow us to work for God's sake"—without enquiring as to why the hopeful people are roaming about. Nobody cares to provide them a sitting place or even a glass of water.

When confronted with the job of getting some laboratory investigations done, the patient's relatives face another volley of hostilities. The sweepers and ward attendants are nowhere to be found and their work is allotted to the attendants of the patient, out of expediency, encapsulated in 'patient's interest'. After depositing the requisite fee for the tests, the relatives wander in search of the laboratories and its ingenious workers. When they turn up in the evening to discuss the report, the replies usually are 'the blood was clotted—send it again' , 'culture sterile' or 'shows growth of no significance', 'NAD'. If any figures are reported, they look to be imaginary and often do not seem to have any semblance to the reality of the situation. Repeat samples are sent every day, fees are deposited daily, but nobody bothers about the reports—if they have come and what they are like! Is it due to the overwork? Overwork has something to do—but not all.

The other area of contact between the patient's attendant and the staff, especially the nursing staff is over the implementation of 'drug administration schedule'. While the medicine is entrusted to be given to the attendants, the problem arises over the administration of different types of injections or drip of blood, glucose, saline, etc. While the relative is supposed to keep a close supervision over the execution of 'drug administration' if he points out any failing he is accused of over-stepping his jurisdiction and told not to step in the shoes of a doctor.

The callers to the hospital, either in their anxiety to enquire after the welfare of the patient or just to mark their attendance as a gesture of goodwill, come under heavy fire. While it is a fact that too many visitors are a menace to the hospital cleanliness, environment or even administration of services to the patient, all the same it is a necessary evil. Wherever a human being is confined to bed, those known to him would come. If their visit could be cut short, but made more comfortable, it would be a better management. Merely shouting at them will not solve the problems. Let them meet him, explain to them briefly and then they can be asked to bow out. Their visit may satisfy the emotional needs of the patients and hence may help in the treatment.

3.11.1 Child Visitors

The practice is to strictly curtail visits by young children to a hospitalized parent. But infants and children may visit a hospitalized parent as an integral part of the treatment plan (Levai, 1968). The organization of a play-room in the hospitals for visiting children has been described as a recent innovation (St. Vincent, 1978). Such facilities are convenient and a step forward. Some hospitals have relaxed restrictive visiting rules for children for a number of years with no ill-effects, and obvious benefits. Notable are improved morale of the hospitalized parent as separation from and anxiety about absence from normal parental role functions are diminished. Moreover, the presence of a child actively counters the potentially morbid tone of a hospital environment for other patients infusing the milieu with vitality and a future orientation. The exclusion of children intensely magnifies the stress of a brief separation imposed by hospitalization.

3.11.2 Information Exchanges

One unfortunate aspect of contact between the nurse and the patient is the barrier in information exchange. While the attending physician often shirks to listen to the visitor's narration about the patient's condition or his progress, they do not like to divulge anything about the patient's condition; diagnosis, prognosis or the plan of treatment. That stone silence in response to the visitor's questions give rise to misgivings about the outcome of hospitalized patient. It would be proper to listen to some of the visitors and give them brief resume of the patient's condition. Though, such an exercise is time-consuming yet not time-wasting. If the relevant facts of the patient's progress or otherwise are given out briefly, it would exhibit staff's involvement in patient's care and allay the anxiety of the relatives, etc. The patient would get a feeling of reasonable attendance and the chances of law suit against the hospital for alleged negligence, would minimize.

3.11.3 Facilities for the Attendants

The attendants involved in patient's care, require organized management for their stay to facilitate their work. After all they are a resource in the patient's treatment plan. If this aspect is ignored they would tend to crowd around the bed of the patient, or the corridors, spread the eatables as well as their body excretions on the floor, look unkempt and fatigued, hence more irritable to the staff—thus polluting the environment and hindering the administration of various services.

Attached to each ward, there should a visitor's room, where they can sit—when not on duty with the patient, use the toilet facility and give respite to their legs. Then for the stay of attendants of such patients, who require round the clock care, a room must be made available in the hospital serai. Such room should be generously/abundantly available on the nurse's recommendation. The physician may not be bothered with this aspect. To look after the needs of such attendants, provision of a canteen and recreation room on the pattern of a hostel is essential. They should be given the impression of being a wanted lot and involved in patient's care, rather than being pushed around or shunted out. If they are well looked after, their level of involvement in the patient's treatment plan would be high.

3.12 Politicians' Role

Politician confronts the hospital administration at every-stage and in a big way, i.e., the conception of the hospital, its setting up, management and its day-to-day functioning. During day-to-day functioning he may appear to be interfering and taxing. Those in power, be it a politician or a bureaucrat, tend to seek a special attention of the hospital services. This may mean seeking advice (either for himself or others recommended by him) for a minor ailment, which could be easily attended outside (by a dispensary doctor or a private general clinic or jumping the queue in a matter of availing various services, e.g., a private room, laboratory tests, consultations, discussion with the concerned physician (which is often unnecessary), etc. Some might interpret it as a nuisance and burden and might treat it as a problem to be dealt with. In fact, the politician cannot be shunned away, from its negative or positive role, either in the management of the hospital or its planning and development. In a democracy you cannot put barriers for any section of society, let alone the politician, who wield power and influence in the government as well as society. However, hanging around the residences or offices of the politician/bureaucrats to unduly please them in a bid to get personal gains at a cost of hospital efficiency and the dignity of the staff, can be ruinous for the functioning of the hospital and prove counter-productive for the hospital administration. The role of a nurse cannot be over-emphasized, to deal with the politician-bureaucrat combine, so that their nuisance can be reduced and they can be made a resource for the hospital.

3.13 Professional Patients

Professional patients are a great menace and an avoidable burden, on the hospital services. Such patients tend to seek repeated and perpetual hospital attention, either in OPD or wards, out of their anxiety and neurotic traits, addiction, malingering, poverty, insecurity, VIP connection or fun-sake.

They devise ways and means and adopt new strategies by virtue of their knowledge and experience of the hospital systems and connections with the staff. Then they manipulate their stay to be longer and longer. Thus, they deprive others who are in dire need, from the services and attention of the physician and nurses. A nurse should try to analyze and understand the underlying cause of request for the hospitalization of such patients and try to help them out of the hospital by neutralizing his resistance tactfully. Whereas, certain factors prompting him to seek hospitalization, e.g., anxiety or phychomatic factors should be dealt with sympathy, others should be resisted. Tact and politeness will always be necessary, since such patients can be a source of adverse publicity, public agitation or even legal suits.

4. NURSING INFORMATICS

In every aspect of patient care, the nurse constantly assesses, diagnoses, and determines the appropriate action, and then evaluates and communicates it to the doctor above and patient below. Effective nursing management depends on acquiring, analyzing, interpreting, and generating relevant information. Not surprisingly, nurses spend their large portion of time on the mechanics of gathering, recording and communicating data. Such findings spurred hospital administrators to try computer-based information systems as a mean to controlling and improving patient care by reducing the time nurses spend on paper work and freeing them to give direct care.

In India such innovation has not developed for want of resources and stereotype and inferior role a nurse enjoys here. There is hardly any growth or development in the area of informatics for nurses. It will take a long time, before management of data comes in the hand of nurses. However, information processing is integral to nursing care. It is inescapable that information system will have to be adopted in nursing practice.

The essentials of management in nursing practice are:

1. Using data, information, and knowledge to deliver and manage patient care.
2. Defining and describing data and information for patient care.
3. Acquiring and delivering knowledge for patient care.
4. Investigating new technologies to create tools for patient care.
5. Applying patient care ergonomics to the patient-nurse-machine interaction.
6. Integrating system for better patient care.
7. Evaluating the effects of nursing information systems.

The newness of the field of nursing informatics and the consequent unfamiliarity of many nurse scientists with the field necessitate explicitness in the examples of types of research needed in an area. Critically examining nursing practice from an informatics perspective reveals knowledge gaps that impair practice and can be filed by research in nursing informatics.

4.1 Research Needs and Opportunities

Although nursing practice is information-intensive, it is just beginning to be studied from the perspective of information science. Research in nursing informatics can enhance nursing science by illuminating nurses' use of knowledge and information to care for patients, articulating nursing knowledge and making it more explicit and creating systems to monitor the effectiveness of care and using the findings to increase the nursing knowledge. Research in nursing informatics can also support the quality and cost effectiveness of nursing practice by providing the means for nurses to accurately and efficiently plan, document, communicate, evaluate, analyze and understand their care. Traditionally, clinical nursing data have not been a useful resource for research. They have not been collected consistently, as their reliability and validity have not been demonstrated. Finally, research specific to nursing needs and applications is needed to create, integrate, and evaluate information technologies.

4.2 Information-based Patient Care

- Identify types of decisions, judgments, and skills involved in delivering patient care.
- Identify information needs in relation to users (nurses, patients, and families) and uses (decisions, judgments, and skills).
- Identify differences among individuals, settings, health conditions, or other factors that influence the relationship between information and decisions, judgments, and skills.
- Create and maintain data based on nursing diagnoses, interventions, outcomes, and resource consumption, and analyze relationships among them.
- Determine relationships between the processes and effectiveness of decisions, judgments, and skills.
- Develop, implement, and evaluate information systems in support decisions, judgments, and skills.

4.3 Applying Patient Care Ergonomics to the Patient-Nurse Relationship

- Assess the effects of bedside workstations on nurse decision-making, interventions, and patient outcomes, and on the relationships between nurse and patient, and nurse and other health professionals.
- Examine the work patterns of nurse in a variety of settings (including identifying patterns that could be improved through the use of appropriate technology), design or select information technology to facilitate the work, conduct demonstration projects, and evaluate the effects of the technology on psycho-physiological comfort and functioning, organizational functioning, and quality of services to patients.
- Establish standards for data to record nursing diagnoses, interventions, recourse expenditures, and outcomes.
- Develop first prototypes and then working systems to track nursing diagnoses, interventions, resource expenditures, outcomes; and link them to one another and to calculations of staffing needs, quality, and productivity.
- Develop prototypes and then working models of networks and workstations that deliver to the nurse clinician or manager the variety of information needed for effective decisions: patient care information, bibliographic information clinical and research databases and data analysis packages, electronic main and messages, and other aids.
- Develop evaluation methodologies that assure valid and reliable results in studying the effects of complex informatic systems on nursing practice; measure the contribution of information system to nurses' clinical decision-making; measure, if possible, the

contribution of information system to patient outcomes; and provide measurable, dependable predictors of nurses' optional use of automated information system.

5. NEWER PERSPECTIVES: NURSE LED PRIMARY CARE

Government policy in the west has emphasized the need to examine the skills among nurses, so as to break down existing demarcations between medical and nursing roles. There is a growing body of research evidence that suggests that these nurses can offer care that is similar in quality and cost to that of doctors in a number of settings. So there is a move to entrust the captainancy of patient care to a nurse, in place of a doctor (who has traditionally been the captain). This is happening without sufficient attention on establishing agreed competencies or standards or training. However, there is in-built hostility from doctors as well as society, to this change of roles, even in the west. In the quack ridden Indian society, the role of doctor may not be transferred to a nurse, since people accept a quack as medical care provider, but not a qualified nurse who is always thought to be an assistant of a doctor.

A new infrastructure is required to support new nursing roles. In particular, more clarity is required over the competencies, training and quality assurance of nursing practitioner services. Nurses perceive that they had received little in the way of support from their professional bodies.

6. WHO EXAMINES THE ROLE: NURSE IN PATIENT CARE

The Director-General, WHO, while addressing the global advisory group on nursing and midwifery, stated the following: During this time, we have been examining the role of nursing and midwifery skills in the different health systems of our world. We have examined ways in which nurse-midwives can contribute to health outcomes and health system performance.

You have responded to Member-States concerns about their nursing and midwifery services. These have been expressed forcefully on several occasions, most recent last year's World Health Assembly. Member-States have repeatedly stated the important contribution that both nurses and midwives can make to health outcomes. They are at the core of any health system. They are extremely concerned about global shortages.

Together, this provides us with a strong platform for advocacy.

We know that nursing and midwifery plays a key role in practical efforts to respond to millions of death each year from infectious and non-communicable diseases. This also means that nurses and midwives are key to the sustained success of the public-private partnerships for health.

6.1 Nurses are at the Forefront

We should show how nurses and midwives are at the forefront of the collective response. They are committed to the delivery of first class health care for all, regardless of ethnicity or gender, in a manner that is both effective and efficient. Their leaders through their involvement in human resource planning; in pursuing optimal work conditions; and in promoting equitable health outcomes.

Our challenges are to: Harness and enhance nursing and midwifery efforts to patient safety; Place nursing and midwifery as a top priority on the health and development of decision-makers; Leverage the contribution of nurses and midwives to addressing risks to her, how they can be mobilized to promote healthier behaviour and to the role model to the population they serve.

6.2 Numbers are Inadequate

The number of qualified nurses and midwives in many developed and developing countries are inadequate and new recruits are insufficient to replace them. Current efforts to encourage the training, recruitment and retention of a skilled nursing and midwifery workforce, and of ensuring their motivation, are not working well enough. Low pay rates and hazardous working conditions are real barriers to retention. As about lack of career development, professional status and anatomy. Severe shortages of nursing staff have lead to the closure of essential health care facilities, including emergency. Shortages also make those who are working more likely to be affected by ill-health.

By launching the Strategic Directions for Strengthening nursing and Midwifery nurses, we have made a first step towards assisting countries deal with these issues. This will help us to implement these directions and help countries with developing their nursing and midwifery service provision.

We have a strong and committed alliance, held together by common purpose. The International Council of Nurses, the International Council of Midwives and the common network of WHO Collaborating Centers for Nursing and Midwifery Development, will all help to define the role of nurses and help to develop nursing services.

7. NURSE-PATIENT COLLABORATION

The theory by Peplau generates an opportunity for nurses and patient to work collaboratively to meet goals. Peplau's role of nurse gives insight and direction for nurses in any field of practice. The concepts of anxiety in relation to goal attainment give direction for specific health care outcomes based on identification of unmet needs.

7.1 Peplau's Concept

Peplau's theoretical concepts include the nurse-patient relationship, roles of nursing situations and the impact of bio-psychological experiences. The descriptive relationship of the concepts promotes therapeutic nursing of the individual in the need of health care. It also provides the nurse the opportunity to relate the correlation between their personal and professional development and the influence it has on the therapeutic and interpersonal relationship. The interrelationship creates a different, unique perspective of the nurse-patient relationship which is her main focus. The society/environment factors are not directly addressed. This theoretical limitation weakens the ability to deal with individuals with certain characteristics such as comatose patient. The theoretical relationship create meaning as they support their purpose through describing relationship stages, explaining nursing roles and predicting outcomes based on psychobiological factors. The theory goes from general to specific, for example, the patient's vague somatic symptoms become more specific as she identifies the emotions causing vague bodily complaints. They concepts examined individually aid in expanding nursing perspective. The collaborative effects of the theoretical relationships allow nurses to approach each individual as a unique biological-psychological-spiritual-sociological structure. Peplau's relational concepts allow the nurse and patient to work together toward goal attainment. The nurse cannot provide services to the patient, in isolation, without the patient's cooperation, collaboration and active involvement. An active collaboration leads to a better outcome, than a situation of "surrender" by the patient to seek one side service.

7.2 How to Evaluate?

Criteria for evaluating a model of collaboration can be based on the following:

(a) Does it promote the well-being of patients?
(b) Does it respect patient autonomy?
(c) Does it protect professional integrity?
(d) Does it sufficiently acknowledge the factual professional and institutional realities.

7.3 Indian Model

The time honoured model, which is prevalent in India entails: The nurse is "mother." She works under the authority of physician (father) for the good of the patient. Her obligation is to respect authority and established procedures; to obey. Her unique contribution is the humanization of the hospital; providing care in addition to the care provided by physicians, i.e to "mother" sick patients.

The so-called new western model treats a nurse as "autonomous professional." Here the nurse brings her own technical competence to the health care enterprise. She shares authority and responsibility for caring with physician or in place of a physician. In this care she assumes the role of a physician for the patient. In a desirable model, the nurse acts as "patient's advocate." It reflects a recognition that patient relationship to health care is one of inequality. Hence the nurse sides with the patient for empowering the patient by providing information, understanding, and representation. She takes up the care and problems of the patient for redressal by physician and others.

Traditionally, efficiency in hospital requires that "inferiors" obey "superiors." It is taken for granted that physicians alone have the necessary knowledge to care and heal. Only nurses can provide the "care" that patients need.

7.4 New Western Model

Those arguing in favour new western model and against the traditional 'mother' model say: This model is based on sex-role stereotyping and outdated understanding. It ignores reality of modern nursing, i.e. nurses have taken on new responsibilities.

We advocate the possibility of a conventional model of nursing, i.e. (i) a partnership between physician, nurses (and other health professionals) (HPs) and patients, (ii) It recognizes that nurses have professional expertise essential to curing and healing, under the "superior" expertise of the physician, (iii) It assures that nurse is well placed to represent patients in an institutional context and can advocate for him. This concept continues hold onto "care" dimension of "traditional" nursing. The captainancy remains with the physician, with nurse continuing to provide 'care' under supervision, with her own skills.

8. NURSE AND HER PATIENT: HOW TO COMMUNICATE

We know one may be reluctant to discuss personal health, intimidated by needles and pills, wary of complex information, or afraid to find out what's wrong with you. But we also know one need a good relationship with nurse in order to get best possible care. This is especially true for people with cancer, an illness that demands special attention from nurse and patient alike. Cancer patient usually visit more than one hospitals and other health care specialists. Information from so many sources can be complex and confusing. That's why we think it best for you to choose one facility as your primary source of knowledge someone you can always feel comfortable approaching with questions and concerns. Remember: your care is ultimately in your own hands. Your doctor may be responsible for providing medical advice and the nurse to give 'care'. It's upto you to select the doctor-nurse team and to make certain you understand each other.

8.1 Patient's Attitude Matters

It depends on the attitude of the patient "when he finds mud tracked on carpet, he may not want to know how, when and why it happened or he may just want the carpet cleared." If he feels the same about his illness he may ask his nurse to tell him how to get better without explaining the inner workings of the body. Simply ask what to do and what to expect. But if he is the type who would want to know exactly what happened to the carpet, he may want to learn all about his illness as well. Ask the doctor and nurse for details—everything he or she can relate. "It may be useful, if patients are advised to care. Prepared for meetings. It may help to write down questions for your health team before your appointment instead of relying on memory after you arrive."

Since you need to be specific when describing symptoms, take notes about them in advance so that you can present them clearly and accurately. When you make your appointment let the receptionist know it you think you will need more time then usual to talk with your doctor first and then take clarifications with a nurse. It's easy for a patient to forget much of what is said during a visit. If you fear you may not remember everything, bring a friend or relative along to listen and take notes with you. Also avail the help and guidance of the nurse to seek clarifications and ask for repetitions.

Don't be ashamed to have your nurse explain medical terms and concepts in language you can understand. Pictures may work even better. Be sure to ask questions about symptoms to watch for, how the illness usually progress, what you need to do the benefits and risks of your treatment, what side effects you may experience, and what you can expect in the future. Repeat or write down anything important your doctor/nurse says. Make sure you understand what you are supposed to do and get written instructions to rely on in case you forget. Be polite and not hostile when asking questions. If the discussion wanders, bring it back to your concern.

8.2 Doctor and Nurse Team in your Friend

- "Never hold back information from your nurse. She is your 'Mother' as well as advocate. Do whatever is necessary to maintain clear communication and a good professional relationship."
- Here are some ways to improve conversation with your doctor/nurse:
- Don't be afraid to ask for more details after your doctor explains something that you don't fully understand. It may help if you rephrase your original questions.
- If you want an active role in your treatment, enter your appointments with as much knowledge as possible so that you can pinpoint your questions and avert the need for long general explanations. Remain clam. Anger hinders communication. Always be polite, but make it clear that you need answer.

Good Relationship is Mutually Beneficial.

9. NURSING CARE AND INDIAN CULTURE DIVERSITY

In Indian set-up, the nursing care "culture" must accommodate not only persons from diverse cultures, but also diverse systems of health care. This fundamental need requires nurses to move quickly to develop cultural competency as individuals and to provide leadership for this system-wide change. Such competence is important when using complementary and alternative systems of nursing (CAM).

Nurses currently work within a health care system that reflects modern philosophy and practice. On the other hand, our patients live in increasing number of diverse cultures that have their own health beliefs, values and practices. These may conflict with those of Western medicine. The challenge for the nurse is to become knowledgeable about diverse cultures and to bring about greater cultural sensitivity and competency while working within the modern health care system. Cultural competence at the system level will result in improved health outcomes and greater satisfaction for patients and providers. Understanding cultural diversity will also lead to a greater acceptability of health care practices.

Cultural diversity has been an integral part of life in India since its beginning. Not only are different castes, religions, regions and economic strata as the barriers, but the level of education, differentials of wealth and diversity of languages and rural-urban divide also prove obstacles to be overcome.

9.1 Holistic Approach

In recent years holistic system of care is gaining greater attention. Many Indians are using complementary or alternative medicine (CAM). They began turning to CAM to deal with chronic pain, other symptoms, and to aid in lifestyle changes. They are also turning to meditation and prayer. Biomedicine is only one system among many and being open to other cultures and their health practices is imperative. This (Allopathy) makes it necessary for nurses to have a working knowledge of other system of care as well as the diverse peoples they serve in our current health care system. Lack of awareness that a nurse may have values and health practices that differ from biomedicine's may come as a surprise. When this lack of awareness is compounded by an assumption of superiority, serious problems for both patients and providers can result. "Attitudes towards Western medicine constitute one of the biggest barriers to transcultural communication between a nurse and patient. Indeed many nurses feel that the biomedical system is the best (and even the only) approach to patient care . . . They may view other health belief systems with suspicion and even contempt, refusing to acknowledge that another's approach might have some merit."

A culturally competent nurse will possess a knowledge base, skills and abilities to provide health care to diverse groups and to achieve high levels of patient and community satisfactory among diverse cultural groups.

In this age of information, nurses have easy access to information that will give them a basis understanding of other cultures.

Awareness of the use of CAM and routinely asking about its use is an essential step in working with patients and families from diverse backgrounds. Determining, however, the compatibility of herbs with biomedical treatments is also critical. Nurses need to become familiar with the practices used by their patients. The Internet can be a ready resource for this purpose.

9.2 What is CAM?

The increased use of CAM by our public is an opportunity for nurses to inform them about what the nursing profession offers. Nursing itself can be conceived as an alternative approach to biomedicine. Nursing's roots are in holism and health. Nurses know that their care fosters the patient's inherent capacity to restore health. The body "knows" how to heal. Nurses know how to support the body's innate ability to heal and maintain health. Many of the CAM traditions are holistic with natural practices that are designed to prevent illness as well as restore health. Nutrition, exercise, and spiritual healing are but some of these modalities common to both CAM and nursing. Nurses need to look carefully at the potential for inclusion of CAM in their practices and to develop their ability to provide culturally competent care in offering these CAM without the benefit of solid research, knowledge of efficacy or safety. Nursing can be a force to clarify these practices.

10. CARE IS THE CORE OF NURSING SERVICES

A number of factors may determine the quality of care delivered by nurses to patients, e.g. nursing competence, use of research, communication skills, care management and organization of workload, provision of health education and health promotion, and creative thinking. There is evidence to suggest that although nurses may be capable of providing quality care and know what constitutes quality care, their performance in practice may be affected by factors such as decreased number and the resulting reduction in available time, which can prevent the delivery of quality nursing care. 'Care' is the core of nursing services and without care nursing services are meaningless. In our big hospitals in the Government sector, it is often seen that nurses are overburdened by work and extraneous interests. They provide all other services to the patient in the ward or OPDs, but fail to provide 'care' for patients and their attendants.

10.1 Traditional Pyramid is Crumbling?

The traditional pyramid of health care with the physician as the "captain" of the team, assisted by nurses, responsible for all medical care of a patient, is not as solid as it once was. The modern labyrinth of roles and responsibilities can create problems and concerns for both the supervising and supervised care-givers, especially in terms of communication and decision-making. While nurses have ceased to be earnest assistants. They are neither capable of taking independent responsibility, nor willing to take the burden. This is an appropriate time to re-examine the essential characteristics of a successful team, without standing on ego crutches.

10.2 Supervision Leads to Success

No doubt appropriate supervision is the central principle behind successful and competent teamwork. The supervising physician bears both the authority and responsibility for the acts. While the question of superiority may be left unaddressed, the question of care can't be. The care entails mutual trust and respect. The nurse is a representative of the physician, treating the patient in the style and manner developed and directed by the physician. The nurse in our set-up is not expected to work in isolation or at cross purpose of what physician holds good for the patient. Mutual respect: It is important for both the physician and the nurse to have professional respect for each other. This means supporting each other with patients, office staff, and colleagues. Disagreements or differences, if any, should be ironed out in private.

A good mutual communication is important to avoid obstacles that impede access to discussion of patient care.

11. A STUDY IN NURSING BONDS: PATIENT FIRST

Compassion, truth, respect, knowledge, and responsibility are traits commonly associated with nursing care. In a pilot study of University of Pitsburgh, a registered nurse Lucke discovered three common threads in what people valued most about the nurse-patient bond: (i) being treated as a whole person rather than as a patient, (ii) feeling that their care was tailored to their individual case, and (iii) sharing the responsibility for decisions about their rehabilitation plan with their nurse.

11.1 Nurses are the Allies of Patients

Traditionally, doctors hold all the decision-making power in determining a course of action for the patient, with nurses overseeing the doctor's plan. The patient's concerns are frequently overlooked or not taken seriously. Although this system is well-intentioned and usually beneficial, it can alienate patients, who have little say in mater that can literally mean life or death to them. In the last decade and a half, health care professionals have been trying to develop a model of patient care based on the notion of autonomy, which Lucke as well as other researchers define as "a state of sensing and recognizing the ability to freely choose behaviors and courses of action on one's own behalf and in accordance with one's own needs and goals." In other words, no one knows more about a patient's situation than the patient. In this new approach to patient care, nurses are no longer merely executors of the doctor's wishes; they are patient's allies, helping them make reasonable choices and gain control of their own health care.

11.2 Associate the Patient in Management

It is not valueless to associate the patient in his own care. No doubt, it is the physician, who knows the best, but it is the patient who is suffering his symptoms the most. It is not undermining or challenging the authority of the physician, it nurse and patient also have a say in the management of his problem. This will be an individualistic approach and would be better than the group-management approach. It is the nurse, who will help the physician in this approach, without unduly impinging on his time.

12. NEW SKILLS: PATIENT SATISFACTION

To provide the best care to the patient it is necessary that nurse interviews the patient and his attendants, first of all and achieve the following in consultation with resident doctor and the consultant:

(i) Preparing the environment and oneself;
(ii) Opening and greeting;
(iii) Eliciting the full range of problems;
(iv) Choosing a priority problem and negotiating what will be addressed during the visit;
(v) Encouraging the patient to tell his or her story in his or her own words;
(vi) Encouraging elaboration about the life context, occupation, and risks of the patient;
(vii) Explaining procedures and examinations;
(viii) Summarizing findings;
(ix) Discussing diagnostic and treatment findings; and
(x) Negotiating plant for care.

However, those with low on health education, were less permeable to advice and treatment.

Patients with low literacy are less knowledgeable about colorectal cancer and more dubious about screening, especially with endoscopes. In cases of diabetic patients, low literacy correlated with less knowledge about signs of hyperglycemia or hypoglycemia, treatment of hypoglycemia, foot care, glycosylated hemoglobin, the value of exercise, or the complications of diabetes.

A heart failure disease-management educational program can reduce morbidity and hospitalizations.

In the near future, efforts to continually improve communication skills will be as important as the skill and knowledge of clinical practice or engaging in regular continuing medical education activities. These skills of communication will be monitored as part of quality control, and that learning will be widely available on the internet. Medical and Nurse Practitioners who work on their communication skills will be rewarded by greater patient-satisfaction with each encounter and with practice overall, and they will find their practice to be more competitive, efficient, and safe.

13. A FRESH GRADUATE NURSE: NEEDS EXPERIENCE TO COPE WITH DEMANDS

A fresh nursing (or Medical) graduate's inability to convert professional, bureaucratic work organizational conflict into positive experiences, can affect patient care. Since they lack time management and also skills and ability to provide continuity of care. Graduates may also neither possess skills nor experience to deal with unplanned events or patients. Coping strategies which are lacking may increase if the graduates are guided into turning these emotional experiences into learning experiences.

There also exists wide scope for evaluation and research into the actual "quality or care" administered by graduates in their first three months of work. This is an important area, as patient care is the ultimate aim of nursing, and it is the nurse's responsibility to be accountable for adequate care. It is possible for nurses to survive the initial "reality shock" and continue to function and learn with support and supervision from seniors. Any kind of discouragement or leg pulling or ridicule has no place in learning or confidence building.

References

Anand, R.C. *et. al.* (1983), Role of Medical Social Workers in a Big Teaching Hospital, *Journal of Hospital Administration.*

Baliant, M. (1957), The Doctor, His Patient and the Illnesses, London.

Baliant, M. *et al.* (1966), 'A study of Doctors', Tavistock Publication, London.

Berlow, B. (1960), Hospital Topics, 38:51, 97.

Berne, E. (1961), Transactional analysis in Psychotherapy, New York.

British Medical Journal (1968), Why Not Child Visitors?

Browne, K. and Freeling, P. (1967), The Doctor-Patient Relationship, E & S Livingstone Ltd., London.

Catwright, A. (1967), Patients and their Doctor: A Study of Feneral Practice, Routledge and Kegan Paul, London.

David, M., Peter, A. (1985), Community General Practitioner, Lancet, Nov. 16, 1985, 1114.

Cass, L.J. and Culran, W.J. (1965), Lancet, ii, 783.

Ellis, A. (1962), Reason and Emotion in Psychotherapy, New York.

Frank, J.D. (1961), Persuasion and Healing, John Hopkins Press, Baltimore.

Greco, R. (1966), One Man's Practice, Tavistock Publication, London.

Gremillion, D. (1980), The Child Visitor, A Hospital Hazard, 7, Commentary.

Higgins, P.M. (1963), The Practitioner.

Karl, S.V. and Cobb, S. (1966), Health Behaviour, Illness Behaviour, Silk Role Behaviour, Arch of Environmental Health.

Kuppuswami, T.N. (1975), "Patients and Hospitals", *Journal of Hospital Administration*, Vol. 12, Nos. 1-2.

Lane, K.E. (1964), *J. Coll. Gen. Practitioner*.

Levai, M., Pinsker, H. (1968), The Value of Permitting Children To Visit on Wards, Hospital and Community Psychiatry.

Mangal, J.K. and Makashir, S.D. (1972), "A Sociology Study of Attitude of Patients Towards Hospitalization", *Journal of Hospital Administration*, Vol. 9, No. 1.

Matorin, S. (1985), Child Visitors and Creative Hospital Administration, Hospital Topics.

Meador, C.K. (1965), The Art and Science of Non-disease, *New England, J. of Med.*

Appendix

RESTORING THE SANCTITY OF THE PATIENT-PHYSICIAN RELATIONSHIP

By Joel R. Cooper, The Medical Reporter

" After all, what oath, promise, or pledge did we ever make, either as individuals, or as a profession, that obligates us to restrict care? We pledged, instead, to provide care."

—Jerome P. Kassirer, M.D.
The New England Journal of Medicine

There was a time in this country when patients trusted their doctors completely . . . trusted them with their lives and listened to them and heeded their advice and friendly consultation. You could talk to your doctor in privacy behind closed doors and you felt entirely confident that what he or she recommended was 100% in your best interest.

There was also a time doctors thought of little else but treated and caring for their patients, and doing everything in their power to offer their patients the best medical care known to science. They trained long and hard in medical school and took an oath to provide the best care possible to their patients, regardless of cost, and make their own selfish interests secondary to their chosen vocation of healing and doctoring.

But something happened in the United States of America. A wedge was driven between patient and doctor. For one thing, our society became increasingly litigious. Doctors, fearing lawsuits, frivolous or otherwise, began practicing defensive medicine—they became a little more detached and self-protective. And patients, having once perceived their doctors as friends, advocates, and teachers, begin seeing dollar signs and spiraling health care costs. Were doctors practicing medicine to line their pockets? Were they in it for their patients or for those fancy European sports cars, exclusive country club memberships, and frequent vacations to various tropical paradises? Could anyone really tell?

Did "fee-for-service" medicine create a perverse or corrupting set of financial incentives for doctors? Why in heaven's name were they ordering so many diagnostic tests? Why were they using so much high tech equipment? And why were there so many coronary bypass operations, hysterectomies, and cesarean sections in this country, anyway? Had good, old-fashioned vaginal birth gone out of style?

To make a long story, people started keeping close tabs on health care expenses. It was determined that spending close to a trillion dollars a year on health care was too much . . . that it was bankrupting the country, and that even with such immense expenditures, many Americans still weren't receiving the medical care they needed. (For example, infant mortality is higher in the U.S. than in other industrialized nations). People were failing through the cracks in the system, even with Medicare and Medicaid. The U.S. health care system was said to be broken and in dire need of repair. Enter the politicians. Health care became a political issue. Strike that, Political hot potato is more like it.

The Clinton Administration banked on comprehensive health care reform. But the issue was more complex and controversial than anyone expected. Americans, it turned out had pervasive fears of big (and inefficient), government involvement in their health care, and throngs of well-healed loyalists roundly and soundly defeated health care reform in Washington, D.C. The hot potato as subsequently tossed back to the states. The health insurance companies, threatened with their own possible extinction under nationalized health care delivery and a government-run single-payer system, breathed a deep sigh of relief.

Now we're left with managed care. And managed care is marching forward in most markets throughout America largely unchallenged, largely backed by huge corporate entities with extensive financial resources and consequently, largely unstoppable. Everyone seems to be buying into managed care, even before we know for sure, if it's good or bad for individual patients or for the health of American, collectively considered. No one, except the very rich individual who can afford to pay for medical care out of pocket, is immune from this progression. Even senior citizens, who could long depend on Medicare for their health care in their aging years, are now being herded into large HMOs to contain costs.

Some say the relationship between patient and physician has been further compromised, further weakened, under managed care.

"The doctor-patient relationship, once considered the basis of therapy, has been subverted by technology, by the medical education system and, more dramatically, by the intrusive demands of managed care," said Elizabeth De Vita, associate editor of *American Health Magazine,* in a recent article.

What is managed care? It's basically a system that attempts to control health care costs by carefully managing how, when, where, why and by whom care is provided. To call it "rationing" would be going too far. But its effect is to prevent needless unnecessary utilization of health care services . . . to keep people away from doctors they don't need to see, and out of hospitals—which, when compared to hotels, are pretty expensive places to stay . . . even for one extra day.

The buzzword in medicine those days is "capitation." The word is reminiscent of a similar word which brings to mind the swift descent of a guillotine blade, followed by the sound of someone's head going "plop" into a bucket. Actually, capitation means doctors are paid one set fee per month for each patient. And if they can't manage their patients' medical care for this set fee. It's likely to be the doctor's heads winding up in the bucket.

"Under capitation at the provider level, the patient becomes a cost center rather than a customer," said Joseph C. Nichols, Jr. MD, President of the Washington State Orthopedic Association. "There is a disincentive to provide care, and the sickest patients who need health care the most become pariahs of the system. The focus in this methodology becomes cost containment, and patient illness becomes a burden to cope with."

"The potential for under-utilizing services is a real concern", continued Dr. Nichols. "Those claims that the fee-for-service system cause physician to inappropriate over-utilize must recognize the potential for those same physician to inappropriately withhold services when they are given incentives to do just that under capitation."

Withholding services may become the "default position" under many evolving scenarios of managed care. In these cases where a bad legal outcome isn't anticipated, without holding services.

May be easier for doctors to do, considering how time-intensive and aggravating it is for them to argue with managed care companies. It's also true that doctors who fight managed care companies. It's also true that doctors who fight managed care companies can be cut from their provider panel. This can hurt doctor's incomes, sometimes seriously enough to jeopardize their practices.

> ". . . many physicians in a captivated system may not provide all the services they should, may not always be the patient advocate, and may be reluctant to challenge the rules governing which services are appropriate."
>
> —Jerome P. Kassirer, M.D., writing in *The New England Journal of Medicine.*

One big problem is that, despite a veritable cornucopia of clinical guidelines available to practically every doctor, nurse, physician assistant other physician "extenders" in the system today, no one really knows at this stage in the game what constitutes under-utilization or over-utilization. That missing bit of information is being worked out by hundreds, perhaps thousands of experts in a burgeoning industry called "outcomes research."

Researchers hope to amass data on what procedures or treatment really improve the lives of patients by helping them to live longer, live more comfortably, or be happier or more content with the quality of the medical care they received. "Medical quality" is another one of those vague and fuzzy terms that the experts have yet to define satisfactorily. For in 1995, when we can track the cost of health care down to the fraction of each penny spent, we don't know what medical quality really means. In broad terms, it probably has something to do with whether you get better or not—with whether you live or die. But many doctors are losing the ability to make that judgment call. What care is "appropriate" and covered, and what is not, is often defined in a seemingly arbitrary manner by managed care corporations and fashioned into hard-and-fast health insurance policy—which is the insurance industry's equivalent of legal gobbledygook. Have you ever been able to read an explanation of covered benefits booklet given to you by a health insurance company and really understand it? Didn't think so. And guess what? There's probably a reason for that which works to the benefit of insurance companies—not health care consumers.

By now, you've probably heard the terms "corporatization" of medicine or "market-driven" medicine. What this means is that health care, and the delivery thereof, becomes a commodity subject to the same laws of the marketplace as soda pop, breakfast cereal, used cars, toaster ovens, and personal computers, for that matter. Is cheaper always better? Are there principles nearer and dearer to as than just saving a buck? Has our emphasis on cutting costs resulted in cutting some very important corners?

"Health care is not toilet paper," said Barbara R. Reed, M.D., President of the Denver Medical Society, in an editorial published in the Denver Post. "As physicians we know that all too well, but we had better spark that realization in others."

She's right, of course. You can easily replace one roll or ten thousand rolls of toilet paper. But when you lose that special, trusting relationship between patient and physician, you've lost something truly irreplaceable, unique, and desirable—yes, desirable.

The relationship between you and your family doctor, for example, is the cornerstone of your health care. Your family doctor knows you, knows your medical history, knows your lifestyle preferences, and knows and understands the context of your familial and other social relationships. There's value in that. Not just medical value, but something that transcends the measurable clinical benefit. "Continuity of Care" is the term used to describe an ongoing relationship with your doctor. It can be one of the single most valuable tools you have in the preservation and maintenance of your health. It's something you should insist on. And be willing to fight for.

But with marketplace medicine, what's happening is that health plans are competing with each other to deliver care at the lowest cost. This, in turn, is being driven by employers who want lower health care premiums. Corporations used to buy health care insurance for their employees as an added incentive for their employees to work for them . . . and stay with them. But, as health care costs increased, those health care premiums became an increasing liability to corporations trying to stay competitive. They became, in effect, a real drain on the bottom line.

Companies nowadays, many of which are operating in a lean and mean "downsized" mode to begin with, show little allegiance or loyalty to their employees . . . or to the companies from which they purchase their insurance. If they can save some money, offer a more favourable report to their shareholders or investors, they will do so. These are the ways of corporate business.

Yet each time a company changes its health plan, employees typically wind up with a new panel of, "providers"—the doctors participating in that particular managed care plan. In many cases employees have to select a primary care physician who participates in their company's health plan.

If they want to stay with the doctor they already use, they typically must pay more—or pay out of pocket. I've heard doctors tell me that their patients leave them regularly just to save a few bucks under a new managed care plan.

This is really sad. In cases of financial hardship, it's certainly understandable, but sad nonetheless. Wouldn't we be better off with a system where we are free to stay with the doctor we already have? If you have a doctor you like, how you believe is a good doctor and who has taken good care of you in times of need, doesn't make sense to stick with that doctor?

Corporations should contract with health insurance plans which allow their employees to maintain their existing relationships with doctors, if they so choose, without penalizing them financially. Allowing employees to keep their doctors may result in healthier and happier employees, which can only improve their productivity and motivation... and the corporate bottom line.

What about the argument that managed care is a good thing because it saves money and prevents needless procedures, and that under the old fee-for-service system doctors really were making too much money anyway?

The real question is this: should health care be treated like a commodity, like an item to be bartered, bought, traced and sold?

Managed care in and of itself isn't the bad guy. HMOs, for example, emphasize preventive medicine and regular check-ups for their patients to rule out disease or detect it early on when it's most highly treatable. They also do a terrific job educating their patients to help them minimize the risk of serious disease in the first place. Under traditional indemnity insurance, such preventive services may not be covered, since patients typically need a presenting complaint (or sickness) before insurance kicks in. In this context, managed care is unquestionably a good thing.

What's potentially hazardous to our health as health care consumers, however, is the underlying set of financial incentives inherent to certain forms of managed care. Serious gaps may exist between the care you need (and which your doctor deems medically advisable) and the care which managed care is willing to pay for. "Medical necessity" is a term that's open to interpretation, and managed care organizations have been known to use it as a weasel word when they don't want to pay or when they want to delay claims processing and payment. As an enlightened health care consumer, you need to ask yourself this: who should be deciding what is or is not medically necessary for you and your family—your doctor or a managed care clerk somewhere?

In the old fee-for-service system physicians and hospitals made their money on the basis of the procedure, text, or treatment given—and on the length of "inpatient" hospital stays. The sicker patients were, and the more surgeries and procedures patients needed, generally speaking, the more money the physicians and hospitals made. This was really a "sick care" system, because people profited from other people bad health. The system was driven, in many cases, by physicians and hospitals, who were paid for their services by insurance companies or, in the case of Medicare or Medicaid, by the U.S. government.

Today, financial risks have shifted back onto the doctors and hospitals and other health care providers. Under global capitation, with doctors getting a set amount of money per patient per month to deliver care, the incentive scheme changes dramatically. Under this scenario, the more care that doctors provide and the sicker patients are, the less money they make. Thus, doctors have a financial incentive to have healthier patients to begin with, and to keep these patients' health. (The insurance industry long ago turned "cherry picking", or selecting the healthiest patients with the lowest risks as health plan subscribers, into a near art form). The danger is that doctors may now limit care in an effort to preserve a bigger piece of the capitation money pie for themselves. Some doctors receive bonuses at the end of the year based on their patients' utilization of medical services. The less care they provide, the bigger bonuses they get. Now, doesn't that just fry your goose—the thought that your doctor will get more money at the end of the year because he or she limited care to you and your family? Does that make you trust your doctor more or less?

In most cases, simple human greed isn't the motivating factor. Fear is, Doctors may limit care because they're afraid that if they provide more care, or more expensive care, than their medical peers, they may be cut from managed care panels. Since managed care contracts often represent a sizable portion of total practice income to many physicians, doctors may be reluctant to "rock the boat." This is especially true in heavily managed care-penetrated urban areas, you have less to fear from managed care now, but the experts say this could change dramatically in the near future.

Some health system analysts fear that the unchecked expansion of managed care may alienate physicians, undermine patients' trust of physicians, and expand the population of patients without health care coverage.

"Physicians will be forced to choose between the best interest of their patients and their own economic survival", warns Dr. Kassirer.

How can this sort of economic climate in the medical profession help to engender trust between patient and physician? Patients expect doctors to advocate of their behalf, to look out for their best medical interests in times of sickness, vulnerability, and need. They need to be able to trust their doctors completely, and know that their medical care is in good hands. Doctors expect to step forward, to help and to heal. They aren't taught in medical school to withhold care that is medically necessary or advisable.

Under fee-for-service medicine, with its underlying financial incentives to do more to make more money, all medicine was not always necessarily in the best interest of patients. Medical tests and procedures, after all, can have side effects. They can leave a patient worse-off than before because of complications or adverse outcomes. Sometimes, less care (instead of more care) is actually better for the patient. That having been said it's also true that too little care, or care given too late, can be ill-advised and dangerous. Consumers need to know they are getting the care they actually need—no more and no less. Their physicians are most qualified to find the right balance and make sure they are cared for properly.

Consumers who sign up with an HMO or otherwise trust their health and well-being to an insurance plan may expect that all care will be provided for them, under all circumstances. They must view the situation more realistically. For many health care consumers, particularly those whose health plans selected by highly cost-conscious employers, the free-rolling and romping days of getting all of the care they want, and letting someone else pay for it are over forever.

People should be more conscious of health care costs, and be more responsible for their own health by adopting healthier behaviours and reducing their personal health risks. Few would dispute that, the risk we face in market-driven health care, however, is that cost-containment will eclipse quality, and pleasing investors will take precedence over patients.

In the short-term at least, managed care will continue to put increasing pressure on doctors and hospitals to keep costs down, driven by employees who are pushing managd care plans to offer greater value for each premium dollar spent. Corporations who are providing health insurance coverage for their employees are always looking for ways to cut costs and shore up the bottom line. The interests of employers in selecting a health plan are not necessarily the same as those of employees and their families.

Sometimes corporations, in their desire to save a few bucks, unknowingly push their employees into health plans that may or may not be in their employees' best interest. Having to switch doctors frequently is more than likely not in one's best interest, health-wise.

Insurance companies and managed care firms have succeeded largely through sales and marketing efforts. They must sell themselves effectively to large employers to get the sizable premium generating contracts. They must also sell doctors, hospitals, and other health care providers on participating in their plans and offering their services at a reduced, or discounted rate. Insurance companies make their money from limiting care to patients and by obtaining increasingly large discounts on services from doctors, hospitals, and other care givers. Insurance firms spare no effort to curtail the amount of money spent on patient care, and yet they have no qualms about huge profits and paying their executives outrageously high salaries.

"The nation's big for-profit health maintenance organizations had a banner year in 1994 by doing what they are set-up to do, squeezing every penny possible out of the fees charged by doctors and hospitals," said Milt Freudenheim, writing in *The New York Times*. "But as they put pressure on health-care providers to cut costs, the HMOs were rewarding their chief executives with sizable pay packages. The cash and stock awards to the chief of the seven biggest for-profit HMO's averaged $7 million in 1994."

Many doctors are forced to participate in managed care plans, whether they believe in their underlying philosophy or not simply to stay afloat financially. Some doctors regard it, as a necessary evil, other regard it as a game. Managed care companies keep careful tabs on doctors, not only on their individual practices and care-utilization patters, but also on whether or not doctors are "managed care friendly"—that is, whether or not they are cooperative, easy to work with, and whether or not they speak favourably of managed care, especially in public.

I've heard accounts of doctors getting cut from managed care panels because they spoke out against managed care in newspaper editorials. This, if true, is not right. Doctors should have the right to say what they will about anything their stands to have such a far-reaching effect on patients, patient care, and health care delivery in this country. After all, doctors will be the ones giving the care, or most certainly spearheading the teams giving the care. In our democratic society, we have always had the opportunity to question, analyze, and speak out against something if we think it may not be right. If doctors want to question managed care in the newspapers or on the Interact, for that matter, that should be their right and privilege. It should also be the right of managed care organizations to voice their opinion, should they desire to do so.

Accordingly, The Medical Reporter will give equal time to physicians and managed care organizations to voice their opinions about some of the issues mentioned here. The Medical Reporter stands for patient advocacy, education, and support. We will be watching managed care organizations to make sure they are not violating the rights of health care consumers in any way. We will also be watching all other groups and organizations that play a role in the provision of health care today. And I am assure you of this; the various World Websites and health care media to which we are linked will be watching as well.

We believe it is time to bring back trust to the practice of medicine and to restore the sanctity of something long cherished and truly invaluable; the patient-physician relationship.

For, in the final analysis, as Elzabeth De Vita so sagely pointed out, "Doctors and patients need each other to survive."

Nurse and Doctor Relationship in Hospitals: To Decent Staff Services

The nurse-doctor relationship is a complex relationship. It is shaped by several issues, such as gender, education, training, responsibility, accountability, salary disparities and national economics. It is also shaped by social and professional issues. Everyone recognizes that collaboration is the desired goal, and this goal of collaboration has been longstanding. The challenge is to establish a collaborative relationship while continuing to work independently. However, this challenge will be greater for those who are in a mode of confrontation and less of an issue where goodwill and common sense prevail.

I. GENERAL

From the medieval times, care of the sick and dying was undertaken by religious establishments. The decline in human goodwill and greater demand for organised care led to the establishment of schools of nursing. With this a more systematic approach to nursing the sick and dying emerged. This served to enhance the image of the nurse as a profession. Medicine has seen a progressive movement towards mutual recognition of the unique skills of the two professions (Doctors as well as nurses) brought to health care. This meant a relationship of partnership and satisfying patient care. Collaboration according to the Oxford Dictionary means simply "to labour together", or to work jointly. Why? Because collaboration in critical care units leads to improved patient outcome. Collaboration should improve productivity, increase job satisfaction and create enlightened spirits, reinforce self-confidence and self-worth. In a properly functioning team, mutual support and consensus develop as information brought to light by both parties is reviewed and discussed. Finally, a less positive reason to collaborate is that one has no choice.

CHART 8.1

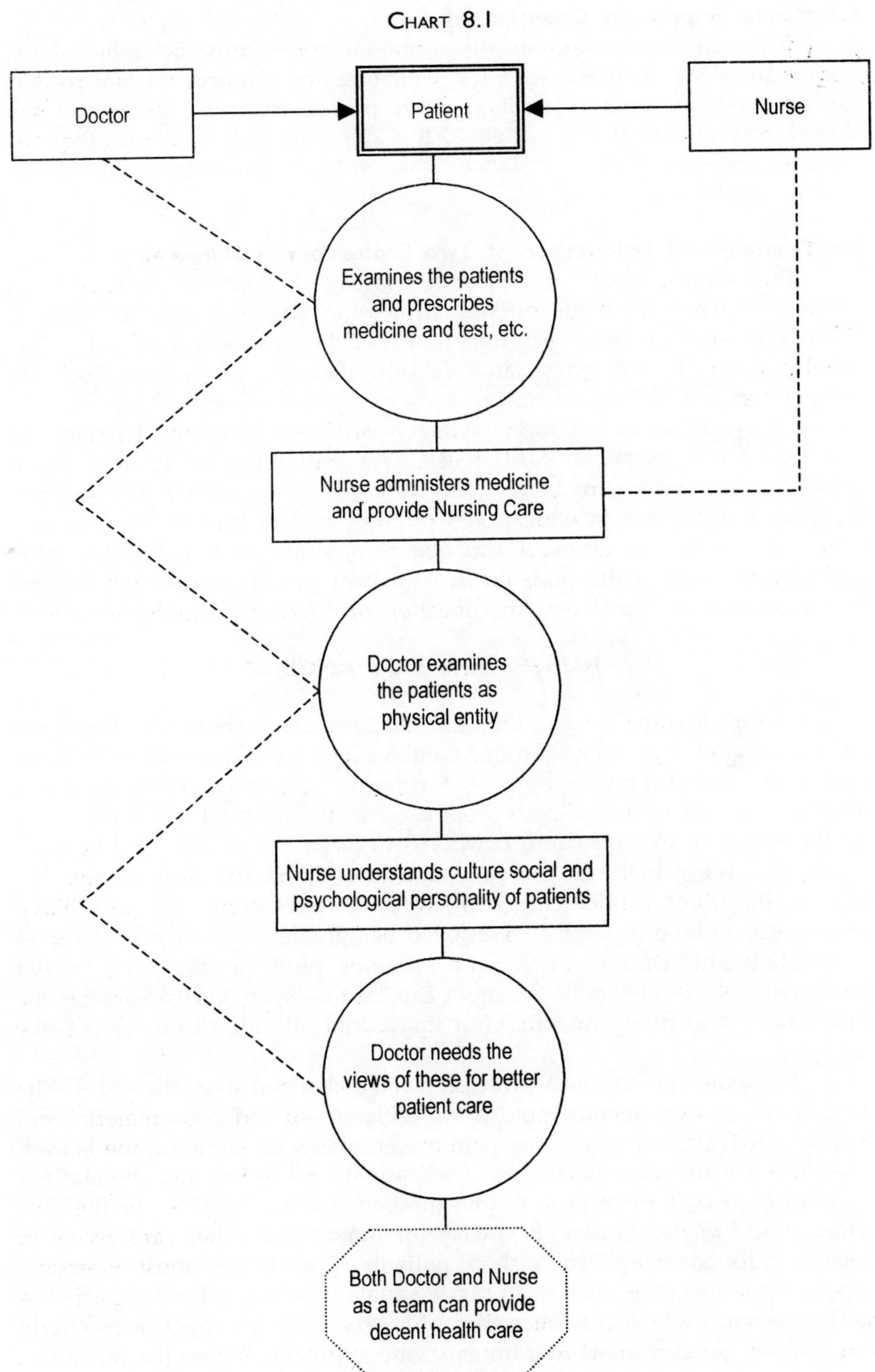
Doctor
Patient
Nurse
Examines the patients and prescribes medicine and test, etc.
Nurse administers medicine and provide Nursing Care
Doctor examines the patients as physical entity
Nurse understands culture social and psychological personality of patients
Doctor needs the views of these for better patient care
Both Doctor and Nurse as a team can provide decent health care

1.1 Mutual Support is Essential

The activities, communications and decisions must be done jointly, even if the decision processes vary. Collaboration requires mutual respect for each other's unique abilities, both professional and personal, and shared accountability. Nevertheless, this does not deny the fact that the ultimate decision in many instances falls on to the physician who may be held accountable.

1.2 Training and Orientation of Two Professions is Different

Physicians study in a culture-oriented towards science and intellectual freedom, while nursing profession has been service-oriented. The two professions have been moving closer, but the balance of power has usually been in the physician's favour. This at times can leads to competition, conflict and distorted communication. Little needs to be said about gender/culture issues, which can also present barriers to collaboration. Economic disparity exists between the two professions and it may lead to a feeling of being "less valued" as a member of the team. Significant difference in educational philosophy has been that physicians have been trained to be exact and objective, while nursing holds a more extended view of health and illness. However, health care is increasingly a system built on teamwork, the question of inferiority should not arise.

2. NURSES ARE NOT ANGELS?

"From the time I was a little girl, all I can ever remember wanting to be, was a nurse. I graduated from Miami Valley Hospital School of Nursing and have worked there ever-since. During my 34 year career in nursing, I have worked on virtually every floor/unit in the hospital and have cared for thousands of patients, from newborns to those in their 90's and beyond. I love providing bed side nursing care and doing the little things like shaving the older gentlemen, giving welcome back rubs, and just taking time out or to hold a hand. I have loved being able to touch people's lives in positive and caring way", said a senior nurse at the time of her retirement. No doubt, only an angel can bestow such liberal care on the sick, smelly and dying humans. But that is not all, not all nurses act like angels.

"Nursing services and profession have changed over the years. The educational process spends more time on classroom and book material and less on actual patient care. There is more emphasis on climbing the ladder. Hospitals are run like businesses. The patients are sicker and the staffing is shorter, so that there is less time to spend at the bedside. In this fast paced world of health care, it is easy for nurses and other care givers to become "disconnected" from their patients. This is the most worrying aspect of nursing care services in big hospitals like PGI at Chandigarh. The selfless service, which was once like a blessing from an angel or motherly nurture has got converted to a bureaucratic approach, where the nurse has transformed herself into a robot, with no sense of care, human touch, concern, sympathy or accountability. While they stand on their ego, matching with physicians in perks and social expectations, they do not exhibit responsibility of even an ordinary good person, who can be trusted to look after a human being in distress, notwithstanding the degree of clinical or intellectual quotient. This has put a question mark over the training of nurses as health care personnel. Let them be human first.

2.1 Nurses are essential Health Managers

While their touch and care, if and when really available, makes them, second to no angel, the earnestness on their part is often found lacking. Similarly, commensurate wages and 'look after' of nursing personnel has also been found wanting. Status and earnings of nursing services managers are not high, but long work hours are common. There is a great demand for nurses all over the world, but they are treated as menials, in many set-ups, despite long and ardous training and nerve breaking nature of work.

Health care is a business and, like every other business, it needs good management to run smoothly. The term "medical and health services manager" encompasses all who plan, direct, coordinate, and supervise the delivery of health care. Nurses enjoy a pre-eminent position in terms of inputs. Large facilities usually have several assistant administrators to aid the top administrator to handle daily decisions. In a hospital set-up, most of the grass-root administration is handled by nurses at various levels.

Even in smaller facilities, nurse administrators handle the details of daily working operations. Doctor have more specific responsibilities than nurses in government hospitals as well as private set-ups. A small group of 10 or 15 physicians might employ one sister incharge as an administrator to oversee billing and collection, budgeting, planning, equipment outlays, and patient flow. Such systems may contain both in-patient and out-patient facilities and offer several patient services. As administrator, many of them are excelling, but the 'humane and care' approach is diminishing.

2.2 Working Conditions

Most nurses work long hours many work around the clock. These managers do not get to work in comfortable offices; may share space with other staff. They may spend considerable time walking, to consult with or supervise co-workers. There are no holidays or vacations.

Nursing service administrators usually are among supervisory registered nurses with administrative abilities and a graduate degree in health services administration. These managers often are responsible for lakhs of rupees of equipment and hundreds of employees. To make effective decisions, they need to consider different opinions and be good at analyzing contradictory information. Motivating others to implement decisions requires strong leadership abilities. Tact, diplomacy, flexibility, and commitment are essential because these managers spend most of their time with others. Thus, the model of nurse physician team is key to providing high quality and cost effective care under Indian conditions.

3. PARTNERSHIP OF QUALITY MEDICAL CARE

Managed care works best through partnerships between the doctor and nurse on the one hand and between managed hospitals and the individuals whom they serve, i.e. patients. An important ingredient in managed care's success is the encouragement of all participants. But promoting improvements in our systems that are patient-centered, we will ensure that managed care remains responsive and accountable and not merely a money spinning game.

3.1 The Following are the Essentials for Quality Medical Care

1. Free and open communication between patient and doctor, nurse, or other caregiver regarding all aspects of health care.
2. Complete information on services available and given in easy to understand language.
3. Ready access to the services you need and which are available.
4. Clear information about what to do when you need a specialized care.
5. To make it easy for you to find out which drugs or other services like tests or surgery are reimbursable from employer or insurance.
6. Personnel, facilities, and systems which are available to you.
7. Payment mechanisms for the treatment you avail.
8. A willingness to display performance against the practices of the 'best institutions', in the area of patient care, to make it transparent and trustworthy.
9. What to do if you have complaints and use the complaints to make systems more responsive.
10. Ways to measure satisfaction of community with hospitals, physicians, services and health plans, as well as health outcomes.

3.2 What is Expected from Members of Community and Patient?

1. Read through newspaper and health plan about services and procedures available in hospitals of your area.
2. Know when you and your family members should have regular check-ups; immunizations, and tests.
3. When you leave your doctor's office after a visit, know exactly what you need to do about medications or a follow-up visit. Be sure you or your family members follow the instructions given.
4. If you're not satisfied with your physician, change them. It's

your right to have a team nurse or choice. But do not do it on whims, ego, flimsy ground. You may lose a good physician friend or a good nurse-doctor team.

5. If you see another doctor or other health care professional on your own, make sure your primary care physician receives necessary information from them.
6. Be as informed as you can be, about a particular disease or condition you may have. Seek additional information from reliable sources.
7. If you have a complaint, follow the procedures established. Remember that you have a right to a timely response.
8. Do your best to follow advice about diet, exercise, and a healthy lifestyle.
9. It is good to get a health policy or mediclaim policy from an insurance company.
10. Be an informed consumer.

4. DOCTOR IS THE CAPTAIN

During the twentieth century, the nursing profession has undergone immense changes. Nursing has progressed from an occupation to profession, with members that provide a broad range of services independently, and in a variety of professional relationships with other providers. This evolution has changed, how nurses are educated, clinically prepared, and how they perceive their role. In the early years of the nursing profession, it was generally believed that nurses served and cared for their patients by assisting physicians. During wars and times of crises, nurses worked with the physicians conducting surgical procedures, diagnosing cases, and prescribing treatments and drugs. The role of the public health nurse, as it developed earlier in this century in the west, was often independent, with nurses working with families of patients with tuberculosis or other highly contagious diseases and providing a broad range of services.

Intrinsic to nursing is the collaborative process: nurses and physicians working together and independently assessing, diagnosing, and caring for patient by preparing histories, conducting physical and psychosocial assessments, and reviewing and discussing their cases with other health professionals to determine the health status of each client.

Nurses and physicians have to understand the importance of this overlap in scopes, practices, and patient care. In India, we are at cross-roads in defining the area of nursing services. They wish to be treated like physicians in every manner, except in education, training and accountability. It will be ideal if they continue to be humane like nurses, but help, share supplement and complement the work of physicians, in a manner of collaboration.

4.1 Avoiding Conflict: A Background

In the context of professional regulation, nursing scopes have always been structured to include narrowly defined independent functions and to mandate a dependent or complementary role. Physicians, as the first category of health care providers to gain registration, always attempted to incorporate all aspects of diagnosis and treatment into the definition of medical practice. Nurses, recognizing the limitations created by medical practice, attempted to act around the physician imposed limitations to create a nursing scope of practice. At that time, the medical profession was virtually all male and nursing almost all female; divisions and attitudes toward and between the two professions often reflected these gender differences.

With the evolution of nursing practice and speciality practices, the nursing profession tried to expand and redefine nursing practice to reflect actual independent practice, and not the restrictive regulatory model. This effort to enlarge their role, which implied stepping on the toes of the physicians, without adequate padding (training and legislation) had the potential of conflict among individuals as well as professions.

Emphasizing the realities of nursing roles, education, and how nurses collaborate with physicians and other professions, nurses began to see an emerging trend involving the incorporation of collaboration into statutory definitions of practice. To a large extent, this trend reflected the compromise that emerged in the face of organized physician opposition to the expansion of nursing roles. However, the nurses were willing to accept the compromise if it included official recognition of their expanding roles.

4.2 What is the Best?

Nurses have always practiced in collaboration with other professionals, e.g. doctors, other nurses and a wide variety of other health care providers. Arguably more than any other category of health care professional, nurse have understood that good patient care depends on the contributions and interactions of various providers. Even physicians who maintain private practices refer to and consult with specialists, or use practitioners for emergency back-up. Also they associate/employ a nurse to manage their private practices.

If collaboration is the norm in professional practice, why should nurses object to it? Determining what kind of relationship is needed with other professionals, and what form it should take are questions of professional judgement. Because "collaboration" is rarely defined and is often used as a euphemism for "supervision" by the physician, which the nurses do not accept and try to plough a lonely furrow, despite their understanding the futility of such an attitude.

In its testimony before the Physician Payment Review Commission (PPRC) in 1993, the American Nurses Association (ANA) explained its concerns about statutory requirements for "collaboration:" Advanced practice nurses are, as are all registered nurses, independently licensed and accountable for their actions. They are able to deliver services independent of their relationship with physicians or other health care providers. Collaborating with and referring to other health providers is a matter of good professional practice. Regardless of practice setting or supervision requirements, advanced practice nurses, like most health professionals, generally maintain a network for referral to and collaboration with other professionals and maintain a means to access emergency back-up. This shows resentment against a dependent and hierarchical relationship, in the name of collaboration.

4.3 US has a Different Model

In US there are twenty-seven states with joint regulation of advanced practice (ANA, 1997). Likewise, there are forty-eight states with some form of statute authorizing nurse prescriptive authority. Some states define collaboration in a manner akin to supervision, while others instead define and compel supervised practice arrangements. While there is a turmoil among the medical and nursing professionals in US over the demand of nurses to gain the authority of prescription and reimbursement, in India the tussle is in the form of under-currents of opposition to dominance of physicians. While no formal demands for freeing them from under the yoke of doctor is made, the resentment of their supervision is palpable.

US Federal Law defines "collaboration" as it applied to advanced nursing practice. For example, Section 1861(s)(K)(2), which refers to Medicare Part B reimbursement of professional services provide by nurse practitioners and clinical nurse specialists, requires that such services be delivered "in collaboration with a physician" to be eligible for payment. Section 1866 provides this definition of collaboration. "A process in which a nurse practitioner (or clinical nurse specialist) works with a physician to deliver health care services within the scope of the nurse practitioner's [or clinical nurse specialist's] professional expertise, with medical direction and appropriate supervision as provided for in jointly developed guidelines or other mechanisms as defined by the law of the State in which services are performed."

Leaders of American Medical Association (AMA) and American Nurses Association (ANA) met during 1993 and 1994 in an effort to reach agreement on the dimensions of nurse physician professional relationships, and specifically to establish a mutually agreeable definition of "collaboration." After lengthy discussion and negotiation, a joint AMA-ANA task force arrived at the following definition: "Collaboration is the process whereby physicians and nurses plan and practice together as colleagues, working interdependently within the boundaries of their scopes of practice with shared values and mutual acknowledgement and respect for each other's contribution to care for individuals, their families, and their communities."

Members of this task force took the definition back to their respective organizations. The ANA Board of Directors adopted it in 1994. The AMA, however, has never adopted it.

4.4 Doctor's Supervision is Essential

Under the early nurse practice acts, all nurses worked under the supervision of physicians. Along with regulation and growth in the profession, registered nurses developed an independent scope of nursing practice. Physician groups often imply that medical supervision of advanced nursing practice is necessary, because they believe nurses always function as agents or employees of physicians, and as such, do not practice independently. To provide effective and comprehensive care, nurses, physicians and other health care professionals must collaborate with each other. No group can claim total authority over the other. Each profession exhibits different area of professional competence that when combined together, provide a continuum of care that the consumer has come to expect. The definitions of collaboration reflect compromise, and are conditioned and tailored to limit competition. So the need of supervision for the 'care' which a nurse offers is being intensely felt even in US. In India, allowing the nurses to independently treat cases, will open the floodgates of quackery, which is already rampant in our polity. In fact, everyone needs supervision and collaboration, even senior consultants in speciality or super-specialty practices. Why not nurses be supervised and why should not they collaborate in patient's interest?

4.5 Gender Sensitization

Previous research on the doctor-nurse relationship has characterized it as 'partriarchal' and a 'dominant-subservient' relationship with the usual male and female gender split found to be of considerable importance when explaining the relatively subservient position of nurses. Historically the situation was even more extreme. In Florence Nightingale's era, for example, good nursing care was equated with efficiently carrying out doctor's orders. The cardinal rule of 'the doctor-nurse game' was that open disagreement between the players had to be avoided at all costs. Nurses communicated their recommendations without appearing to make recommendations, and physicians requested recommendations from nurses without appearing to ask for advice from them. However, there is some change in the mind-set and 'on the ground' that has led to gender sensitization.

4.5.1 Covert Game

The important point about the doctor-nurse 'game' was that doctors and nurses collaborated and it remained relatively covert. The medical profession is still largely male and medical authority is largely equated with male authority. For a long time, physicians have been coded as males in the minds of nurses as well as patients. So a male physician may still appear more normal and acceptable than a female physician to most people, including other health care personnel. Bluntly put, those who work with a female physician could experience the dilemma of having to choose between treating her a member of the medical profession or as a woman. Female doctors often find they are met with less respect and confidence and are given less help than their male colleagues.

4.5.2 Less Help to Young Female Doctors

A third of female doctors surveyed complained they got less help and assistance from nurses than male colleagues. For example, if nurses are assisting a female physician, they will immediately turn to help a male doctor, if he joins the scene. But it is mainly the younger female physicians who felt they received less help. While 40 percent of those under 35 years of age reported this, the corresponding figures were 29 percent of the women aged 35 to 44; 17 percent of those 45 to 54; and only nine percent of women aged over 55.

4.5.3 Intriguing Finding

One explanation for this intriguing finding is that perhaps the older female physicians are established in higher positions in the medical hierarchy. The status differences between them and female nurses are thus bigger than those between young female doctors and nurses, which could translate into a higher probability of getting the assistance they ask for. The female doctors also complain that nurses show a lack of respect and confidence in their decisions. It appears that gender hugely influences a doctor's relationship with nurses. The female doctors surveyed saw the nurses attitude to them a strategy by which the nurses were trying to cut doctors 'down to size'. Nurses were targeting women physicians because, being of the same sex, they saw themselves as a more equal match.

4.5.4 Flirting Potential

The female doctors also reported that nurses find the doctor-nurse relationship more attractive if the doctor is a male because of its potential for flirting.

4.5.5 The Strategies that may Work for Female Doctors

(i) Making friends with nurses by actively courting them. The disadvantage of this tactic is the difficulty of being a friend on the one hand and gaining respect on the other.

(ii) Relying less on nurses by making oneself more independent of them. Sixty percent of female doctors as opposed to only eight percent of their male colleagues—thought female doctors asked for less assistance than male counterparts.

(iii) Clearing up after procedures in ways that male doctors tend not to. This usually helps to 'get on the good side' of nurses.

(iv) Being more efficient than male doctors—when nurses request something, doing it straight away.

(v) Asking nurses advice more often than male doctors do, and 'aiming to follow nurses' suggestions more.

4.5.6 Common Experience

While female doctors experience greater irritation and resentment over the differential treatment male doctors receive at the hands of female nurses, it is important to understand that there are possibly deep sociological reasons, partly linked to the history of the two professions.

5. COMMUNICATION IS THE KEY: DON'T LET THE EGO BLOCK IT

Communication is a key tool that doctors and nurses must use to elicit cooperation among themselves and other individuals in the delivery of health care services. It can be described as exchanging information. Differences between their perspectives can interfere with exchange of necessary information. The communication can increase awareness of a health problem, affect attitude to create support for individual, demonstrate skills, reinforce knowledge, attitudes, or behaviour. Close liaison between doctor and nurse entails individually interacting to achieve a common good, i.e. the health and well-being of patients. For example, it can be an ongoing dialogue about a patient's concern, behaviour, attitude, or diagnosis.

A second assumption about human communication is that it is transactional, which means that both individuals in an interaction are affected by and affect each other. Human communication is based on relationship dimension. The relationship dimension defines how doctor and nurse are connected to each other, e.g. 'send this specimen to the laboratory.' The message refers to how the doctor and nurse are affiliated: to the doctor's status, the relationship to the nurse, the physician's attitude toward the nurse, the nurse's attitude toward the physician, and their feelings about one another and to that of the patient.

5.1 Behaviour and Response

Dominant or submissive behaviour usually stimulates the opposite behaviour in others. More explicitly, doctors who act dominantly usually stimulate the nurse they are interacting with, to act submissively. Hateful or loving behaviour usually stimulates the same behaviour from others. Physicians in health care settings often assume or are placed in the dominant role, while nurses are placed in a submissive role. It is this role model of nurses, which tends to rebel against dominance and the reaction is not based on any realization of merit in the independent status.

5.2 Gender Role Models: Mindset

Gender divisions are of primary importance in the assigning of roles and relationships between doctor and nurses. Within the patriarchal doctor-nurse relationship, parallels between husband and wife can be drawn. The nurse's role in this set-up is looking after the emotional environment, while the doctor decides the patient's diagnosis and the method of treatment. Traditionally, female nurse takes on a subordinate, non-professional role in the dominated medical division of labour, demonstrating the importance of gender ideologies in the caring professions. The idea of care is seen as an extension role and less privileged in status: working/middle class nurses *versus* upper class doctors, hence the subordination of nursing.

It is reported that doctors avoid working with male nurses, implying that the aspect of doctor-nurse relationship in which nurses service the needs of the doctor, still remains heavily dependent on the feminine identity of nursing. With the deterioration of public esteem for doctors, recognition of their fallibility and increasing number of female doctors and male nurses joining the patient care, the element of gender role dominance is being negated. The value of nurses as doctor's assistants or handmaidens is acknowledged all over the world, and so is the reaction to their authority and role.

Nurses are found to be largely responsible for the categorization of patients, history taking and observation, often indicating the likely course of treatment before the patient is seen by the physician. However, diagnosis is still formally recognized as the primary task of the doctor, although younger, inexperienced doctors rely immensely on experienced or senior nurses for advice and assistance. So a lot of mutual collaboration occurs *'de-facto'* but *'de-jure'* nurses resent supervision and doctors persist with dominance. Some techniques one can use for communication include: effective speaking, effective listening, feedback, alert to non-verbal signals, emotional effect, assertiveness, and handling conflict.

Any person's emotions, knowledge, and past experiences initiate a particular response. Some common styles of response by listeners are withdrawing, judging, analyzing, questioning, reassuring, and paraphrasing. Withdrawing can occur when the topic of discussion creates uncomfortable feelings. It usually is interpreted as lack of concern or callousness. Judging almost immediately extinguishes open communication. Judgemental responses can be damaging to relationships, especially when someone is judged negatively. The judged person has to defend his opinion, belief, or behaviour, placing the person in a position of rejection of or resistence to the judge.

Analyzing is similar to judging. It explains to a person why they reacted as they did. This leads to the person becoming defensive and less willing to reveal thoughts and feelings. Questioning can either enhance or inhibit communication. Helpful questions are always welcome. These questions usually encourage people to communicate rather than become defensive. Reassurance indicates acceptance of the person.

5.3 Non-verbal Responses need to be Analyzed

Effective communication requires that one is alert to the many non-verbal cues expressed by listeners. These include posture, gestures, facial expression, tone and inflection of words, personal dress, and personal space. It reflects the Individual's personality and culture. For example, how a person stands as you talk? In general, moving close to you indicate an interest in you or the discussion. Keeping a distance may indicate uncertainty about you, or a dislike of or disinterest in your topic. Walking away means, total rejection of the dialogue.

Watch the person's hands as you interact. Even though the person appears calm, nervousness is often revealed through hand activity. The classic sign of folded arms over the chest may indicate that the individual may be feeling defensive. Usually, a non-verbal message is more accurate. It is easy to control our words, but more difficult to control tone of voice, facial expression, posture, and other non-verbal signals. Emotions include feelings, physiological changes, and a pattern of overt expression. Even people who have difficulty verbally expressing their emotions can display them through their facial expressions and body language.

Communicating assertively is the use of honest, direct communication that maintains and defends one's right in a positive way. People who are assertive express their points while at the same time respecting the right of others.

5.4 The Doctor-Nurse Game

Sources of conflict have been reported between physicians and nurses. The "doctor-nurse game," first described in the 1960's, is a stereotypical pattern of interaction in which female nurses, while appearing to defer to the doctor's authority, learn to show initiative and offer advice.

In the former years, physicians were described as freely conferring with other colleagues, but consultation with a nurse seemed inappropriate. Many doctors felt threatened when they exhibited signs that they were not completely independent and totally in control of the health care situation. Medical training gave doctors feelings of omnipotence in preparation for a world of unwieldy responsibilities and a physician dominated doctor-patient relationship.

The nurse had accepted the position of defence to the physician and other authority figures. She was described as docile, subordinated, and deferent, with a traditional reputation of fulfilling a role of blind obedience rather than one of autonomous professionalism.

Many physicians still view the nurse's role as primarily carrying out their orders and reporting the patient's progress to them, when physicians are asked for suggestions for improving nursing care, they typically equate good nursing care with fulfilment of their orders and demands. In playing "the game", as long as nurses comply with physician's wishes, they are acceptable. Other factors that cause communication problems between nurses and physicians are the physician's lack of understanding of the functions and goals of the nurse, and the nurse's lack of insight into the scope of the physician's responsibilities.

5.5 Physical vs. Psychosocial

Traditionally, nursing students and medical students do not have the same classes, nor are they aware of the studies of the other group. But both are expected to work together for the well-being of the patient. Nurses place a greater emphasis on the patient's psychosocial needs. Physicians feel that nurses ignore the patient's physical needs in their effort to serve the patient's psychosocial needs. Conversely, the nurses believe that physician does not recognize the patient as a person and instead treats him as a subject. This area has been a major misunderstanding between the nurses and physicians. Also wide ranging educational preparations among nursing personnel has been confusing to physicians. With the addition of the nurse practitioner in various specialties, the role may appear to be threatening to some physicians. Generally in hospitals two systems of authority exist. The nurse, in her ambiguous role, not only receives order through the hospital administrators but also from physicians.

Since a majority of nurses entering the profession are women, it may be perceived that the primary emphasis of their employment is temporary because of the vision of women valuing marriage and motherhood over a permanent committed position. This decision to place their family before their career goals could have severely diminished respect for nurses by physicians, and it could have greatly contributed to their lack of communicational professional commitment.

5.6 Mutual Observation

Physicians and nurses are in a position to observe one another's performance, at least to the degree that their functions overlap. This role has caused much stress on both professions in the health care arena. It has been suggested that because the nurse is the only one to observe the physician's work, she has been kept in the subservient role and thus unquestioning to the errors made by a physician. Traditionally, it has not been unusual for nurses to be subjected to the outrages of physicians (often in front of patients) about the quality of their work. The second role of the nurse can be an observer of the physician providing a below standard quality performance. The nurse's ethics are called upon to surface. Will the nurse challenge the medical decision of the physician?

Another source of contention within the medical profession is physicians resenting nurses stepping into the realm of medicine. This steams from the concept that the medical society perceives itself as the authority in all medical care. Organized nursing and organized medicine have been in opposition on numerous issues. One of the ways in which nurses have asserted their independence has been in their attempt to describe nursing as entirely separate profession from medicine. In Indian conditions this is untrue. Nurses work only in big hospital set-ups as a part of physician led team. She is expected to provide 'care' under supervision, but it is the doctor who is fully accountable for her words and deeds.

5.7 Tradition is giving Way to Modernity

Traditionally, subordination is the interpretation of physician nurse interaction which involves nurses not questioning their obedience to medical orders, and demonstrates complete absence of nursing input into decision-making. For example, a medical order is given without prior consultation or explanation, nurses carry out that order without further negotiation and no alternative explanation could be given for the subservience. Nurses thus display unquestioning obedience. This model is now undergoing change. In non-teaching hospitals the atmosphere is easier, more relaxed, and characterized by an informal working atmosphere, while in large teaching hospitals the atmosphere is more formal and competitive, and often interfered with working relations. The obstacles that interfere with working relations are unequal balance of power and practice constraints. The unequal balance of power between physicians and nurses are perceived to arise principally from differing education levels among the two disciplines. With increased nursing knowledge and autonomy, the power between nurses and physicians may be altered. However, functioning of the doctor-nurse team as a cohesive and unified unit is important for proper care of the patient and image of health care professionals in general.

5.8 Hospital Environment Induces Sullen Behaviour: Keep Cheer Intact

The daily task of facing seriously ill, chronically suffering and perpetually dying people is not easy. Nurses must assist patients in maintaining their courage to live through another day. Fresh graduate nurses are not prepared in school with skills and abilities to face the many stresses related to hospital environment. Even seasoned nurses often experience frustration from the numerous non-nursing task imposed upon them. These task many times impede the nurse from performing routine nursing care, cause work overload and consequent fatigue. Emergencies frequently occur in which nurses are required to accept more responsibility than they can reasonably manage within a given period of time. In addition, nurses are often expected to perform multifarious duties in numerous departments.

The distinctly separate educational experiences of physicians and nurses often lead to a lack of insight into one another's roles and responsibilities and consequent interpersonal conflicts and lack of communication.

If a professional don't communicate, how can patients receive quality care services?

An increase in territorial disputes is another problem created by lack of understanding. Nursing roles have expanded immensely, leading to confusion as to which professional has expertise in a particular area. When roles overlap, one professional might perceive that the other person is trying to take over his or her powers and responsibilities. This action can result in unproductive competition. Physicians have considerable latitude in their actions in professional practice, while nurses are limited in their autonomy. Discrepancies in degrees of autonomy among professionals can led to interpersonal tensions.

5.9 Cooperation and Assertiveness Go Hand in Hand

Collaboration requires both cooperation and assertiveness, and involves fully recognizing others concern while not sacrificing or suppressing one's own. Collaboration requires energy and hard work Collaboration may be more difficult for nurses and physicians until they spend more time together in face to face interaction; and until they acquire a better understanding of the kinds of problems the other group faces.

It consists of sharing in planning, making decisions, solving problems, setting goals, assuming responsibilities, working together cooperatively, and communicating openly. Usually with Cooperation the results are positive because both sides win: communication is satisfying, relationships are strengthened, and negotiated solutions are frequently more cost effective.

Cooperation implies respect for each other's roles and responsibilities. Generally in a professional environment, physicians and nurses have reduced cooperation skills in reference to patient care. Both professions must be aware of and be respectful to each other's roles and responsibilities. A nurse may feel offended when the physician ask that the nurse to write down some verbal orders clerical work. Interrupting the nurse's professional responsibilities. To perform the duties of a clerk may not be pleasing to the nurse, and the nurse might perceive that the physician feels her role to be inferior. They should accept and share their differences to increase mutual understanding. This openness can reduce role confusion and territorial disputes.

There are indications that the old hierarchical way of cooperation between nurses and physician is changing. Physicians are increasingly depending on nurses expertise and skill in critical care settings and emergency departments, as well as in community settings, residential care settings, and home care services. The quality of care can only be enhanced through cooperation and good decision-making.

6. INTERACTION THROUGH EDUCATIONAL INTERVENTION

This section reports the results of an educational intervention to improve attitudes among nurses and physicians. During this study, the researchers paired each medical student with a nurse during one (8 hour) shift, with the consent of both participants.

Physicians are not with their patients all day long. Physicians cannot watch everything that happens in the hospital. Part of their success is due to the help of nurses. Additionally, nurses have access to information useful to the physician about how the patient is doing and how the patient is feeling that is not available from anyone else. Likewise, the physician has information that would allow the nurses to carry out their roles smoothly and achieve their objectives more completely. When this information is shared and when each does his/her best in a coordinated and deliberate manner, the patient is the winner. Many studies support nurse physician collaboration as a major contributing factor in positive patient outcomes.

A few medical schools in U.S. have introduced programs in which medical students and residents spend time with nurses as part of their academic curriculum. These programs provide opportunities for future physicians to understand and appreciate the roles of the nursing staff and to observe directly how optimal patient care can be fostered through positive working relationships among nurses and physicians. One important rationale for providing such an experience early in medical education is to shape attitudes before more negative (doctor-nurse) stereotypes become ingrained. Educators suggest that introducing collaboration into an actual practice setting is likely to be the most effective approach. Comments by medical students included the following: "I am amazed at the variety and range of things nurses need to keep track of," "I never realized exactly what nurses did," and "Patients say things to nurses that they never say to physicians."

In the study mentioned above Medical Students' comments were grouped into four themes: range of nursing responsibilities, nurse-patient relationships, physicians' orders, and overall satisfaction. In the area of nurse-patient relationships, students commonly expressed the view that because nurses spend more time with individual patients, patients became more comfortable sharing personal concerns such as their discomfort or emotional state. Students recognized and appreciated nurses' compassion for and emotional support of patients. Because nurses had important insights into patients' emotional state or ability/inability to perform activities of daily living, many students expressed their intention to solicit input from the nursing staff to provide better care for their patients in future. Medical students gained a better appreciation for the range of nursing responsibilities and articulated many qualitative observations on the differences among nurses' and physicians' styles of communication with patients.

Many students expressed genuine appreciation for nurses' tasks and responsibilities, conveying understanding and respect, and healthy attitudes that are essential to collaboration. When these students become practicing physicians and physicians' assistants, they may be more inclined to solicit and incorporate nurses' perspective and expertise, which can have a positive effect on patient care decisions, discharge plans, and patient education. Medical educators should emphasize the value of collaboration among health care providers as one important component of high quality medical care and develop curricula to foster collaboration.

7. MEDICAL COMPLIANCE IS *SINE QUA NON*: NURSE HAS A GREAT ROLE

Medical Compliance is defined as an action in accordance with a command from a doctor and the tendency to submit easily by the patient. It is based on the premise that the physician knows the best and that the patient would follow the command and that in doing so all will be well.

In this model, the patient is expected to willingly submit to the physician's authority and expertise, and comply with the treatment regimen. Non-compliant behaviour is seen as problematic, it contravenes professional beliefs, norms, and expectations regarding the proper roles of patient and professionals. A nurse has an important role in achieving medical compliance from the patient.

Medical compliance is an essential element in effective medical management. Nurses expend enormous amounts of energy and valuable time educating non-compliant patients of the dangers of their actions. Sometimes these efforts are no avail, and sometimes the consequences are dire. Patients being treated for hypertension were found in a study to have non-compliance rates in excess of 50%, whereas non-compliance in heart transplant recipients was found to be considerably lower—as many as 50% of heart patients discontinue cardiac rehabilitation within the first year. Greater variation is found when specific aspects of non-compliance (e.g., diet, smoking, activity) are also individually analyzed.

If a nurse exhibits conflict with the clinical accumen or authority of a physician, the compliance will fall. So the medical compliance is give *qua non* to the successful patient care and the cooperation and role of a nurse is key to achieving compliance.

8. BRIDGING THE VOID IN TREATMENT: THE MANAGED CARE CREATES DISTANCE

What is essential is an understanding of how to establish or re-establish an environment that will facilitate the development of trust and healthier coping mechanisms, thereby replacing power, conflict, and non-compliance with cooperation and mutual involvement. Because of managed care, with its restrictions and cutback, an unfortunate distancing between patients and physicians and his team has taken place. Physicians have less time and opportunity to develop the relationships with their patients. This leaves a void in the treatment process. The aim of the medical team should be to make the patient feel that he or she is a valuable member of the treatment team. Providing an environment of cooperation begins with the patient's first encounter with the medical team. The ways in which physicians and nurses talk to patients about their illness, treatment, and outcome and well serve to create the foundation from which their relationship will develop. The communication void is not always the result heightened emotional state or an intellectual defect in the patient, it can be a lack of rapport.

Physicians have long standing feelings about what they represent and how they should be treated. Although in reality their position of importance does not appreciably change with patient being a partner the feelings evoked in them may not correspond. It would not be surprising that a difficult adjustment to the idea of the patient as a member of the treatment team may take place. These feelings need to be acknowledged and understood if physicians are to appreciate their influence on the patient and effectively help patients resolve issues of non-compliance.

It is important to remember that the power to make decisions lies with the patient. The goals of the medical team are only supportive. So it is the physician, assisted by nurse, who has to make adjustments with the needs and demands and aspirations of the patient and not to force himself/herself on his wishes and resistance.

9. NON-TRADITIONAL NURSING ROLE

How does the role of an Infection Control Nurse fits into a collaborative scheme? First, she starts with some inherent advantages. The role is less service-oriented and more observational. Infection Control Nurses have a broader view of the health care continuum, one that is whole of hospital-wide than patient, or ward-oriented. The person is less "nurse-like", and more physician-like. In fact, the person may not come from a nursing background at all. The person often has formal training in the field, and has a substantial knowledge-base—often more formal training than even the physician in Infection Control. He or she also has daily learning opportunities. He or she often has prior experience and maturity that lends credibility to the practice.

9.1 The Infection Control Nurse

In a complementary fashion, most Infection Control Physicians are well aware of the Infection Control Nurses level of expertise and the utility of their knowledge of the institution's functional operation as well as their valuable observations. An astute physician appreciates the value of a "second pair of eyes and ears." However, the knowledge and experience of the nurse can also be the ground for competition rather than collaboration.

9.2 The Infection Control Team

The advantages of a team approach is that the playing field is more level in this relationship. The disadvantage is that the playing field is smaller. But a well functioning team is synergistic, mutually supportive, innovative and efficient. The team should be creative and innovative, collegial, sharing decisions and accountability, supportive—with respect for each other professionally and personally; and functional, with an appreciation for each other's professional roles.

9.3 The Goal is Infection Control

The ultimate goal of Infection Control team is to function as a unit with recognition of and respect for individual skills and expertise. Collaboration is the key, which promotes initiative and pride in the team's endeavours and improves patient outcomes. Nothing can match the feeling of pride and initiative that results when true collaboration occurs. Collaboration is not a static process but one that must be "constantly nurtured, reinforced and reflected on." It is goal that should be sought by health care professionals and in the life as a whole.

10. PRIVATE SET-UP CASE REPORTS: THE SUPERVISION AND COLLABORATION ARE ALL IMPORTANT

Lack of close supervision of a nurse/assistant can lead to malpractice suits targeting the Doctors.

Most mistakes concern diagnoses, and the strategies of the plaintiffs attorney in the two cases in US, detailed here are obvious: He simply puts a primary—care physician on the witness stand who will say, "Any careful physician would have recognized the correct diagnosis from the signs and symptoms the patient presented. So, the doctor's failure to check on the nurse's work while the patient was still in his office, was instrumental in causing this tragic outcome."

(i) Death of Seven Month Old: A US Report of Assistants' (PA) Negligence Leading to Suit against Doctor

A typical example of the malpractice risk created by PA's is demonstrated by a case that was settled several weeks ago for $175,000. Payment was made to the parents of a seven month old infant who died of bacterial meningitis in July 1995. A clinic, consisting of three family physicians and two assistants was the defendant.

In the early morning of July 23, 1995 the decedent child became ill with a low grade fever, irritability, some vomiting and a reluctance to nurse. The next morning, his mother took him to the defendant clinic, where he was seen by an Assistant of the physician. Following his examination, the assistant told the mother the baby had a middle ear infection, prescribed an antibiotics and told her to return if the infant was not improved by the next day. The night the baby slept poorly, and by morning, he had developed projectile vomiting. He was feverish and more irritable, and was taking fluids poorly. The mother took him back to the defendant clinic in the early afternoon, where the child was seen by another PA. He was retching, and the PA felt he was somewhat dehydrated. His temperature was 103.5. A nurse gave him a tepid bath, which brought down his temperature, and he was sent home with a prescription for Suprax. As before, the diagnosis was a middle ear infection. There was no indication that meningitis was considered by either PA. At 7 o'clock the following morning, one of the clinic physicians phoned the mother and asked about the status of the baby. She told him the baby was still vomiting, was lethargic and dehydrated, and would not nurse. The doctor told her to bring the child back to the clinic immediately. He examined the patient and referred the mother to a local hospital emergency department, where the baby was seen by a pediatrician. About two hours were consumed in evaluating the infant, accomplishing a spinal tap, establishing the diagnosis of bacterial meningitis, and then initiating therapy. The patient was then sent by helicopter to a tertiary-care facility, but he experienced a cardiac arrest enroute and died.

Had the cases been tried, the plaintiff would have concentrated on the theory that the assistants were inadequately supervised. Particularly with the second clinic visit, when the patient was evaluated by the second assistant, one of the family physicians should have examined the baby. (It was contended that at least one of them was at the clinic at the time). While the chart entries had been countersigned by a physician, only assistant saw the baby on each of the two visits.

(ii) Second Case: Negligence Charge when Assistant Erred

In another case on the night of Feb. 5, 1988, on Friday, the five month old patient developed a fever and became very irritable. The mother said she telephoned her pediatrician early Monday morning. She said she told him she lacked a Medical sticker for the visit, and he refused to see the patient. According to the doctor, he did not recall the telephone call, and he would never have refused to see a sick infant for any reason.

Later on Monday morning, the mother took the baby to an urgent care facility. She was directed to an examining room, and a man in white coat came in. The mother said she assumed he was a physician, but in fact he was a physician assistant (PA). The PA's record entry indicated the baby was irritable and febrile, with a runny nose, for two or three days. A moderately elevated temperature was recorded, but there was no reference to other vital signs. While the ears were noted to be "clear", there was no comment about an examination of the nose or throat, and there was no observation about neck flexibility. The impression was "vital infection" and the direction was: "Observe, give Tylenol p.r.n." The mother was given no written instructions, and nothing was written about the indications for a return visit. The mother testified the PA told her this was a virus infection which would have to "run its course." The PA recalled telling her to bring the child back if she became worse.

The defendant general practitioner was in the buildings, but he did not see the baby. However, since the PA worked under his supervision, he did review the record some time on Wednesday, two days after the patient's visit. He testified he felt PA's entry was inadequate, especially since there was no recording for respiratory or heart rates. But this did not prompt him to telephone the mother.

The mother testified that on Wednesday evening the baby's suck was poor, and she again called her pediatrician. She said the doctor told her to take the baby to the emergency room or to see him at his office in the morning. The pediatrician denied receiving the call. He said he would not have given this advice when presented with the infant's history. The pediatrician was an excellent witness. The jury felt he was an emotional person, and they had no difficulty in accepting his testimony.

On Thursday morning, Feb. 11, the mother brought the baby to the pediatrician's office. The diagnosis of bacterial meningitis was quickly established and appropriate treatment was given. The child's residual disability is moderately sever mental retardation, paralysis of the right arm and weakness of both legs, requiring braces. There is sever expressive aphasia. It is estimated that her future employment potential is very limited.

At trial, it was brought out that the PA had been working at the urgent care center for the last three months. A PA's scope of practice is limited to what is usual and customary for the physician with whom he is associated. Furthermore, there must be written instructions to the PA, defining the range of his functions. But in the three months of his employment, the general practitioner had never given the PA any written instructions, and the office seldom had infants less than six months of age as patients. Thus, it was contended the PA was acting outside the scope of his certification by rendering care to this patient.

As noted above, the plaintiffs expert witnesses were critical of the PA's causal approach to the case, his failure to have a follow-up appointment and the absence of a record entry detailing instructions given to the mother. The doctor's recognition of the inadequate record, and the fact the mother were criticized by the plaintiff's experts, but this was not a point that was emphasize.

As it turned out, the jury regarded this as the most important evidence in the trial. They accepted uncontradicted testimony that the weakness of suck on Wednesday meant that meningitis would have been examined on that day.

It was the defense position that the clinical picture on Monday, when the patient was first seen, did not suggest meningitis, and the impression of an ordinary viral infection was reasonable. By the time the general practitioner reviewed the record on Wednesday, it was asserted the meningitis probably was sufficiently established to limit the effectiveness of therapy if begun at that time.

The jury's $2.4 million award was unanimous after 12½ week trial.

In Indian conditions, nobody other than physician is expected to make a diagnosis or prescribe a treatment for any patient. However, physician bears the brunt of any vicarious liability imposed on him, due to the act of omission or commission of nurses, attendants, ward servants, etc. So the physician must clearly define the role of a nurse working under his supervision and issue unambiguous instructions about the area of her 'patient care'. The task of injection or pill administration, dressing or any other intervention on behalf of the doctor, must be done on specific instruction only.

Patient's Rights: Doctors and Nurses have to take care

1. What is the Patient's Statement of Rights?

The patient's statement of rights is a list of what a patient has the right to know and ask from his/her attending physician which includes treatment, medication, prognosis and possible consequences of his/her treatment.

2. What are these "Rights"?

There are four main categories of a patient's rights and each of this category is guided by several principles. The four categories are:

1. Right to adequate health care.
2. Right to information.
3. Right to privacy and confidentiality
4. Right to self-determination.

3. What are the Principles that Fall under each Main Categories?

A patient has all the rights of a human being, and thus, should be accorded with the following:

(a) "considerate and respectful care",
(b) "reasonable continuity of care", and
(c) "reasonable response for the patients' request for service."

4. The Right to Information

(a) Patient should never be embarrassed if he asks questions regarding his:
   - ❑ Doctor's advise.
   - ❑ Medicines prescribed, dispensed and given by a doctor, nurse, and pharmacist respectively.

(b) Patient has the right to information necessary to enable him to give an informed consent prior to the start of a treatment regimen.
(c) Patients has the right to know the names of a person responsible for the procedures and treatment to be carried out.
(d) Patient has the right to obtain information as to any relationship of his hospital to other health care and educational institutions.
(e) Patient has the right to examine and receive an explanation of his bill regardless of source of payment.
(f) Patient has the right to know existing hospital regulations that apply to his conduct as a patient.
(g) Privacy concerning his own medical care program.
(h) Case discussion, consultation, examination, treatment and tests should be conducted discreetly.
(i) Patient right to the advice, if the hospital proposes to engage in or perform human experimentation affecting his care and treatment.
(j) All communications and records pertaining to his care should be treated as confidential.

5. The Right to Self-determination

Patient has the right to refuse treatment contrary to his beliefs, e.g. against blood transfusion and bear the medical consequences of his beliefs.

6. *Regarding Confidentiality, can a Doctor or Nurse be Held Liable in Case, he Divulges Care?*

Yes, a patient can hold his doctor or nurse liable regarding any unwarranted leakage of his medical problem and treatment. This is embodied in the Code of Ethics of medical profession. Even the pharmacist can also be accountable in case he disclose information on patient's medications without consent as provided for in their own Ethics. Any violation shall constitute unethical and unprofessional that can be sufficient ground for reprimand, suspension, or revocation of his license.

7. *Drug Costs and Consumer Rights*

Under the declaration of basic policy of the Consumer Act of the Phillippines patient has five fundamental rights:

1. Right to access
2. Right to choice
3. Right to information
4. Right to redress
5. Right to safety

Doctors who receive drug information from the industry, the regulators and management should relay the relevant information to the patient.

Giving the consumer the relevant cost information requires a dual approach "a system for establishing drug pricing and regulatory mechanisms, and a willingness to acknowledge price in the drug decision." This would protect the interest of the patient and enable consumer organizations to explain the part played by costs in the decisions process.

Acknowledging that price is an issue does not destroy the trust in the doctor-patient relationship, but informs the patient who, as taxpayer, is footing the bill and seeing that the money is spent to the greatest possible benefit for everyone.

8. *How should Drugs be Stored to Ensure Potency and Safety?*

Excessive heat, light or humidity may cause your drugs to spoil. A few tips to ensure potency and safety of your medicines:

1. Designate a separate closet where to store your medicines.
2. Tablet and capsules should be stored in separate containers with desiccant (non-edible drying crystal) to absorb moisture and the container properly labeled and identified. Keep containers closed.
3. Some drugs, such as eye and ear drops, injectables get spoiled quickly when exposed to light. Only indirect light should enter the storage closet.

4. Keep storage are a clean and free from pests. Remember to check expiry dates before giving any medications. Do not use any discoloured, fragmented or cracked tablets/capsules. Keep any medications out of children's reach!

(A Phillipine Model: Deptt. of Health)

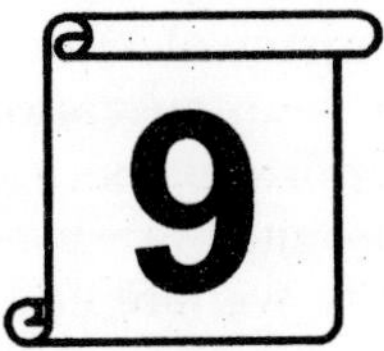

Health Education to Patients in a Hospital: Role of Nurses

Health Education is the sum of experiences which favourably influence habits, attitudes and knowledge relating to individual, family and community health.

Health Education has been an integral part of the functions of Nursing personnel since time immemorial to educate the people pertaining to factors which influence their health. We have been engaged in the 20th century in finding out new technology and medicines to tackle the problems of health. That is why super-speciality hospitals have come up in a big way. However, we have ignored the role of health education in preventing killer diseases resulting from faulty lifestyle, use of alcohol, smoking drugs, etc. Let us analyse these health hazards which are causing great misery to individual, families and society and role of nurses in preventing them.

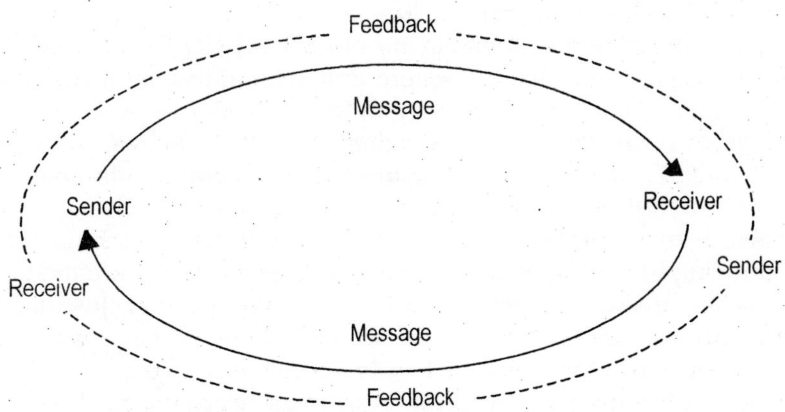

NURSES ARE EFFECTIVE HEALTH EDUCATORS

It need not be over-emphasised that it is the nurse, who is most of the time with the patient and his attendants and relatives in the hospital. She has the best opportunity to impart health education to the patient and those attending to him. The impact of education given by her will have lasting effect. She may educate them on various subjects depending on the need of the patient and the opportunities available to her. She may begin with personal hygiene, environmental cleanliness, deitics, preventive measures against diseases, family welfare and planning, etc. of course, this can be done effectively if she bears in mind the principles and practices of health education as it is already being competently executed by her sisters in the field of public health.

I. *(i) Dietary Lifestyles*

Muhammad Al-Khrateeb[1] in his Article "New Lifestyles' New Diseases" rightly remarks that Recent Social development—such as bigger incomes and greater availability of a wide variety of commodities—have led to changes in lifestyles that threaten health. Coronary diseases are on the increase because of changes in diets; people are eating more fats, carbohydrates and animal proteins; fast-food restaurants offer hamburgers, hot dogs and fried chicken intake of salt from canned food is rapidly increasing; access to transport facilities reduce physical exercise; and stress is common in their daily life, Nurses must educate the people about change of lifestyle.

(ii) Non-availability of Balanced Diet

There is a large population in the developing countries especially India which is suffering from a number of diseases caused by malnutrition and under-nutrition. Some of the diseases are protein-energy malnutrition related diseases e.g., low birth weights, Iodine deficiency disorders, Vitamin A deficiency disorder, iron deficiency, Anaemia, etc. These diseases do not require super specialists' interventions but timely Primary health care and education of mother and simple medicinal interventions by Nurses

The International Conference on Nutrition (ICN) in 1992 enunciated the following goals: (1) reduce severe and moderate malnutrition among children under five years of age by half of the 1990 levels, (2) increase the percentage of newborns having an adequate birth weight (2500 grams or more) to 90%, (3) reduce to less than 10% and possibly eliminate iodine deficiency disorders, (4) eliminate Vitamin A deficiency and its consequences including, blindness, and (5) reduce iron deficiency anaemia.

Drawing up an integrated national strategy for the prevention of non-communicable diseases is both advisable and economically, justifiable. But prevention of such diseases cannot be achieved through the efforts of health officials alone. Health education has to be made accessible to the entire population and non-health institutions and various mass media should be mobilized to this end. Research data yielded by national as well as international studies show that early intervention can make the prevention of diseases possible.[2]

2. Use of Excessive Alcohol, Smoking and Drugs

World Health, July-August, 1995 has published figures about prevalence of alcohol, tobacco and drugs which are quite alarmings.[3] In developed countries, typically 70-90% of adults consume alcohol. Studies in a number of industrialized countries suggest that 5-10% of drinkers are dependent on alcohol.

For several diseases, including cancers of the mouth, Oesophagus and pharynx, as well as for many forms of injury including motor vehicle accidents, industrial accidents, drowning, falls, suicide and homicide, the contribution of alcohol is well known, the risk increasing steadily with the amount consumed.

World-wide, there are about 1100 million smokers with 800 million in developing countries and 300 million in developed countries. About 6000 million cigarettes are smoked every year. In developed countries, about 41% of men and 21% of women regularly smoke cigarettes. In developing countries, about 50% of men and only about 8% of women smoke.

Tobacco causes about 3 million deaths a year now, with about one-third of them in developing countries. If current smoking trends persist, tobacco is likely to kill approximately 10 million people a year in 30-40 years time, with about 70% of them in developing countries.

If current smoking trends persist, about 500 million people currently alive (about 9% of the world's population) will eventually be killed by tobacco, and half of them will be in middle age when they die, losing about 20-25 years of life.

In many developing countries heroin and cocaine use is becoming more common and increasingly problematic. In several countries heroin use is increasingly replacing traditional patterns of substance use including opium smoking.

In many developing countries drug injecting is becoming increasingly common, and in these countries injecting often means the sharing of injecting equipment, with the risk of HIV, hepatitis and other infections.

One crude estimate suggests that, world-wide, between 160,000 and 210,000 deaths every year are associated with drug injecting.

Norman Sartorius in his Article "Putting a higher Value on Health" in *World Health,* June 1986 has cautioned about the negative effects of the use of these horrible drinks in excess. To quote:[4]

"The abuse of psychoactive substances including alcohol, tobacco and narcotic and psychotropic drugs causes enormous damage to the health and productivity of nations. It undermines the quality of life of individuals and their families, and threatens the welfare of communities. The health consequences of abuse are also grave, and range from violence and delinquency to liver cirrhosis, brain damage and lung cancer."

Dr. H. Mahler, Former Director General of World Health Organisation in his Article "Smoking or Health: The Choice is Yours" rightly stated,[5] "Smoking increases the risk of lung cancer, heart disease and respiratory infections of all kinds. In fact, many of the diseases associated with smoking have become current only in the last few generations, when the habit of smoking factory made cigarettes became widespread."

The latest report of South-East Asia Region on Health situation in 1994-97 has clearly brought out the consequences of the use of these substances. A major problem with the use of alcohol is its impact on the health and well-being of the family. A study carried out in India in 1996 reported that drinking families from lower income groups spend from 15% to 45% of their income on alcohol. A high proportion of hospital beds are occupied by the physically and mentally damaged victims of alcohol dependence. Many beds occupied by accidents affected patients are because of alcohol.

The causal relationship between tobacco use and diseases such as cancers, cardiovascular diseases, and chronic respiratory disorders is increasingly being studied in most countries of the Region. In India the number of avoidable cases of chronic heart and obstructive lung diseases have been estimated at 12 million per year. Cancer incidence data reveal that almost 50% and 25% of cancers in men and women respectively are related to tobacco use. The incidence of oral cancer caused by chewing tobacco is estimated to be one of the world's highest, at about one-third of all cancer cases. Annually, tobacco-related conditions are reported to cause 635,000 deaths in India.[6]

The basic question is how to tackle these non-communicable diseases? How to motivate the people using these substances not to do so? What can be done by health experts? The only answer to these questions is the need of strengthening Health Education intensively. Muhammad Al-Khateeb[7] suggests that drawing upon integrated national strategy for the prevention of non-communicable diseases is both advisable and economically justifiable. But prevention of such diseases cannot be achieved through the efforts of health officials alone. Health education has to be made accessible to the entire population, and non-health institutions and various mass media should be mobilised to this end. Research data yielded by national as well as international studies show that early intervention can make the prevention of disease possible.

Achieving 'Health for All' requires much more than just setting up a health centre in every district and providing a high standard of medical care within easy reach of everyone.

A key element in the primary health care approach to Health for All is health education, which seeks to bring about a change in behaviour patterns by making essential health information available to all people in a simple, direct and effective manner. It is hoped that people will thus be motivated to evaluate their habits and practices, and will modify them according to the requirements of health protection and promotion.

Behavioural change, however, is too complex a process to be initiated simply by providing a set of facts. The motivation to break a habit must be much stronger than the force of habits or the pleasure derived from a certain practice. The spiritual dimension can be highly influential in this process of behavioural change.[8]

In spite of overwhelming evidence linking tobacco consumption and various diseases, including cancer, the consumption of cigarettes in nearly all countries of the world is increasing. The rise in tobacco consumption is especially seen among women and the youth. Non-smoking campaigns over the past years have been less than successful. This is mainly because of the aggressive advertisements and counter-attacks by the tobacco industry and the fact that nicotine is addictive. Moreover, most governments are reluctant to take a strong stand on this issue considering that tobacco is a source of revenue and of foreign exchange.

The need for heightened global advocacy for tobacco control has been stressed by Dr. Gro Harlem Brundtland, WHO Director-General, in her statement to the Fifty-first World Health Assembly in May 1998. To quote her:

> "I am a doctor, I believe in science and evidence . . . Tobacco is a killer, Tobacco should not be advertised, subsidized or glamorized."

Of late there is a move to ban Tobacco companies from sponsoring Sports events in India leading to a major debate as to whether it would be at the cost of the Sports activity and so on.

MEANING, NATURE AND SCOPE OF HEALTH EDUCATION

The most important aim of Health Education is to alter behaviour which may have directly or indirectly influenced occurrence of spread of diseases in a given cultural setting. A culturally relevant health education programme can be planned only after understanding the behaviour in all its manifestations. One of the best definitions of Health Education was offered by Wood in 1926: "Health Education is the sum of experiences which favourably influences habits, attitudes and knowledge relating to individual, community, and racial health."[9]

Different authorities have differently viewed the aims of health education. According to one source:[10]

> "The aim of health education is to help people achieve health by their own actions and efforts. Health education begins therefore with the interest of people in improving their condition of living, — and aims at developing a sense of responsibility for their own health betterment as individuals and as members of families, communities or government."

Another source[11] highlights that, "Health education aims at promoting the greater possible fulfilment of inherited powers of the body and the mind and the happy adjustment of individual to society. It is the educational approach to health problem and as such is concerned with practical measures for the promotion of health and the control and treatment of disease."

Unfortunately, the experts and development planners have failed to improve the lives of the people as they do not understand properly the science to communicate effectively with each other or with the people they are trying to help. Most of the people in authority today, who are guiding the people in this field, have not realised the urgency of such education and the benefit it can generate; consequently governments have not taken any substantial steps in this direction.

Health education does not mean merely removal of ignorance. On the contrary, it involves four important things:

- (i) It provides a person with appropriate knowledge to enjoy decent health and also the knowledge about the occurrence and spread of disease thus enabling him to adopt relevant preventive measures;
- (ii) It creates in him an interest in his own health and well-being;
- (iii) It even creates in him an interest for the health of other members of his family as well as of those living in his surrounding; and
- (iv) It creates in him a desire to support health education programmes in his area.

Besides, Health Education should make the people understand the benefits that they can derive from modern medicine. K.S. Sanjive, Professor of Medicine has said:

> "It will not be an exaggeration to say that the paramount step in the effort to take modern medicine to every corner of the country and every citizen is health education. Health education in its widest sense of getting every one to understand what moden medicine can do to diminish disease and death and to be properly motivated to utilise this knowledge in their daily lives, requires the simple quality of sincerity more than highly specialised techniques."[12]

Neglect of health education is one of the main reasons why scientific medicine is not taking root in the country and people are steeped in ignorance and superstition.

ESSENTIALS OF HEALTH EDUCATION

Health education would be possible only if the health educator and the receiver are in constant dialogue with each other. It is not wholly correct that the purpose of health education is to manipulate the receiver. What might be more appropriate is a circular diagram in which the parties to the "Communication Contract" as it is sometimes called, function dually as senders and receivers.

This model would avoid the possibilities of misinterpretation. We know that even well-planned campaigns can end in failures if there is no proper monitoring or feed-back to make sure that the wrong effect is not being created by the communicator, however innocently.

In a democratic society, the dynamic power which impels governments to action is the voice and enlightenment of the people. People can only pressurise their executive or legislative machinery to undertake suitable health measures when they themselves are aware of the means of warding-off disease and promotion of positive health. This knowledge (Health Education) is therefore a pre-condition and prerequisite to creating the demand for health and setting the pace of implementation of environmental sanitation and the total health policy.

FUNCTIONS OF HEALTH EDUCATION PROGRAMME (See Chart 9.1)

No health education programme can function in isolation. A health education programme has to be an integral part of various other development programmes. Functionally, a health education programme should aim at bringing about the following changes:

1. A Change in Knowledge

The most important need which health education programme can serve is to provide appropriate knowledge about health and diseases to the people. This knowledge should be provided in such a way that the recipients do not find it hard to accept it. How to provide this knowledge in an acceptable way? This is the first challenge faced by a health educator. Meaningful responses are relatively easier to learn than the meaningless ones. The health educator can do a lot better by making his demands on the response of receivers which are meaningful. For instance, the health educator who gives a big lecture to the mother on the value of practising family planning without indicating its benefits to her as an individual would be showing inadequate understanding of this principle, for she has to look into her own benefits first. Vigorous efforts would be required to proliferate suggestions that are realistic and meaningful.

2. A Change in Attitude

A change in attitude is possible only when the knowledge offered is acceptable to the recipients. Its utility should also be well known to them. Normally, provision of appropriate knowledge should lead to formation of positive attitudes not only towards a person's own health but also towards the health of other members of the community.

CHART 9.1

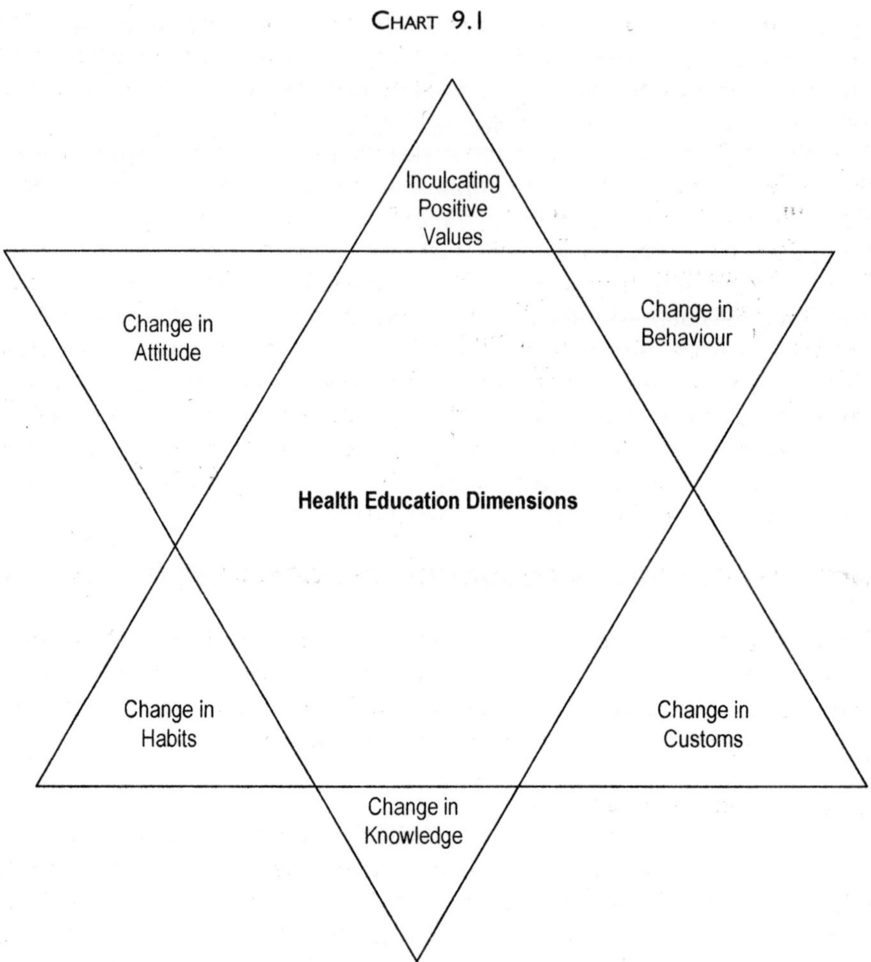

3. A Change in Behaviour

Once positive attitudes are formed, these must reflect in the behaviour of the recipients. They should not only become mindful of their past behaviour but should also avoid doing things which can in any way influence occurrence or spread of diseases.

4. A Change in Habit

The change in the behaviour of the recipients must lead to habit formation. A habit can be formed only when the behaviour becomes repetitive. If proper habits are formed, not only the individuals concerned but the whole community will be benefited. Habit formation, however, is a slow process and it has been well said, that 'habits die hard'.

The persuasive communicator or health educator should be interested both in the long range effects of his messages and in their initial effects. As a matter of fact, he should be interested in turning the learned responses into habitual ones. What are the other principles that guide the establishment of a response? First, the probability of response will increase with the increase in the number of rewarded repetitions. As long as the stimulus with reinforcement following each correct response is not adequately repeated, it will not become a habitual response. Many messages are short-lived because of lack of reinforcement and are likely to become extinct. Second, in order to establish habit patterns, it would be necessary to have a shorter interval between response and reward. Third, habit formation is easier when stimuli are presented in isolation. A nutrition message when unaccompanied by another message such as sanitation message facilitates habit formation. Fourthly, timely increase in reinforcement will further strengthen habit formation. Fifth, receiver's original level of motivation will also influence her habit formation. The mother having a better level of motivation from the beginning will find habit formation much easier. Sixth, providing timely information about receiver performance, would lead to further improvement in performance. Providing selective information to a mother on the positive aspects of her performance will also improve her performance. Thus, communication of health ideas can yield the desired result if the above principles are followed religiously.

5. A Change in Customs

Acquisition of positive attitudes leading to appropriate habit formation must sooner or later, evolve into customs. Only when a substantial number of people in a given cultural setting start behaving in a customary manner, one can say that behaviour has become a part of their customs.

Don Palmer in his article "Social Health: A True Story, Culture and Tradition as Medicine" in the *Daily Tribune* dated 26th January 2000, rightly stresses the need of health education. Modern urban life, devoid of the goodness of social health, can be particularly tough for young indigenous inhabitants of developed countries. Some kill themselves, while many more drift into drugs, alcohol and crime. Now a prison programme is helping in rehabilitation of aboriginal offenders by reintroducing them to their cultural traditions."

It needs to be re-emphasised that health education is a slow process and that it proceeds gradually—a part of the process may get established without any problem but additional efforts may be required to complete the whole process. This process may be directed towards the following important programmes: (See Chart 9.2)

(a) Personal hygiene.
(b) Knowledge of modern medicine, i.e., use of health services.
(c) Nutrition.
(d) Mental health.
(e) Prevention of communicable diseases.

CHART 9.2

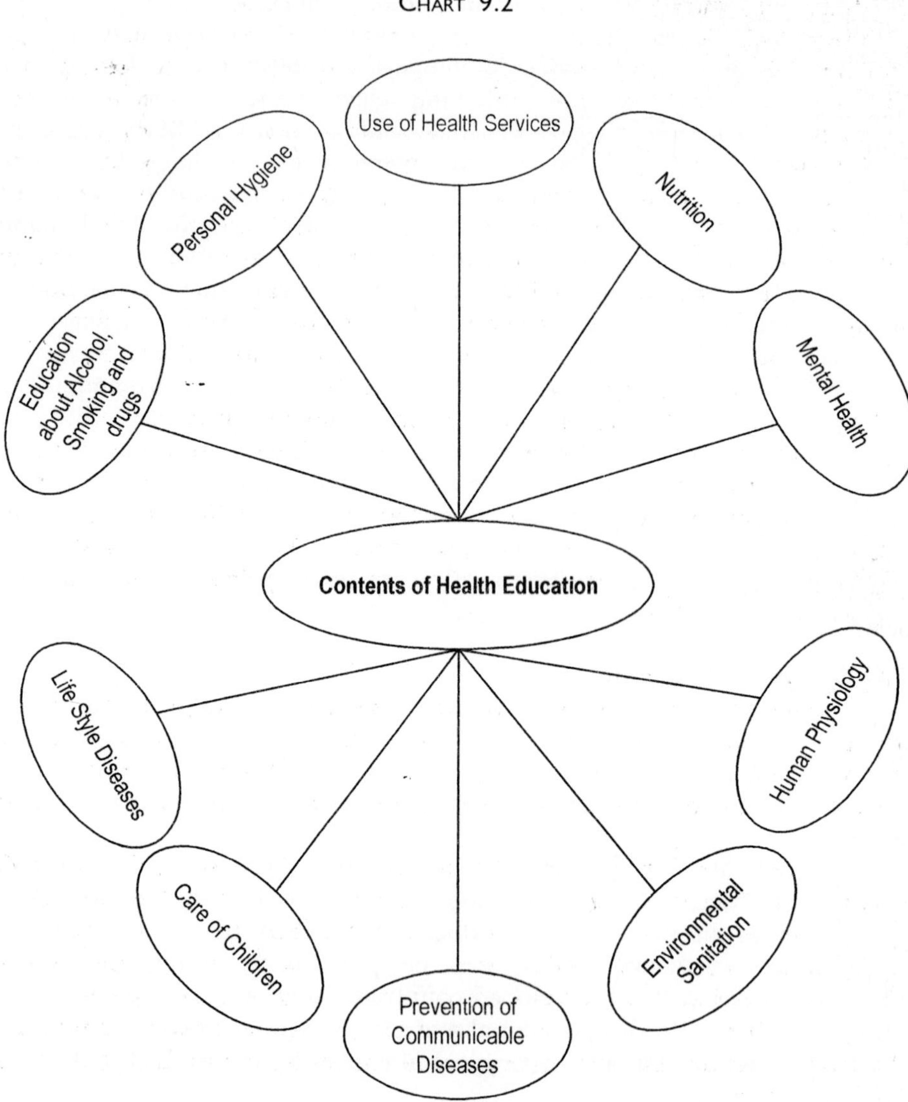

(f) Care of children.
(g) Environmental sanitation.
(h) Human physiology.
(i) Lifestyle diseases.
(j) Education about Alcohol and drugs.

Health education must be imparted keeping in mind latest developments in the field of health. Life is changing fast and the individuals must be educated in the new technology—its role and limitations. Mr. V. Tatochenko, a member of the WHO Expert Panel on

Maternal and Child Health in his Article on "Education for Health" said, "Rapid changes in lifestyles and the evolution of views on health and disease call for new departures in health education. A quick glance of health education material of even one generation ago will show how fast it tends to get out of date. Medical facts, it has been estimated, get outdated within a decade or so. Effective health education, therefore, requires a continuous stream of knowledge, development of the people's ability to absorb it, and decisions taken on the basis of a constantly changing body of information.[13]

METHODS OF HEALTH EDUCATION

Health organisations are set-up to promote positive health. A good health organisation must establish environmental linkages—points of interactions with the environment. These can be classified into four categories: enabling, functional, normative and diffused. The enabling linkage ensures and protects the organisational authority to operate, its access to resources and its power to achieve results. Functional linkage is to link the programme with the task environment. Normative linkages try to modify the behaviour of the people into the existing value system of the society. Diffused linkages imply reaching the clients through public relation (health education).

Sociologists have categorised diffusion process which leads to a widespread acceptance of the programme into five critical stages: awareness (the individuals first introduction to a new idea or practice), interest (the stage at which he actively seeks further information and background data), evaluation (the stage of assessment on critical grounds), trial (a limited phase of experiment), and finally acceptance or adoption. These processes have been occurring for centuries. The need of the present day health administration is to accelerate adoption of the health programmes and to control diffusion process in a short span of time to achieve effective implementation of health programmes.

Changes in knowledge, attitudes, behaviour, habits and customs can be brought about by 'personal' as well as 'impersonal' methods of health education. These methods have certain advantages and disadvantages. While personal methods involve face-to-face interaction, the impersonal methods do not require such a close personal contact. Personal methods are indeed more convincing and generally more successful. However, the success of personal methods greatly depends on the establishment of a good rapport between the health educator and his recipients. The impersonal methods are relatively simpler and even less time-consuming. The radio, the newspapers, the posters, and the pamphlets, etc. can all play an important role in imparting health education. Experience with personal and impersonal methods of health education have revealed that if both the methods are used simultaneously one can obtain better results than simply using one or the other method. The most important aspect in the adoption of the programme is the use of inter-personal relationships. Alastair Metheson, Deputy Director of UNICEF's division remarks on the basis of his research that:

> "To get people to act in ways that conform to new values almost always requires that mass communications to be reinforced by personal influence."[14]

Thus, we see that communication, i.e. dissemination of information is only an important element in health education. The adoption or acceptance may not take place simply by Communicating health information. A study conducted by United States Public Health Services has revealed that, "Unfortunately knowledge alone does not motivate a person to act in accordance with it. He may well know the correct answers to questions without really believing and accepting such information as the basis for his own action."

Dr. Gisela Gastrin, a Finnish physician mentions in his article, "How Education Helps"; "People Can be motivated to adjust their outlook towards health and disease, but before this can happen their negative attitudes have to be countered with factual information. Education needs to be a part of a comprehensive programme in which responsibilities involving the health authorities and others are clearly delineated and resources allocated."[15]

For effective health education, people's involvement is essential.

Eric R. Ram[16] in his article, "Information is Power" in *World Health*, rightly says that making people aware of their rights and responsibilities helps them to determine their own health priorities and take part in solving their own health problems, a step so essential in the process of empowerment of the people. We have to employ all credible channels of communication, including the traditional methods of story-telling and drama, in order to reach all people. Films, radio and television whenever available can be useful, but we have to recognize their limitations; they are useful in creating awareness among people in their communities, but to bring about a real change in health practices, people have to decide for themselves and take responsibility for their own health.

It was mentioned by Dr. E. Berthat in his article, "A New Role for Teachers" that besides information and motivation, action is indispensable. He said that "Information and motivation are not enough; it remains for governments to ensure that a good health infrastructure is available to all the people. Health education has to convince the men and women who are responsible for taking decisions that health is a basic raw-material for their country's eventual social and economic development."[17]

A health educator, as a persuasive communicator can make the best possible use of the personal methods of health education. But he has to see that the messages which he is delivering get mentally registered with his recipients. Actually, he can present his message and then wait until he gets the requisite response from his recipients. D.F. Skinner has distinguished between two types of approaches to the learning situation, as 'operant behaviour' and 'respondent behaviour'. The two situations have also been described as involving instrumental learning and conditional learning. In 'instrumental learning situations', which involves 'operant behaviour', the health educator will present his message and then wait for the receiver to make a correct response. When the receiver makes this response, the health educator will attempt to fix the response by the appropriate award or reinforcement. On the other hand, in 'conditioned learning situation' which involves 'respondent behaviour', the health educator presents his message in such a way that he elicits the response that he wants from his recipients and thus the stimulus that originally served to elicit the response becomes the reinforcing or rewarding element in conditioning. Undoubtedly, conditioning is much more efficient than instrumental learning. It is, however, necessary for the health educator to be aware of both kinds of situations since the condition for using 'respondent behaviour' may not be present in the persuasive situation. The health educator has to be aware that the recipients of his messages differ in the ways in which they learn a given response. They may give different responses essentially in the same situation because of certain specific reasons.

Gone are those days when people used to feel frightened at the thought of going to a hospital. Hospitals were considered as sordid places where people waited for death. Today, the image of hospitals has vastly changed. People expect hospitals to be well organised so that all the services offered by them are well received by the clients. Somehow, the modern hospitals, both teaching and non-teaching, continue to attach the highest importance to providing curative services. The teaching hospitals, in particular, assign a great prestige and value to medical education and research activities. Thus, the medical scientists remain 'wedded to curative medicine rather than to preventive medicine.' A developed country, like the United States of America, had a couple of decades back, recognised the need of combining curative aspects of diseases with preventive aspects. Such a recognition had led to the opening of some of the best schools of hygiene and public health in the world in some of the prestigious American Universities like the Harvard, John Hopkins, North Carolina and California. Thus, for a developing country like India, there is not only a need for combining curative services with preventive services but there is also the need for introducing effective health education programmes in the teaching as well as non-teaching hospitals.

In February 1977, India organised a national workshop with WHO's collaboration on health education in hospitals which was attended by sixty hospitals and health administrators and health educators. This is going to be extended to cover other hospitals in the country. The efforts of Sri Lanka are noteworthy in this direction. Most of the country's larger hospitals have accepted health education as one of their functions. Each of these hospitals has been equipped and the staff have been trained in health education.

Educational work is undertaken in wards, clinics and out-patient departments. These activities are coordinated with those in the communities.

The functions, which the teaching and non-teaching hospitals can perform in the modern times need to be defined properly. At present, no effort has been made to study the functions of these hospitals in relation to the needs of the people. Even among the staff members of these hospitals there is a great deal of confusion about individual's role, perception, role expectation and role performance. The health administrators have differently perceived the roles of the different members of the teaching hospitals. These hospitals, no doubt, can play a significant role in imparting health education to the patients because they have certain basic facilities available to them in the form of staff members like physicians, nurses, social workers, photographers, and artists and they also have various audio-visual aids.

The object of health education, as defined by WHO is to help people attain not just freedom from disease or infirmity but a state of complete mental, physical and social well-being. If this object is followed seriously then the hospitals cannot escape the responsibility of organising relevant health education programmes with the help of experts in the field of health education. The hospitals provide an extraordinary opportunity to the medical staff to communicate modern concepts and ideas about health not only to the patients but also to their relatives who accompany them to the clinic for moral support. In fact, health education can be provided at the out-patient departments in the special clinics, in the wards and even at the registration counter. The Departments of Obstetrics and Gynaecology and Pediatrics can play a special role in organising suitable health education programmes for their clients when they come to them for ante-natal and post-natal care. Actually, the immunization activities can also be combined with certain well-planned health education activities. At the Primary Health Centre level too, there is a great scope for imparting health education to the patients and their attendants, but unfortunately, the medical staff there rarely uses this opportunity to educate them by providing certain basic knowledge about prevention of diseases. Similarly, the in-patients provide a tremendous opportunity to the medical staff to talk to them about various health protective, preventive, and promotive measures. If these situations were utilized properly to educate people who come to the hospitals for seeking medical care, the general health of the Indian people would have been much better than what it is today. As long as the specialists and the super-specialists working in the teaching hospitals will not realize that they themselves have to become health educators rather than leave this task to the paramedical only, one can hardly hope for a positive change in the health status of the Indian people in the near future. The specialists like the general surgeons, orthopedic surgeons, obstetricians, pediatric surgeons, eye surgeons, dental surgeons, plastic surgeons and the like can all, in their own distinct ways, play an exceedingly important role of providing specific disease-related health education to the patients when they come to them for treatment. No one can deny that a person involved in an automobile accident can understand the value of wearing a helmet much more quickly if he is told about it by an orthopedic or plastic surgeon to whom he has approached for the treatment of his head injury. Similarly, a pediatrician, treating a case of neo-natorum tetanus can use this opportunity of educating the mother about the devastating effect of the traditional practice of applying cowdung on the umbilical cord.

The kind of value and respect which the patients attach to the word of a medical specialist is virtually beyond the domain of a para- medical like the present day community health workers who just have a three-month training at a health centre. Unfortunately, not many teaching hospitals provide good examples of working in teams. The specialists succumb to a certain tendency of working in their own closed compartments. Thus, the higher the specialisation, the greater the possibility of compartmentalisation. Health education can have its impact only when it becomes the responsibility of the entire team of specialists. If all of them equally realise the importance of health education, they can create a desirable preventive atmosphere in the hospitals. The most frequent complaint against the hospital administration are lack of sympathy and courtesy on the part of medical and administrative staff. This is particularly the case in the OPD's and Emergency Ward as the patients and their attendants are already in a state of agony and tension. It is suggested that the medical and administrative staff must spare some time to console the patients and their relatives. This would provide a great psychological and moral satisfaction to patients. The hospital authorities must foster goodwill, trust and understanding among the patients and their relatives. This would operate genuine climate and real situation where health education can be imparted to the people. In this way the functioning of the hospital would not be limited to its four walls but would infiltrate in the whole community served by the hospital. This would create a good relationship between the hospital and the community it serves.

In order to improve the functioning of the administration of health education at the Union and State levels in India, the following facts and suggestions may be taken into consideration:

1. Effective Role for Hospitals in Health Education as Patients are Amenable to their Advice

Hospitals within the country are not serving as agencies of health education. Health education can be imparted to mothers when they come to hospitals with their babies. During their stay in the hospital, mothers can be taught how to care for their children during sickness and how to feed them correctly. The mental field is also full of promise. Hospital physicians can do much in this direction by their own attitude to patients, give them simple instructions and, above all, treat them as persons rather than cases.

2. Modernise Health Education Institutes

Those very institutions responsible for imparting health education courses are lacking in standards for sanitary facilities. It is difficult to see how the concepts of sanitation can be effectively imparted among trainees under such conditions. The curricula and contents of health education need careful planning. The educational methods for health education used in a country or community should be regularly evaluated and revised in line with socio-economic development. Health education should be oriented to health consciousness and not disease consciousness.

3. Constant Research and Evaluation

There is the necessity of research in behavioural sciences for the improvement of health education. Dr. B.S. Sehgal, Director CHEB, New Delhi, said, "It was essential to conduct research on the behavioural sciences, in order to build up a body of knowledge for meeting the challenges posed by the health programmes."

4. Special Attention to Training of Trainers

Training for trainers needs re-orientation and re-examination. We should supplement classroom-based academically-oriented training strategy in health education with the actual practice based on models of social change. The emphasis should be on learning by doing and not by listening alone. To quote a UNICEF/WHO study information dogmatically, as if this alone would bring about a transformation. Inevitably, the outcome has been disappointing. The pattern of existing resources—economic, human and cultural—has been forgotten and this too has contributed to health education's failure."

5. Creation of Womens' Club as in Democratic Republic of Korea (DRK)

Women can be effectively approached only by women workers. The experiment of mother's club has been sufficiently rewarding and useful in the People's Democratic Republic of Korea as agencies of socio-economic development. The process of social and economic development is a process of human development for people is the target as well as essential variable in development. Communication being a two-way process, provides for participation at whatever stage of enlightenment the individuals composing a society find themselves. Mother clubs if established in India in right earnest can be the key factors in both the communication and development process since they can be the instruments for getting facts to the people upon which decisions can be based?

6. Understand Local Social-cultural Issues

Before launching any programme of health education, the health educator must assess the local problems and possess the knowledge about the beliefs, conceptions and misconceptions which the people have formed about diseases, their causation and cure. This is possible provided the multi-disciplinary studies of rural communities are encouraged. Such studies would throw light about the cultural background of the people. He can arrange his programmes accordingly and this will save him from antagonism and hostility.

7. Create Good Relations with Mass Media

There is less coordination between health education and the means of mass media communication which needs strengthening on positive lines. It needs to be recognised that most of our health education programmes and activities are so ritualistic in nature that they rarely "education programme is often so deficient that they find it hard to deliver the health education messages in a culturally acceptable manner." It needs to be stressed that the cultural aspect of health education programme is of the greatest importance in the Indian situation. Anthropological and sociological studies in the area of health education are so few in our country that health educators find it extremely hard to understand the many changing aspects of the communities they deal with. There is, thus, an urgent need to study the social and cultural context of health and disease, and to design health services in such a way as will gain the acceptance and support of the people involved. The social scientists can help the health educator in the following ways:

(1) to understand the role of socio-cultural factors in health, including people's beliefs about etiology, diagnosis and therapy of prevalent diseases;
(2) to understand the food culture including people's belief regarding consumption or rejection of various foods on socio-cultural considerations;
(3) to understand people's attitudes towards acceptance or rejection of health education programmes; and
(4) to help them plan and develop culturally relevant health education programmes.

South-East Regional Office of WHO has also expressed its dissatisfaction over the lack of importance to health education in its report, "Health Situation in the South-East Asian Region 1994-97" (p. 72).

Despite these achievements, health education and promotion practices are faced with major constraints—the low priority accorded to health education at the policy level, high illiteracy levels, inadequate resources, poor social status of women, and limited capacity for health promotion research are but only a few examples. To overcome such constraints, new thinking and innovative approaches are required. As we move into the 21st century, the challenges for health promotion go beyond the wider articulation of the concept of health promotion, to building infrastructure and achieving adequate levels of resources, both technical and financial, in order to respond effectively to the increasing demands for health promotion in the Region. "Settings for health" represent the organizational base of the infrastructure required for health promotion.

Partnerships which effectively respond to the health needs of specific population groups, such as workers, women and school children, need to be more vigorously pursued. Healthy public policies need to be developed to ensure supportive environments for individual and community health action, and to protect people from lifestyle-related problems such as those due to tobacco and alcohol. Documentation and dissemination of health promotion outcomes are also critical to the legitimization of the cause of health promotion in the Region.

New health challenges mean that new and diverse networks need to be created to achieve intersectoral collaboration. Such networks should provide mutual assistance within and among countries, and facilitate the exchange of information about which strategies have proved effective. All countries need to develop the appropriate political, legal, educational, social and economic environments required to support health promotion. In this venture of health education, mass-media if properly used can help solve the problems.

Health promoters and educators need to be convinced that the mass-media can operate in the public interest and should play a critical role in social affairs, including health issues. The health concerns of readers, listeners and viewers are very much the concerns of the print and broadcast journalists. The basis of the relationship between the health and media sectors should therefore be one of partnership, not one of user-helper.

Health and media are not naturally inclined to work in unison. Historically, medical scientists trained in the methodical and meticulous search for knowledge have been somewhat skeptical of any effort at popularizing their work. Some doctors even view the media with suspicion and ambivalence. Media people, on the other hand, need to have their source material in language understandable to the layman; they have motive to dwell on technical details, and often lose patience with lengthy scientific papers.

Yet media and health in a close partnership have much to contribute to the public's welfare. Without the involvement of the media, the health sector cannot hope to inform the public on health issues or to help stimulate a community's involvement, which is critical to the success of any health effort. Without the technical input of the health sector, the media cannot fulfil their obligations to serve the interest of the public and these public interests certainly include health.

The complexity of the media, with their obsession for meeting dead lines and their own technical constraints, is little appreciated or understood by health professionals. Those in health who work in partnership with the media need to acquire a rudimentary knowledge of how media works—not in order to become media specialists but to be more empathetic in their dealings with the journalists and broadcasters. This in turn will call for a good hard look at the core curriculum of the training of health promoters and educators.

Whether the health professionals can play their rightful role in battling successfully against lifestyle-related illness—including AIDS and whether health education and promotion practitioners will enter the 21st century adequately prepared for the communication challenges, will depend on the actions that health authorities take now.

In the new millennium, we need to harness all the resources especially the mass-media in a planned manner. This would require active collaboration between media and health specialists. Jack Ling in his article, "Health and the Media" has rightly stressed that the health sector should focus on making technical subjects digestible and understandable to the layman. In particular, the health professionals should identify existing, credible channels of communication, including traditional ones, in order to reach the public. The media offers the public health community more than just access to air-time and newspaper space; they are also a source of communications expertise that is needed to ensure the success of large-scale health promotion campaigns and transmit technical information about health to a mass audience.

What is more useful is the follow-up of media-transmitted message that can be effected by village health workers. For instance, primary health care workers can be an effective channel of communication by delivering in person the same messages that have been delivered to a target audience in print or over the radio, thus increasing the overall impact of the educational drive.

A dialogue has to be initiated between decision-makers in media and in public health. The object of that dialogue should be to heighten awareness among the media personnel about the important responsibility they hold for the health and well-being of their people, and equally to alert health professionals to their own responsibility for ensuring that their health initiatives reach all people. Without this whole-hearted backing from the media in conveying health messages to the greatest number of people, we risk having only Health for Some and not Health for All.

However, the success of health education would depend in the long-run upon the shoulders of the providers of health care to the people. They should be motivated to do this job as a part of their medical duties. S.S. Sooch in his Article, "Revamping Health Care" in the *Daily Tribune* (26 January, 2000) rightly remarks that there is a general feeling that most of the health care providers in the government-run hospitals are indifferent, apathetic and insensitive and a few even outrightly arrogant in their behaviour. A sense of compassion and human touch is simply missing. A series of crash courses should be arranged to expose the entire staff to the art of public relations.

Health Education is vital to provide health to all in 21st century. This is the cheapest and most effective tool of health care. The success of Primary Health Care in 21st Century depends upon the identification of community needs through community needs assessment surveys and later on providing health education, to the community so that they can solve their health problems themselves.

Notes and References

1. Muhammad Al-Khateeb, "New Lifestyles, New Disease" in *World Health*, July, 1989, p. 23.
2. *Ibid.*
3. WHO: *World Health*, July-August 1995, p. 16.
4. *World Health*, June 1986, p. 2.
5. *World Health*, Feb.-March 1980, p. 1.
6. WHO: SEARO: Health Situation in the South-East Asia Region, 1994-97, New Delhi, 1999, pp. 149-51.
7. *World Health*, July 1989, p. 23.
8. Abdulmoneim Aly: Health Education Through Religion, in *World Health*, July 1989, p. 27.
9. John J. Hanlon, Principles of Public Health Administration, St. Louis, 1960, p. 402.
10. WHO, Technical Report Series No. 89, p. 4.
11. WHO, *Ibid.*, No. 156, p. 3.
12. K.S. Sanjive, Planning India's Health, Orient Longman, New Delhi, 1971, p. 64.
13. WHO, *World Health*, Feb.-March 1979, p. 24.
14. UNICEF, UNICEF News, "Communication: A Tool for Development", Issue 84/1975/12, p. 18.
15. WHO, *World Health*, Nov. 1975, p. 14.
16. *World Health*, Jan.-Feb. 1989, p. 9.
17. *World Health*, May 1979, p. 25.

References

Borkar, Health in Independent India, p. 217.

For further details refer to author's article, "Role of Communication in Family Planning: Setting up of Mother's Club in PEN", Family Planning Association of India, Haryana, Branch, May 1977.

Jack C.S. Ling, "The Media its Role," in *World Health*, January-Feb. 1989, p. 25.

Jack Ling, "Health and Media" in *World Health*, March 1986, p. 18.

UNICEF, Health and Basic Services, Keys to Development, *op. cit.*, p. 46.

WHO Technical Report Series, 1954.

WHO, SEARO: SEA/RC 23, p. 88.

WHO, *World Health*, April 1977, p. 20.

WHO: Technical Report Series No. 89, 1954.

Appendix I

CAPACITY PLANNING IN HOSPITAL NURSING: A MODEL FOR MINIMUM STAFF CALCULATION

(A case study of nursing services in 2 hospitals viz. Alvarez Buylla, spain and Norwood hospital, USA)

Nursing Economics, Jan.-Feb. 2002 by Pilar L. Gonzalez-Torre, B. Adenso-Diaz, Olallo Sanchez-Molero—

* An aging population, emerging technology, heightening patient expectations, rising health care costs, shorter patient stays, and growing pressure to improve quality have made the management of nursing resources even more critical today.
* While approaching a model for staffing levels, the authors considered factors such as patient acuity, work redesign, and minimum quality standards.
* The methodology for analysis included estimating the time needed to complete nursing tasks and calculating the average number of tasks per patient.
* With respect to nursing quality measures, the study examined the adequacy of nursing documentation including admission history, assessments, nursing procedures, and discharge report as well as nursing-driven outcomes such as fall and phlebitis rates.
* Lastly, the authors determined the theoretical number of staff needed to provide nursing care according to quality standards.

Today, the appreciation of the important work of nurses in the sound running of hospital institutions, is growing (Silva and Aderhodlt, 1989). At the same time, with in the public budget devoted to health, the cost of staff is also a main concern. The successive cutbacks in staffing result in an increase in staff workload, especially in nursing services, where quality issues are also an important concern. This can lead to increased dissatisfaction of staff and a notable increase in the risk of professional errors (Hendrickson, Doddato, and Kovner, 1990).

To design a model that permits the determination of the number of nurses required to cover minimum levels of quality, it is necessary to define several prior steps including (a) patients must be classified (not all patients require the same nursing care), so as to subsequently identify the different tasks that nurses carry out in their work; (b) discover a way of determining the time taken to carry out each nursing task, (c) identify the desired levels of quality in the hospital, (d) establish the relationships between the theoretical staff and quality levels, and (e) establish the procedure for calculating staff.

The purpose of this article is to present an efficient methodology for capacity planning in the case of hospital nursing, the ultimate aim being to determine the minimum staff needed to carry out all the functions corresponding to a nursing unit, bearing in mind the quality of the service provided.

The Problem of Capacity in Nursing

Managing nursing staff in hospitals is a complex task, not only because of the characteristics *per se* of staff management in whatever activity in the service sector, but also due to the social and economic importance of the work that these professionals carry out (Shullanberger, 2000). An urgent need exists to match patient needs with the health resources available. In recent years, both medical and nursing staffs have grown notably without an excess of available resources (Visser, 1997). The present study focuses on nursing staff.

In the United States, the management of nursing has been considered worthy of extensive, in-depth analysis. For instance, a study conducted in a hospital with six different specialized units (Hendrickson *et al.*, 1990) concluded that on average nurses only spend 31% of their working time directly with patients, devote 45% of their time to clinical, indirect care, and spend 10% of their shift on non-clinical activities. At the same time, nurses spend 10% of their working day directly preparing therapies and spend an additional amount of time (5% estimated) on indirect tasks (correcting mistakes, checkups, counts, verifications, etc.). The results also indicate an average of 1 nurse for every 4.8 patients on the day shift and 6.9 on the night shift.

In Europe, hospitals are faced with a considerable increase in demand for health care, high patient expectations to improve service and quality, and tighter and tighter budgets and greater restrictions on the availability of resources (Visser, 1997). This provokes imbalances between the service offered to patients and hospital management since their respective objective levels of use of hospital resources differ (among which we find nursing staff grouped with the number of beds and operating theaters available). This situation is even more adversely affected by the following current tendencies in these services (Visser, 1997; Vries, Bertrand, and Visser, 1999).

* The present demand for care is growing as a result of the changes in population structure (more elderly).
* Through research, new therapies and techniques are appearing. Some of these technologies replaced previous outdated technologies, but many are new systems to be included alongside already available therapies and treatments. That is to

say, the introduction of a new technology will simply lead to a new demand and not to the substitution of an old technique to cover one and the same treatment.

* Normally, patients do not wish to wait more than 15 minutes for a specialized consultation or for a checkup. Neither are they willing to go to the hospital twice for the combination of a visit to a specialist and a checkup, if they can do both in 1 day. In the case of having to be admitted to hospital, a previous appointment is preferred for admission or at least 1 week's prior notice. This requires greater organizational effort and frequently the use of more resources.
* The costs of health care must be controlled at a national level to maintain a competitive position with respect to other countries. This means that hospitals face heavy reductions in their budgets.
* The stay of patients in hospitals is being shortened due to the greater turnover of treatments of hospitalized patients, and to treatments at health and day care centers, all of which require the use of new technologies and increased specialization within the health system.
* Moreover, pressure is also building to increase the quality of services, and to reduce waiting lists and times within the process.

Faced with this situation, the aim of every nursing administrator is to balance the needs of offering patient services and the capacity of available human and material resources. To do so, a method should be defined to measure the seriousness of the patient's condition on admission, on the basis of which nursing care needs are generated. Given the diverse combination of treatments that a patient may require, it is essential that the topic of patient classification be tackled so as to ascertain the specific needs of each of the possible types of existing patient and, thus, make the problem at hand manageable.

Classification of patients

A number of systems have been proposed at an international level for classifying patients that, on the basis of the category to which patients have been assigned, permit the estimation of the care activities that they will require, and which may thus be provided to them during their stay (or at least while their state does not vary, leading to the subsequent change of class or category). A patient classification system consists, therefore, of a set of tools for grouping together patients in such a way that each group receives equal or similar care. This has been used to assign nursing staff to shifts, normally in line with budgeting considerations, so that the needs of each patient may be covered by the available staff (Poulson, 1987).

In the last 40 years, patient classification has taken on more relevant significance for nursing administrator. Patients are classified according to the evaluation of seriousness of their illness, the severity of the symptoms they present, and the dependence on the nurse and/or the interventions required on the part of nursing staff (Rosendall, 1983). Traditionally, these systems for classifying patients have been based on others already predefined for the medical field and thus had to be redesigned in accordance with the particular characteristics of nursing for their subsequent application in this field. Furthermore, these tools are also a basis for evaluating staff productivity.

At the same time, measuring workloads in nursing is not a simple task. The time needed to carry out certain care depends on several factors, such as the place where it is carried out, the actual patient who receives the care, and even the person who carries out the practice. In general, it may be said that two strategies exist for measuring or evaluating the workload in nursing (Giovannetti, 1979):

1. One based on the estimation of the average time needed to carry out the care treatments for each patient category, which requires having previously decided on the patient classification system to be used.
2. Another based on the times of standard care treatments for specific nursing procedures.

Among the most commonly used systems for evaluating nursing workloads are GRASP, PRN, and Medicus. All of these systems have in common the measurement of care treatments individually required for each patient, and the load imposed on the nursing staff due to activities other than direct care (for example, the filling out of the patients' nursing records or other administrative tasks). Therefore, the measurement of the total care received by a specific patient is not easy to calculate, since many indirect activities are intermingled for different patients or are tasks pertaining to the management of the unit (Williams, 1977).

Of all of these, Medicus is the system finally employed in the capacity model proposed in this study, since Medicus is the one that best adapts to the characteristics of the hospital subject to this empirical study. The desired time of care treatments is revised annually and adjusted to needs. With this methodology, different types of levels of dependence are established according to the nursing care required, and the relative workload is estimated for each. Then, depending on the patient's dependence level, multiplying this value by its relative load provides the total load of each level of care. This value, multiplied by the desired amount, gives the hours of care required per day of each type. The total is reached by adding up the hours of each level of care.

The greater accuracy of this type of measurement allows an objective evaluation of the care to be given, which makes it possible to know the nursing resources needed quite precisely. This presents, among other advantages, the assignment of tasks to each professional without work overloads, which improves his/her job satisfaction, thus contributing to an improvement in both the working environment, and (even more relevant) the quality of service perceived by patients and their families.

Proposed Methodology of Analysis

The model proposed for determining the minimum capacity of hospital nursing services requires six successive steps—

1. Estimating the times needed to execute the different nursing tasks. The starting point consists in ascertaining as exactly as possible the real times of execution, under normal conditions, of each of the different tasks that the nurses carry out in their day-to-day work in a specific unit. Among the possible alternatives for carrying out this phase are those of time study using a stopwatch, laboratory experiments, or the Delphi methodology.
2. Calculating the average number of activities per patient. To calculate the theoretical staff, once the execution times of each of the different nursing tasks are known, it is necessary to ascertain for each type of patient (dependence level) how many activities of type I are carried out on average per shift.
3. calculating the theoretical staff based on historical data. The theoretical staff is calculated for each of the months for which registers are held, using a system of workload evaluation (the hospital's own or an adapted one).
4. Calculating the historical ratio. Subsequently, a ratio is determined which represents the quotient between the real number of staff on the ward and the theoretical number calculated previously.
5. Consolidating the quality results in accordance with the ratios. Next, the quality results obtained in accordance with the historical data collected are analyzed. Subsequently, these data on quality are consolidated on the basis of the ratios.
6. Calculating minimum staff. The proposed model relates the available capacity to specific quality indexes, thus evaluating how the number of staff affects the quality of the services offered.

With the information obtained in the prior step, grouping together the quality indexes into a single one by means of a specific function, it is possible to estimate the expected quality on the basis of the values (and therefore on the basis of the theoretical staff).

Thus, given a specific ward on any day, on the basis of the type of patients that are received, it is possible to calculate the theoretical number of nurses on the ward (on the basis of standard times). By multiplying this staff by the specific factor determined according to the aforementioned analysis it is possible to obtain the minimum admissible number of nurses or the ward, bearing in mind the desired levels of quality.

Applying the Model to a Real Environment

The methodology proposed in this study was applied to the Hospital Alvarez Buylla, belonging to the Spanish National Health System-Insalud, located in Mieres (Principality of Asturias, in the north of Spain). The hospital has 202 beds and offers services of hospitalized medical-surgical attention, outpatient consultations, and diagnostic support to the inhabitants of the area.

The hospital was built in 1954 though it has undergone modifications since then; its present structure dating from 1986. The Hospital Alvarez Buylla has a staff of 554 workers, of which 4 belong to the management staff, 101 are doctors, and 295 are nurses and nursing assistants. If the resources of this hospital are compared with the body of the Spanish National Health System, a level of staff slightly lower than the average is appreciated.

Of the different units in the hospital, the one chosen for this research study was internal medicine, since it was considered to be the most representative from the point of view of nursing tasks and, in the particular case of the hospital under study, has the youngest staff, and which is therefore more favorable with respect to obtaining a high level of participation in the study.

Empirical study

Due to the difficulties that the other alternatives presented in this study, it was decided to apply the Delphi methodology to determine the standard times. This type of methodology has already been applied on other occasions within the health field presented an experience using this method, although their aim was to clearly define the professional concept of nursing and the tasks to be carried out on the basis of the patient's dependence level).

The questionnaire used in the first mailing was based on a listing of the different activities into which hospital nursing may be broken down, elaborated in the "Signo" project instigated by the Spanish National Health System (Insalud, 1996). This listing was corrected in accordance with the particular characteristics of the specific nursing unit under study (internal medicine), eliminating the tasks that do not belong to this nursing unit or that are normally carried out by nursing assistants. The panel of experts considered was formed by the nursing staff of the unit under study at the Hospital Alvarez Buylla in Mieres (14 nurses). The distribution of this initial questionnaire was carried out by mail to the homes of each professional on January 14, 2000 and replies were received until February 29, 2000.

Once the initial questionnaires were received, the pertinent statistical values (mean, standard deviation, and interquartilic interval) were calculated for each nursing activity under consideration. As consensus was not reached during the first Delphi round, a second mailing was elaborated only for those activities where a relevant degree of discrepancy had been demonstrated which needed to be justified. Eight of the activities included in the first questionnaire were eliminated from the second, as they were considered by a large number of the experts to belong to the tasks of nursing assistants and not to the nurse, who is the subject of study. The distribution of this second questionnaire was carried out in a similar way to the first; only soliciting the opinion or change in the original response of the expert in those cases where these fell outside the corresponding interquartilic interval. Finally, a number of definitive conclusions were extracted.

It is important to highlight the fact that on comparing the times obtained in this Delphi study with those already existing in the documentation of the "Signo" project (Insalud, 1996), with the aim of ascertaining whether or not some kind of relationship between both studies existed that would indicate the possibility of extrapolating these times to other potential hospital services, and on analyzing the existing correlation between both series, a Pearson correlation coefficient equal to 0.732 was obtained with a level of significance of 0.01. This sample estimator indicates the presence of a high, positive relationship between both. The corresponding simple linear regression analysis was then carried out to determine this relationship precisely.

Subsequently, taking a sample of the patients at the hospital in Mieres as the starting point, the number of activities of each type that are normally carried out were determined as a function of the dependence level of the patients.

The system considers three dependence types:

- Type 1: Autonomous patient
- Type 2: Semi-dependent patient
- Type 3: Patient totally dependent on the nurse

Given the difficulty of managing the previous years' clinical records of the hospital's patients (still not completely automated) and the amount of episodes present in each of these, a random sample of 236 patients was used. Of these, 63.6% were men. Average patient age was 67 years. With regards to the dependence level of the patient, semi-dependent patients predominated (50%), followed by autonomous patients (43.2%). The sample serves as a reference base for ascertaining the number of times that each of the different nursing tasks are carried out each day for a standard patient of each level of dependence.

With respect to quality indexes, nine were handled in the hospital study:

1. *Graphs and therapy sheet*: This is the register of the daily activity for medical monitoring. Among the basic data are patients' pulse and temperature checks (at least twice daily) and daily data on urine, vomiting, and bowel movements.
2. *The nurse's notes sheet*: This includes information on the daily work carried out by the nurse with a particular patient, mainly indicating the time and quantity of treatments and doses received by the patient.
3. *Admission evaluation sheet*: This includes the basic information needed for the sound health attention of patients, both their personal details (age, home address, family and labor status, etc.) as well as their medical characteristics (allergies, vital signs, previous operations or treatments, etc.). It is elaborated on the patient's admission to the hospital.
4. *Nursing discharge report*: This is a document that includes the care received by the patient during his or her stay in the hospital as well as the post-hospitalization care required.
5. *Phlebitis rate*: This indicates the problems of vein inflammation resulting from some of the practices or treatments received by the patient.
6. *Fall rate*: Some patients need more or less attention based on their condition, especially if they are prone to falls. These may include different types: falls from bed, falls when patients go to the bathroom, falls in the corridors when patients are accompanied by members of their family, etc. An attempt should be made at all times to avoid these types of situations, since they can give rise to the worsening of the general state of the patient.
7. *Scab rate*: This refers to scabs or similar manifestations produced in patients as a result of certain treatments. An attempt should be made to avoid them or at least to reduce them as much as possible.
8. *Care planning sheet*: This reflects the specific care plans that the patient must receive as prescribed by the physician.
9. *Urinary infection rate*: This problem presents primarily in patients with catheters.

The last two indices were not employed in the present study because insufficient data were collected (this is a recently introduced index in this hospital nursing service quality control) and no significant differences were found in these data, respectively.

The first four quality indices refer to the adequate completion of several documents that nurses manage in their work, evaluating their percentage of correction. To evaluate them, 6 monthly histories were randomly taken per unit and the completion of a series of parameters was observed. In contrast, the remaining three indices indicate the number of incidences of each event as a function of the total number of patients attended.

The first four indices were evaluated in percentages and the three others as a ratio. To standardize them, the indices were inverted to the correct completion of the documents managed by the nurse. The errors committed by the nurses were calculated in an effort to reduce them.

In evaluating the total quality of the care delivered by the nursing staff, not all the indices described above present the same relevance. Therefore, an overall quality function was constructed where these indices are weighted on the basis of their importance. The values corresponding to the rates of falls, phlebitis, and scabs are linked to the direct care of the patient, as a result of which they are accorded the greater weightings (20%). On the other hand, the remaining quality indices employed are related to the indirect tasks carried out by nurses, but which are also necessary for the adequate development of their work. The weightings accorded to these indices were 10%.

The overall quality function allows the determination of the staffing thresholds with which it is possible to offer the hospital nursing service while guaranteeing certain levels of quality.

One potential problem of data validation appears due to the fact that the majority of the temporary and stand-in contracts are made before vacations and rest periods of permanent staff in the holiday period (June, July, August, and December). There exists the possibility that the service offered to patients during these months is of an inferior quality, thus distorting the results. For this reason, the hypothesis of the equality of the means of the quality indices in the aforementioned periods and the remaining months of the year was tested. No significant difference appears to be confirmed between the quality indices in periods with high levels of temporary hiring of staff with respect to the remaining months of the year.

Conclusions

The present study proposes a model for calculating the minimum staff in a nursing unit, guaranteeing a minimum level of quality care to patients during their stay in the hospital. It is worth highlighting, on the one hand, the social relevance of the sector under study, and on the other, the contribution of this model at a time in which the health sector is undergoing budget cutbacks worldwide, especially in the area of human resources.

The proposed model was studied in a real environment, the Hospital Alvarez Buylla in Mieres (Spain), using a Delphi study to estimate the duration of the tasks (obtaining activity times strongly correlated with other prior contributions carried out by the Spanish National Health System), the study of real staff, the hospital's quality indices, and the register of patients.

The aim of the study was not limited to calculating theoretical staff, but also to determine the minimum levels of quality in the care offered with which the tasks of hospital nursing should be developed. To do so, as well as the theoretical staff determined previously, historical data were collected of the quality indices managed by the Hospital Alvarez Buylla which was the test subject of this method. This permitted the determination of the minimum staff needed to be offered by the nursing service while complying with the minimum levels of desired quality.

Subsequent studies might focus on the computerization of this process of calculation so as to facilitate its implantation in a general nursing unit. Moreover, the results obtained might be extrapolated for implementing the system in other nursing units other than internal medicine. Likewise, a subsequent step to this study should consider a non-homogeneous distribution of the activities among the different work shifts.

The Ratio [DELTA] Between the Real Staff on the Ward and the Theoretical Staff Calculated by the Medicus System Using Historical Data

Month/Year	*Theoretical Number of Nurses*	*Real Number of Nurses*	*[DELTA] = Real/ Theoretical*
October 1998	6	4	0.66
November 1998	7	7	1
December 1998	5	6	1.2

Quality Indices Registered for Each Month (And Therefore for a Specific [DELTA] Ratio)

[DELTA]	*Month/Year*	*Registered Quality Indices*		
		[I.sub.1]	*[I.sub.2]*	*[I.sub.n]*
0.66	October 1998	0.8%	0.0	1.0%
1.00	November 1998	0.5%	0.0	0.0
1.20	December 1998	0.6%	0.1%	0.0

An Extract of the List of Estimated Times for Each of the Activities Employing the Delphi Methodology

Activity Code	*Description*	*Estimated Time (Minutes)*
R01	Administration of aerosols	6.67
R02	Administration of oxygen	3.00
R03	Aspiration of secretions	7.83
R06	Breathing exercises	12.00

A Summary of the Results of the Multiple Regression

- Dependent variable: Insalud (time determined by Insalud study)
- Independent variable: Delphi (time obtained in the Delphi study)
- Pearson's correlation coefficient: 0.732
- Regression line: Insalud = 0.737 * DELPHI + 4.231
- Durbin-Watson value: 1.758

Register of the Frequencies of Execution of the Different Nursing Activities in Relation to the Type of Dependency of the Patient and Calculation of the Times Needed Considering the Number of Patients of Each Typology

Activity	*Number of Times Degree of Dependence of the Patient*			*Times Degree of Dependence of the Patient*		
	Type 1	*Type 2*	*Type 3*	*Type 1*	*Type 2*	*Type 3*
R01	1.65	4.28	2.6	11.03	28.53	17.33
R02	0.21	0.56	0.2	0.62	1.67	0.60
R03	0.10	0.05	0.00	0.81	0.36	0.00
R06	0.03	0.09	0.00	0.41	1.12	0.00
AH01	0.00	0.02	0.00	0.00	0.23	0.00
AH02	0.00	0.00	0.00	0.00	0.00	0.00
AH03	0.00	0.00	0.00	0.00	0.00	0.00
AH04	3.14	1.60	0.8	43.15	22.06	11.00
AH05	0.14	1.49	2.4	2.41	26.05	42.00

Quality Function Designed for this Study

Overall quality function = 0.2 [MATHEMATICAL EXPRESSION NOT REPRODUCIBLE IN ASCII]

[T.sub.1.sup.1]: mean value of the phlebitis rate for the interval [DELTA]

[T.sub.2.sup.[DELTA]]: mean value of the fall rate for the interval [DELTA]

[T.sub.3.sup.[DELTA]]: mean value of the scab rate for the interval [DELTA]

[FH.sub.1.sub.[DELTA]]: mean value of errors in the graphs and therapy sheet for the interval [DELTA]

[FH.sub.2.sup.[DELTA]]: mean value of errors in the nurse's notes sheet for the interval [DELTA]

[FH.sub.3.sup.[DELTA]]: mean value of errors in the admission evaluation sheet for the interval [DELTA]

[FH.sub.4.sup.[DELTA]]: mean value of errors in the nursing discharge sheet for the interval [DELTA]

Comparison of the Quality Index Means in Accordance with the Corresponding Time Period

Holiday Levene's Test Student t-Test and/or [H.sub.0]: [H.sub.0]: Stand-In [[sigma].sub. [[mu].sub.1]= Periods Mean 1.sup.2]= [[mu].sub.2] [[sigma].sub.2.sup.2]

[DELTA]	NO	1.0292	Accept	Accept
	YES	1.0486		
[FH.sub.1]	NO	0.1115	Accept	Accept
	YES	0.1008		
[FH.sub.2]	NO	0.0958	Accept	Accept
	YES	0.0836		
[FH.sub.3]	NO	0.0330	Reject	Accept
	YES	0.0526		
[FH.sub.4]	NO	0.0667	Accept	Accept
	YES	0.0991		
[T.sub.1]	NO	0.0046	Accept	Accept
	YES	0.0035		
[T.sub.2]	NO	0.0266	Accept	Accept
	YES	0.0330		
[T.sub.3]	NO	0.0965	Accept	Accept
	YES	0.0993		

Nursing at Norwood Hospital

Nursing Mission

We are dedicated to providing exceptional care to our patients and families based on the art, science and spirit of professional nursing.

Nursing Vision

To en-cultrate a professional nursing practice environment which empowers nurses through a spirit of inquiry, shared decision-making, and reflective practice.

Schwartz Center Rounds at Norwood Hospital

Our Staff Development Department has a leadership role in orientation, continuing education and professional development of our nurses. We are committed to professional development by providing on-going contact hour programs, development of critical thinking skills and bringing evidence-based practice to the bedside. We are also committed to providing individualized education to our patients.

Norwood Hospital provides its new RN graduates with ongoing support as they transition from student nurse to registered nurse. They work with highly skilled RN preceptors and the unit-based CNS.

Our nurse educators offer a variety of presentations for the continued growth and development of our nurse assistants.

Continuing Education

Based on our annual learning needs assessment and feedback from program reviews, Norwood Hospital offers many contact hour continuing education programs. For example, our medical and surgical units offer morning and noontime lectures on a variety of nursing topics in collaboration with the medical and surgical physicians.

Net-Learning

Our on-line educational tool, Net-Learning provides nursing staff with 24/7 access to mandatory and continuing education opportunities.

Tuition Reimbursement

Norwood Hospital provides full- and part-time employees with a generous tuition reimbursement benefit for continued opportunities of professional growth.

Schwartz Center Rounds at Norwood Hospital

Unique, multi-disciplinary sessions in which hospital staff explore the emotional side of care-giving.

A national program with sites across the country, Schwartz Center Rounds are funded by the Kenneth B. Schwartz Center, a Boston-based non-profit dedicated to advancing compassionate health care.

In a typical Rounds session, a panel of caregivers presents a patient case that brought up interesting and important psychosocial issues. Topics have included: delivering bad news; when religious or spiritual beliefs conflict with medical advice; taking care of a colleague; and losing a patient. Hospital staffs then share their own thoughts and feelings related to the day's topic.

Unlike grand rounds, these sessions are not about clinical problem-solving, but rather about exploring and processing the emotions that come up in the daily work of hospital staff. A comprehensive study of Schwartz Center Rounds has shown them to help caregivers connect better with patients emotionally; enhance their understanding of the effects of illness on patients and their families; improve communication among caregivers and decrease feelings of caregiver isolation and stress. Schwartz Center Rounds are held five times a year at Norwood Hospital.

Practice Model

The Nursing Practice Model at Norwood Hospital is patient-centered. The professional registered nurse (RN) is the coordinator of the delivery of care. The RN uses the nursing process to provide patient care. All patients are assigned to a registered nurse. Ancillary staff assists with the provision of care under the direction of the registered nurse.

Care is provided in a collaborative manner, within a multidisciplinary care model involving all health care team members. The team members develop a care plan that will guide the process of care and achievement of quality outcomes and rounds together every day.

Our Nursing Workgroups—Opportunities to Shine . . . Diabetes Resource Group

The Diabetes Resource Group consists of nurses and dietitians who act as resources for the dissemination of up-to-date information on diabetes for the staff on their units. The group meets quarterly. Meetings consist of educational offerings, medical record reviews, development of policies for diabetes patient care, problem-solving for issues on units, case study presentations and discussion of how to educate nurses throughout the hospital in current diabetes trends.

Among its accomplishments, the Diabetes Resource Group worked with the hospital Pharmacy to provide for the dispensing of new glucometers for patients new to blood sugar testing or in need of an update. The Diabetes Resource Group has coordinated in-services on these meters to provide staff with the knowledge and key points for patient education. Group members also work with the interdisciplinary health care team to improve timing of blood sugar testing, insulin administration and meal time distribution on their units.

Nursing Research Committee

The Nursing Research Committee facilitates nursing research and assists nurses in developing projects to improve patient outcomes, decrease costs and support best practices within a culture of evidence-based practice (EBP).

In addition to supporting nursing research, the Research Committee will:

- Assist in the enculturation of Evidenced Based Practice (EBP) within the institution by supporting research utilization and best practice.
- Utilize and support the relationship with an academic institution to provide an expert researcher at Norwood Hospital.
- Act as a forum for continued support for nursing research at CNH.
- Establish a mechanism to present nursing research conducted at Norwood Hospital to the community.

Establish a venue for nurse researchers from outside the institution to share their expertise and research findings to the community.

Evidence-Based Practice Projects in Process Adequate Nutrition for Patients on Respirators

Nurses in the intensive care unit are actively addressing the problem of inadequate nutrition in patients who are on a respirator. These patients are often on tube feedings and are fed every hour. Past practice has been to withhold feedings if too much liquid nutrition is in the stomach when it comes time to feed the patient again. By determining the maximum amount of food that can be in the stomach before a feeding must be withheld, it is hoped that patients' nutrition will improve. A study of the effects of a change in policy is currently under way.

Family Visiting in the Post Anesthesia Care Unit (PACU)

The PACU nurses are carefully reviewing the literature to determine the advantages and disadvantages of families visiting loved-ones recovering from anesthesia in the PACU. The current policy of a five-minute visit by 2 visitors every two hours is being researched to see if a more liberal policy might put in place.

- 2008 Nursing Journal Clubs
- Cath Lab—monthly
- Diabetic Resource Group meeting
- ICU—monthly, every third Wednesday, 12:15-12:45 p.m.
- Pain Resource Group meeting
- Unit-Based Performance Improvement Resource Group meeting

Wound/Ostomy Resource Group Meeting: 2008 Nursing Research Studies Delirium Nursing Research, Unit 32

Delirium in elderly women and men is not uncommon, especially when they are hospitalized. A research study is currently underway to investigate nurses' use of a screening tool that will allow them to detect delirium earlier, before patients' symptoms affect their safety and that of others.

Emergency Department Nursing Research

In today's health care environment, retaining new graduate nurses is a challenge faced by both large and small hospitals, especially in specialty areas such as emergency care. In response to this challenge, two nurses will soon be researching the experiences of new graduates in the emergency room who recently completed the department's new orientation program. Expected outcomes include a better experience and increased retention as compared to the past.

2007-08 Nursing Research: Highlights of Accomplishments

- Developed a 2007 Nursing Research Strategic Plan (goals)
- Facilitated five Nursing Grand Rounds
  - o *The Hospital Elder Life Program*: An Interdisciplinary Team Working to Reduce Delirium and Functional Decline in Hospitalized Elders
  - o *High Risk/High Alert*: Preventing Insulin Administration Errors, a Peer Review
  - o *Patient Safety*: Effective Communication and Skin Integrity, a Peer Review
  - o *A Reflection of Suicide*: Trends, Assessment, Treatment
  - o Transforming the Culture of Pain
- Implemented evidence-based practice (EBP) and nursing research Net-Learning modules, with more in development
- Reviewed nursing research proposal, Early Identification of Delirium by Nurses
- Developed folder with nursing research/EBP information on MyCaritas nursing web portal

Proposed and developed an all day EBP workshop: Pain Management Resource Nurse Group

The Pain Management Resource Nurse (PRN) group consists of nurses who are especially interested in providing patients, other members of the health care team, and patient family members with the latest in pain management modalities. This group of dedicated nurses is the pain resource for their individual patient units. They have advanced pain management education and are knowledgeable in various pain management modalities.

The management of pain is a core value upon which nursing care is dedicated. The PRN is a unit-based nurse who functions as a resource to other members of the health care team, disseminating information and consulting with nurses, physicians, patients and families to facilitate quality pain management. The PRNs meet with a nurse practitioner (NP) coordinator quarterly tand as needed throughout the year to receive the latest information regarding pain management medications, therapies, and complimentary therapies that may be employed at the bedside.

The nurse practitioner coordinator is available for nursing consults on patient care units as necessary. In the past, the PRNs have taken part in a research project to increase awareness on their units of the PRN role and to increase awareness of effective pain management through a variety of approaches. The PRN is an effective catalyst on the clincial units to introduce new and better means of effective pain management.

Wound/Ostomy Resource Clinician

The Wound/Ostomy Resource clinician functions as a resource to other members of the health care team, disseminating information and consulting with nurses, physicians, patients, and families to facilitate wound/ostomy teaching and management. The resource clinician group consists of nurses, physical therapists, and nutritionists, all of whom participate on the team to improve patient care and outcomes. The resource group meets quarterly to conduct a pressure ulcer prevalence survey by direct patient assessment on six National Database Nursing Quality Indicator (NDNQI) units and an all-hospital survey annually in March. The resource clinician meetings are also an opportunity to review and update ostomy, wound, and skin care standards and policies. On-going education related to wound/ostomy products and care is also an essential part of every quarterly meeting. The wound/ostomy resource clinician also acts as a role model, educator, and change agent bringing new knowledge and up-to-date information to unit colleagues.

Department Overviews

Following is a nursing perspective of the various departments throughout Norwood Hospital.

Nursing staff is comprised of RNs and nursing assistants who work together in a collaborative practice model to deliver patient centered care. Nurses work eight- and 12-hour shifts. This is an excellent environment to develop a set of nursing assessment skills essential to ongoing professional development. Critical thinking skills, flexibility and a sense of humor are essential ingredients for the nursing staff. Staff nurses are given a strong support network in which to learn and grow, starting with a competency-based preceptor program and supplemented with a unit-based clinical nurse specialist. There are numerous clinical resource groups with representatives on each unit who foster Evidence Based Practice at the unit level. Clinical leaders and charge nurses are additional resources for staff on each unit, providing clinical guidance and support.

Adult and Geriatric Medical, Unit 21

Unit 21 is a 24-bed adult and geriatric medical unit. Patients are admitted to Unit 21 from the Emergency Department. A registered nurse is assigned as the charge nurse every shift. The charge nurse functions as a clinical resource with an overall knowledge of all the patients on the unit and oversees patient assignments, physicians' offices, or other in-patient units. The Nursing Practice Model for the unit is patient centered. The nurse is responsible for coordinating the care and services of a group of patients involving multidisciplinary collaboration and discharge planning.

Adult Medical/Surgical, Unit 31 Pediatric Sub-Unit 31 is a medical-surgical adult unit with a pediatric sub-unit. It offers six beds for pediatric medical-surgical patients from two months to 18 years and 16 adult beds. Special services particular to this area include medical telemetry and care of the patient with an acute medical condition or exacerbation of a chronic medical condition. Unit 31 has a dedicated nurse manager who provides management support and planning for all staff on the unit.

Adult Medical, Unit 32

Unit 32 is a 28-bed adult medical unit providing care for patients from age 16 through end of life. Patients present with a variety of challenging specialties, including but not limited to oncology, pulmonary, infectious disease, gastroenterology, nephrology and cardiology. Special services particular to this area include medical telemetry, care of the patient with an acute medical condition or exacerbation of a chronic medical condition, care of the patient with acute alcohol or substance withdrawal, inpatient chemotherapy, pain control, terminal care and geriatric care. Unit 32 has a dedicated nurse manager who provides management support and planning for all staff on the unit.

Adult Psychiatry, Unit 28

Norwood Hospital's Unit 28 is a 12-bed inpatient psychiatric unit. Upon admission, the nurse assesses patients holistically, initiating psychiatric care plans as well as addressing any medical issues. While hospitalized, patients have access to a variety of psychiatric services, including medication management, individual therapy, occupational therapy, and substance abuse treatment counseling.

The small size of Unit 28 offers the advantage of a less stimulating, comforting environment, which serves patients well. The unit functions as an interdisciplinary team working together to provide an individualized treatment plan for each patient.

Geriatric Psychiatry, Unit 35

Unit 35 is a 28-bed unit for geriatric psychiatry. Generally, patients admitted to the unit are over the age of 50. Patients may be admitted with any psychiatric diagnosis. Frequently patients have some degree of cognitive impairment, such as memory loss, difficulty taking care of themselves, or significant changes in behavior.

Patients on Unit 35 are monitored for psychiatric and medical problems. Each patient is evaluated daily by a psychiatrist, and a nurse practitioner is available seven days a week. Registered nurses provide daily and ongoing assessment of the patient's status and response to treatment. Multidisciplinary teams, consisting of physicians, nurses, occupational therapists, and social workers, in collaboration with the patient or the patient's family, determine the plan of care for the patient.

Patients are encouraged to participate in daily therapeutic groups offered by members of the multidisciplinary team. Groups include psychotherapy, cognitive rehabilitation, sensory modulation, and hygiene, and pet or music therapy.

Adult Psychiatry, Unit 36

Unit 36 is a 21-bed acute care adult psychiatric unit. The multidisciplinary team works to provide exceptional care to this challenging patient population, which consists of patients ages 16 years and over. Often our patients have multiple psychiatric, medical, emotional, social, spiritual, and cultural issues.

One of Unit 36's special challenges is helping people with various addictions. We work to promote healthy coping skills in creative ways given the restriction of an acute mental health unit.

Unit 36 has a primary nursing system in place in which nurses and mental health associates take on primary assignments. Teamwork is key to the promotion of the safety and well being of the patients and staff and integral to everything we do. Each of the Unit 36 staff members plays an important role in the care of patients, regardless of job description and hours.

Cardiology Department

The Norwood Hospital Cardiology Department consists of a dedicated nursing staff committed to the heart health of our patients. We work cohesively with all medical and surgical units and primarily with the Emergency Department, Intensive Care Unit, and the Telemetry Unit to ensure optimal care for our patients. Cardiology includes the Cardiac Cath Lab, Cardiac Rehabilitation, EKG services, Stress Lab, and ECHO Lab.

The staff consists of a nurse manager, registered nurses, special procedure techs, including stress, EKG, and ECHO, and exercise physiologists and administrative secretaries.

Patients are referred to Cardiology from within the hospital and by other physicians and facilities. We are proud to offer state-of-the art cardiology services. We have performed emergency angioplasties since 1999. We also offer elective angioplasties through the Massachusetts Department of Public Health's MASS COMM trial on non-emergency coronary artery angioplasty in hospitals that do not perform open-heart surgery. In addition, we perform diagnostic catheterizations, peripheral angioplasties and implantation of pacemakers and defibrillators.

Norwood Hospital Cardiology also offers cardiac rehabilitation classes, such as exercise, nutrition, stress management and smoking cessation programs under the management of our RN health counselor, exercise physiologists and dieticians.

Emergency Department

The Norwood Hospital Emergency Department (ED) is a busy 28-bed unit that provides compassionate emergency care to patients of diverse age groups. We serve about 50,000 patients were treated in the bustling ED.

We are proud to be affiliated with Boston Children's Hospital, whose pediatricians are on site 24/7. The ED serves the local area of Norwood and other surrounding towns and is part of Mass. State Emergency Medical Service Region IV. Our ED uses a collaborative team approach to deliver care. Physicians, nurses, nursing assistants, and administrative professionals are assigned to specific areas of the ED. Each area contains a subset of patients who are triaged to an area, according to their presenting symptoms and acuity.

Areas of care within the ED are Triage, Fast Track, Pediatrics, Psychiatry, and Diagnostic Testing, including CT and MRI.

The ED also uses Life-Net, a computer modem linked system, which allows hospital-based paramedics to send cardiograms to the emergency department prior to a patient's arrival at the hospital. This results in the rapid activation of the Cardiac Catheterization team for emergency cardiac procedures when indicated.

The ED nursing staff members are highly skilled with Basic Life Support, Advanced Cardiac Life Support and Pediatric Advanced Life Support training as a part of their education to emergency nursing.

Norwood Hospital has been designated a provider of Primary Stroke Service by the Massachusetts Department of Public Health. This certification requires that the ED meets strict guidelines for treating individuals with stroke symptoms, including timely treatment of patients with thrombolytics, the clot-busting drugs considered the standard of care for treating certain kinds of strokes.

Endoscopy

Endoscopy Unit consists of registered nurses (RNs) and Endoscopy technicians highly skilled in the delivery of specialized care to patients suffering from disorders of the gastrointestinal tract. The Endoscopy nursing staff is a cohesive and dynamic group of individuals. Each staff member brings individual skills and talents that blend and complement one another enabling us to provide comprehensive care to our patients.

We provide diagnostic as well as therapeutic care to our outpatient and inpatient population. Our procedures include EGD, colonoscopy, flexible sigmoidoscopy, esophageal motility studies, 24-hour ph monitoring studies, liver biopsies, and more.

In the Endoscopy Unit, we are sensitive to the psychosocial and spiritual needs of our patients. Many of our patients are having screening procedures for different types of cancer and/or follow-up procedures for a cancer diagnosis already made. They are frightened and apprehensive and need the emotional support that our nursing staff is exceptionally qualified to offer.

The Endoscopy nursing staff feels fortunate to also provide preventative care to many of our patients. We believe that our department helps to save lives with primary care detection and that our compassion, care, and holistic view of each patient comforts those suffering from gastrointestinal bleeding to those suffering from colon or gastric cancer.

Intensive Care Unit

Norwood Hospital's Intensive Care Unit (ICU) is an 11-bed critical care unit located one floor above the emergency department and just steps away from the operating rooms.

The nursing focus is the care of the critically ill adult and geriatric patient. Highly skilled nurses are trained in both Basic Life Support and

Advanced Cardiac Life support. Round-the-clock physician coverage is provided. Patients in the ICU most often require intense resources and time, as they often require mechanical ventilation, invasive hemodynamic monitoring and management of highly sensitive medications.

A modified Nursing Collaborative Practice Model is used to deliver patient care. A registered nurse (RN) (primary) is assigned to each patient upon admission. This RN is responsible for coordinating the care and services of a small group of patients involving multidisciplinary collaboration and discharge planning and is also responsible for the initial assessment and development of the plan of care.

The RN reviews the plan of care, oversees its implementation, assesses patient progress toward expected outcomes, and revises the plan of care, as necessary. In addition, the RN is responsible for review and transcription of physician's orders, review of diagnostic data, and direct communication with the physician regarding his/her patients. There is a registered nurse assigned as the charge nurse every shift. She/he functions as a clinical resource, has an overall knowledge of all patients on the unit and oversees patient assignments.

Medical Step-down, Unit 22

The medical step down unit is under the same nursing leadership as Unit 22. The medical step down unit consists of four dedicated beds within the unit. The step down unit is indicated for a specific subset of patients that need more care than can be provided on the general medical ward but less than the ICU. Typically these patients may require more frequent vital sign monitoring, nursing interventions and/or non-invasive ventilation. These patients are hemodynamically stable and do not need invasive monitoring.

Surgical Services

Norwood Hospital's Surgical Services department (OR) is staffed by specially trained RNs and scrub technicians. There are seven scheduled operating rooms in the hospital's main OR area.

Based on nursing assessment, diagnosis and a plan of care, the nursing focus is on the intra-operative phase of the peri-operative patient. We are available seven days a week, 24 hours a day to meet the surgical needs of the hospital. Our staff provides services for all types of surgical cases with the exception of open-heart procedures and organ transplant. Support staff includes OR assistants, anesthesia technicians, surgical business office staff and a unit secretary.

Medical/Surgical/Telemetry, Unit 33

Unit 33 is a 30-bed adult and geriatric medical/surgical/telemetry unit. The professional nursing focus on this unit is the care of the adult and geriatric patient with cardiovascular disease.

Patients admitted to Unit 33 may come from the Emergency

Department, ICU, another in patient unit, physician office, or other nursing facility. Criteria for admission include patients with chest pain requiring cardiac telemetry, pre op/post cardiac catheterization, and patients with newly placed pacemakers.

Nursing staff is highly trained and participate in specialized classes for EKG interpretation and care of patients with abnormal EKGs.

A modified Nursing Collaborative Practice Model is used to deliver patient care. The registered nurse (RN) is assigned to each patient upon admission reviews and revises the plan of care as necessary. This nurse is responsible for coordinating the care and services of a small group of patients involving multidisciplinary collaboration and discharge planning. A nursing assistant may assist with a patient assignment under the direct supervision of the registered nurse. There is a registered nurse assigned as the charge nurse on each shift. She/he functions as a clinical resource, has an overall knowledge of all patients on the unit and oversees patient assignments.

Small Miracles Birthing Center, Units 24, 25, 26

Our Small Miracles Birthing Center focuses on family-centered maternity care, with a main focus on parents and baby during their hospital stay. We have six labor and delivery rooms and 18 private post-partum rooms. Our experienced staff is cross-trained and proficient in labor and delivery, nursery care and post-partum care. Small Miracle's management model is that of nurse manager and obstetrics clinical specialist.

We also provide care for women's health and gynecologic services on our post-partum floor. Our affiliation with St. Elizabeth's Medical Center in Boston provides for weekly patient services of maternal fetal medicine and Level II ultrasounds at Norwood Hospital.

Norwood Hospital's affiliation with Children's Hospital of Boston means that there is a Children's Hospital pediatrician in house 24/7 and available to the nursery and labor and delivery units as needed. In addition, our OB unit has 24-hour coverage from our excellent anesthesia group.

Small Miracles also offers extensive childbirth education programs from pre-natal yoga to infant massage and CPR, breast feeding and new mothers' support groups. We also have the "Small Miracles Boutique," which offers products for a new mother's breast-feeding needs.

References

B. Adenso-Diaz, PhD, is Associate Professor, Management Science, Escuela t. Superior de Ingenieros Industriales University of Oviedo, Spain.

Giovannetti, P. (1979). Understanding patient classification systems. *Journal of Nursing Administration*, 4(2), 4-9.

Hendrickson, G., Doddato, T.M., and Kovner, Ch.T. (1990). How do nurses use their time? *Journal of Nursing Administration,* 20(3), 31-37.

Insalud (1996). Proyecto Signo II. Comision Tecnica de Enfermeria, Ministerio de Sanidad y Consumo.

O'Brien-Pallas, L., Leatt, P., Deber, R., and Till, J. (1989). A comparison of workload estimates using three methods of patient classification. *Canadian Journal of Nursing Administration,* 2(3), 16-32.

Olallo Sanchez-Molero, is Nursing Staff Director, Alvarez Hospital, Mieres, Spain.

Pilar, L. Gonzalez-Torre is Assistant Professor, Industrial Engineering, Escuela t. Superior de Ingenieros Industriales University of Oviedo, Spain.

Poulson, E. (1987). A method for training and checking interrater agreement for a patient classification study. *Nursing Management,* 18(9), 72-80.

Procter, S., and Hunt, M. (1994). Using the Delphi survey technique to develop a professional definition of nursing for analyzing nursing workload. *Journal of Advanced Nursing,* 19(5), 1003-14.

Rosendall, R. (1983). Patient classification systems: The ideal vs reality. *Journal of Nursing Administration,* 2, 13, 14-19.

Shullanberger, G. (2000). Nurse staffing decisions: An integrative review of the literature. *Nursing Economics,* 18(3), 124-48.

Silva, N., and Aderhodlt, B. (1989) Computerizing assessment of workload and productivity. *Nursing Management,* 20(11), 49-56.

Visser, J.H.M. (1997). Helping hospitals making the trade-off between service and resource utilization. A production control perspective. Internal report, Faculty of Technology Management, Eindhoven University of Technology.

Vries, J.M.G., Bertrand, M., and Visser, J.H.M. (1999). Design requirements for health care production control systems. *Production Planning and Control,* 10(6), 559-569.

Williams, M.A. (1977). Quantification of direct nursing care activities. *Journal of Nursing Administration,* 10(7), 15-18.

Appendix 2

GLENEAGLES INTAN MEDICAL CENTRE (GIMC), KUALALAMPUR

INTRODUCTION

Malaysia is one of the most pleasant and developed countries in South East Asia. Its warm tropical climate is matched by its equally warm and friendly people. Malaysia offers tourists a vibrant and colourful fusion of Malay, Chinese, Indians cultures and customs. From busting cities to serene landscapes, the world's highest buildings to the region's highest peak, sunny beached to misty highlands, visitors will be enchanted with the character that is positively Malaysia. Here also, the harmonious species-rich tropical forest. Whatever you're seeking, be it adventure shopping, culture, festivals and health care, are here for you.

WORLD CLASS HEALTH CARE

Decades of economic growth and prosperity have greatly elevated the health care standards in Malaysia. Today, 88.5% of the population lives within 5 km of medical centre or private practitioner. The country's English-speaking medical professionals are generally trained in the United Kingdom, the United States and Australia. Some of the world's most advanced medical facilities and treatments may be found in Malaysia. These attractive factors make Malaysia a preferred destination for visitors seeking truly world-class health care.

GLENEAGLES INTAN MEDICAL CENTRE (GIMC)

Step into GIMC and you will be elevated to a world where your health and medical needs are addressed in an environment that truly promotes health and comfort.

Which is why, at GIMC, you will benefit from its medical services delivered with advanced technologies and facilities. Perhaps more importantly, you will be cared for by a team of compassionate medical practitioners.

Our specialist consultants are experiences and skilled. These medical professionals have earned credentials as well as certified and registered with internationally renowned medical colleges around the world. You can be assured that the standards of the medical centre's medical professionals and staff match international requirements according to ISO standards.

FACILITIES

GIMC utilized modern equipment to perform diagnostic tests, surgeries and other medical procedures. Beyond modern technology and equipment, GIMC is very much a medical centre for the 21st century. From the moment you enter the hospital, our aesthetically pleasing interiors make GIMC a warm and attractive environment. We designed our patient rooms bearing in mind that patients recover more quickly when surrounded by comfortable and appealing furnishings. We have paid close attention to the details that will ensure patients are as comfortable as they are well cared for. It may not be home, but you will feel at home here at GIMC.

GIMC HEALTH CARE COST ESTIMATION

Gleneagles Intan Medical Centre* (Malaysia)

Procedure	*Average Cost (US Dollars)*
Angiogram	$1,250
Heart valve replacement	$7,895
Cataract surgery**	$1,053
Coronary artery bypass surgery	$8,000
Removal of brain lesions (craniotomy)	$9,211

* The above pricing is subject to changes without prior notice
**Cost per eye

FOR ENQUIRIES

Gleneagles Intan Medical Centre (KL)
Marketing Department
2nd Floor, Hospital Building
Tel No: 603-4255 2982
Fax No: 603-4255 2980
E-mail: marketing@gleneaglesintan.com.my

EXECUTIVE HEALTH CHECKUP

EXECUTIVE SCREENING PROGRAMME

What is the Executive Screening Programme (ESP)?

The Executive Screening Programme is designed to provide you with an individuated and through medical examination to assess your health status.

Why should you consider an Executive Screening?

With the fast-paced high stress lifestyle of toady, maintaining good health is vial. Preventative health checks sometimes takes a back seat to daily life, but these are essential to our future health.

Early detection of common diseases like Diabetes. Heart Disease, Hypertension and Cancer can assist in the prevention of serious complications and ill-health.

What do we do?

Our premium medical evaluation consists of a complete history, physical examination and screening tests. Our examinations will be tailored to your health concerns as well as meeting the needs of busy executives and their employees.

How do we help?

- By identifying "well" persons with potential health risk factors.
- By identifying asymptomatic persons with early signs of disease.
- By evaluating your health status and early prevention of disease.

Where is the Executive Screening Centre Located?

Our Executive Screening Centre is situated at Suite 116, on the 1st Floor of the Medical Consulting Suites (Opposite the Main Hospital Building)

Preparation for the Health Screening

- You will need to fast for at least 8-10 hours prior to your appointment. If you are thirsty, you may have sips of water.
- It is advisable to refrain from smoking at least 8 hours prior to your appointment.
- I you are on any prescribed medication, please seek advice from the ESP Coordinator before the appointment.
- If a Stress ECG has been arranged, kindly bring along comfortable shoes and clothing, to exercise in.

How long will the screening take?

Our Executive Screening Programme process takes approximately 2-3 hours to complete. A complimentary meal voucher will be provided for your enjoyment and convenience. The doctor will discuss your results in detail with you during a review at a later date.

The Health Report and Review

The complete medical report with results will be complied within 5-7 working days and shall be discussed during a review with your examining doctor. For medical tourists, the medical report shall be prepared and available for review with the patient by the third working day. If one has to leave the country before this time, arrangements can be made for the report to be couriered, at a change to the home country. This shall provide you the convenience to see a doctor of your choice back home for a review.

Screening services are available:

Monday-Friday	:	9 a.m.-5 p.m.
Saturday	:	9 a.m.-1 p.m.

Earlier appointments at 8.30 a.m. are available. Please enquire at the time of booking.

EXECUTIVE SCREENING PROGRAMME (ESP)

Basic Screening ***(Male and Female)*** **RM388.00**
Physical Examination
ECG with Report
Lung Function Test with Report
Chest X-Ray with Report
General Screening Profile 3*

Comprehensive Screening (*Male and Female*) **RM870.00**
Physical Examination
ECG with Report
Stress ECG (Treadmill) with Report
Lung Function Test with Report
Chest X-Ray with Report
Ultrasound Abdomen and Pelvis
General Screening Profile 3*

Premium Screening (*Male*) **RM1,008.00**
Physical Examination
ECG with Report
Stress ECG (Treadmill) with Report
Lung Function Test with Report
Chest X-Ray with Report
Ultrasound Abdomen and Pelvis
PSA (for cancer of the prostate)
CA19.9 (for cancer of the gastrointestinal system)
HSCRP***
General Screening Profile 3*

Premium Screening (*Female*) **RM1,155.00**
Physical Examination (including pap smear procedure and breast check)
ECG with Report
Stress ECG (Treadmill) with Report
Lung Function Test with Report
Chest X-Ray with Report
Ultrasound Abdomen and Pelvis
CA19.9 (for cancer of the gastrointestinal system)

CA15.3 (for cancer of breast)
CA125 (for cancer of ovary)
Liquid-based Pap Test (ThinPrep)
HSCRP***
General Screening Profile 3*

Applicable Test(s) for Ladies Below 40 years: Premium Screening (Female) with Ultrasound Breasts	**RM1285.00**
Applicable Test(s) for Ladies Above 40 years: Premium Screening (Female) with mammogram	**RM1316.00**
Premium Screening (Female) with Ultrasound Breasts and Mammogram	**RM1367.00**

Below are some of the more commonly asked tests, which are available as options to be done with any of the packages

- HbA1C (Diabetes Test)
- Hepatitis C antibody
- Bone Mineral Densitomentry (for osteoporosis)
- Barium Meal (for peptic ulcer disease)
- Virtual Colonoscopy (for colon disease)
- Stool Test for Occult Blood (for colon cancer)
- Liquid-based Pap Test (ThinPrep)
- HSCRP
- Ultrasound Breasts
- Mammogram
- Dietary Advice Referral
- Calcium Scoring (Coronary Screening)
- HIV Screening.

Some Info on tests in the packages

Liquid-based Pap Test (ThinPrep Pap Test)—for cervical cancer screening (At our laboratory, this test is done using the ThinPrep Pap Test method which is FDA-approved and differs from the conventional Pap Smear, in that, after the cells are obtained in the usual manner, the cells are placed directly in a collection vial containing a preservative fluid. A processor in the laboratory separates the cells from other materials such as blood and mucus and the cells are then transferred to a slice to form a uniform, thin layer that is much easier to read and interpret compared to the conventional method).

***HSCRP (High Sensitive CRP) for coronary risk factor
PSA (for prostate cancer)
CA 19.9 (for cancer of gastrointestinal system)
CA 15.3 (for cancer of the breast)
CA 125 (for ovarian cancer)

General Screening Profile 3-Full Blood Test

- o Full Blood Count with PBF and ESR
- o Kidney Disease
- o Screening for diabetes
- o Calcium and Phosphates (for bone metabolism)
- o Gout
- o Liver disease and liver cancer
- o Thyroid disease
- o Cholesterol level (Risk of heart disease)
- o Colon cancer
- o Rheumatoid arthritis
- o Syphilis screening
- o Hepatitis A and B screening.
- o Urine Test

Special rates can be arranged for corporate clients and groups of 20 or more people. Kindly enquire from the **Executive Screening Centre** at **603-4255 2982** or **4255 2983.**

OCCUPATIONAL HEALTH CENTRE

A return on investment for health

Medical surveillance and screening are two fundamental strategies for optimizing employee health. The purpose of surveillance is to detect and eliminate underlying causes (i.e. hazards or exposures) of any discovered trends and thus has a prevention focus. It is the analysis of health information to look for problems that may be occurring in the workplace due to occupational exposures hazardous to health such as; chemicals, workplace ergonomics, etc.

Surveillance may be based on a single case or sentinel event, but is more typically from the group of employees being evaluated to look for abnormal trends in health status or to be performed as a preventive measure to ensure that working conditions are safe. Review of these group results helps to identify potential problem areas and the effectiveness of existing worksite preventive strategies.

- For e.g. according to Occupational Safety and Health (Use and Standard of Exposure of Chemicals Hazardous to Health) Regulations 2000, health surveillance is necessary for the protection of health of employees exposes or likely to be exposed to conditions that maybe hazardous to health. Employer should carry out health surveillance and it must be conducted by an Occupational Health Doctor (OHD).

Definitions

Occupational Safety and Health:

Prevention of injuries by accidents and illnesses at work.

Health:

A state of well-being and free from illness.

Hazard:

Anything with the capability to cause harm (i.e. chemical, electricity, working on ladders, etc).

Risk:

The chance or probability of harm actually being done. It can also be expressed as number of events in a unit of time.

OSH Policy, Organization and Arrangements

The Occupational Safety and Health Act, 1994 places a duty on every employer and self-employed person to prepare and as often as may be appropriate, revise a written statement of his general policy with respect to safety and health at work of his employees and the organization, and arrangements for the time being in force for carrying out that policy and to bring the statement and any revision of the notice of all his employees.

Surveillance Required by Law Factories and Machinery Act, 1967

- Lead Regulations
- Noise Regulation
- Mineral Dust Regulations
- Asbestos Regulations

Occupational Safety and Health Act, 1194

- Use and Standards of Exposure of Chemicals Hazardous (USE CHH 2000)

Why is medical surveillance implemented?

- To indicate the adequacy of control measures
- To identify individuals at increased risk
- Provide baseline for medical data
- Identify and modify disease trend
- Set benchmark for preventive action.

Why is Occupational Health and Safety important?

Work plays a central role in people's lives, since most workers spend at least eight hours a day in workplace, whether it is on a plantation, in an office, factory, etc. Therefore, work environments should be safe and healthy. Yet this is not the case for many workers. Every day workers all over the world are faced with a multitude of health hazards, such as:

- Dusts
- Gases
- Noise
- Vibration
- Extreme temperatures

Components of the Medical Surveillance Programme Include:

- Pre-employment and pre-placement medical examination.
- Biological monitoring and biological effect monitoring.
- Health effects monitoring.
- Investigation of occupational disease and poisoning including workplace inspections.
- Notification of occupational disease and poisoning.
- Assist in disability assessment.
- Return to work examination after medical removal protection
- Record keeping and monitoring.

SCREENING PROGRAMME

PRE-EMPLOYMENT PACKAGE—RM 50

- Physical Examination
- Chest X-Ray
- Urine FEME

BASIC OCCUPATIONAL HEALTH PACKAGE—RM 110

- Physical Examination
- Chest X-Ray
- Full Blood Count
- Liver Function Test
- Renal Function Test
- Urine FEME

Other tests are conducted depending on the types and level of occupational exposure. Kindly contact the Occupational Health Physician for advice at 03-4255 2997 or email **dralaen@gleneaglesintan.com.my**

GENERAL OPTIONAL TEST APPLICABLE TO THE ABOVE PACKAGES

• Treadmill Stress Test	RM 322.00
• Mammogram (For Women above 40 yrs)	RM 161.00
• Ultrasound Breast (For Women below 40 yrs)	RM 130.00
• Mammogram with Ultrasound Breast (For Women above 40 yrs)	RM 212.00
• Ultrasound Abdomen and Pelvis	RM 204.00
• ThinPrep (Liquid-based cytology)	RM 96.00
• Audiogram (Hearing Test)	RM 100.00

OTHER SERVICES AVAILABLE

- Education
- Case management
- Drug screening
- Consultation
- Pre-employment or annual physicals
- Environmental monitoring and safety consultation
- Functional capacity evaluation
- Hearing conservation programme
- Lung function test
- Work place assessment
- Risk assessment
- Medical surveillance
- Rehabilitation and job placement
- Sickness absenteeism

OSTEOPOROSIS

Osteoporosis is a diseased in which bones become fragile and more likely to break. It is often called the "silent disease" because bone loss occurs without symptoms. People may not know that they have osteoporosis until their bones becomes so weak that a sudden strain or fall causes a hip fracture or a vertebra to collapse. Collapsed vertebra may initially be felt or seen in the form of severe back pain, loss of height, or spinal deformities such as hypnosis, or severely stooped posture, If not prevented or left untreated, osteoporosis can progress painlessly until a bone breaks. These broken bones, also known as fractures, occur typically in the hip, spine, and wrist.

Any bone can be affected, but great concerns are placed on fractures of the hip and spine. A hip fracture most often requires hospitalization and major surgery. It can impair a person's ability to walk unassisted and may cause prolonged or permanent disability or even death.

Spinal or vertebral fractures also have serious consequences, which include loss of height, severe back pain, and deformity. According to a WHO report osteoporosis is a disorder affecting nearly one in three women today. Osteoporosis occurs after middle age, and is six times more common in women than men. Loss of bone is accelerated during the post menopausal period due to changes in hormonal balance. Currently, one-half of all women in this group are believed to have a clinically significant degree of bone mass loss.

Our Bone Mineral Densitometry Examination (BMD) is a fast, safe and painless way for us to provide you and your physician with a highly accurate assessment of your bone mass. Early detection of this disease not only improves the effectiveness of certain therapies but it also helps the physician in evaluating the effectiveness of these treatments over time.

If the patient's bone density is low, or decreases at an abnormally fast rate, the patient may be at risk for osteoporosis. Through appropriate changes in diet, exercise habits medication further deterioration of bone can be prevented.

What is the purpose of this test?

- To measure bone density, or bone mass
- To detect bone mass loss
- To confirm diagnosis of Osteoporosis
- To monitor bone loss during chemotherapy
- To monitor effectiveness of medication
- To assess and/or predict risk of fractures

Is the test painful?

- No, this low-dose radiation test is painless

Who should have a BMD?

BMD should be done for the following conditions:

- Women at or post mensopause
- Women on Hormone Replacement Therapy (HRT)
- Early menopause, especially female atheletes
- Elderly men
- Hypogonadism (low testosterone levels)
- Thyroid disorders and pre-thyroid surgery
- Pre-hormone therapy
- Patients undergoing chemotherapy
- Diabetics on glucocorticoid medication
- Family history of Osteoporosis
- Low body weight/weight loss
- Excessive alcohol intake
- Smokers
- Long-term steroid therapy

Is there any preparation involved?

Unlike many other medical examinations, no special preparation is required. However, as in any medical procedure, please inform your doctor if you are pregnant, to avoid any accidental radiation to the unborn fetus.

What is BMD?

In BMD testing, your bone mass is compared to the bone mass of an adult between the ages of 35 and 45. A score is thus determined, thereby measuring bone mass against that which is normal for your age, as some bone loss is normal with ageing.

Bone Densitometry Score Diagnosis (T score)

Above	–1.0	Normal
Between	–1.0 to –2.5	Osteopenia (low bone mass)
Below	–2.5	Osteoporosis
Below	–2.5 with fracture	Service Osteoporosis

How long will the BMD test take?

The test will take 30 minutes.

When will the BMD report be ready?

Specialties and Services

Aneasthesiology
Audiology Service
Cardiology
Cardiothoracic Surgery
Dental Surgery
Dermatology
Diabetes Care Centre
Ear, Nose and Throat Surgery
Endocrinology
Executive Screening Centre
Gastroenterology
General Surgery
General and Vascular Surgery
Gerontology
Haematology
Hand and Microsurgery
Maxillofacial/Facial Cosmetic Surgery
Nephrology

Hospital Floors

7th Floor
—Medical and Surgical Ward

6th Floor
—Medical and Surgical Ward

5th Floor
—Medical and Surgical Ward

4th Floor
—Paediatric Ward
—Rehabilitation Unit

3rd Floor
—Labour Delivery Rooms
—Maternity Ward
—Neonatal Intensive Care Unit/ Nursery

Neurology
Neurosurgery
Obstetrics and Gynaecology
Oncology
Ophthalmology
Orthopedic and Trauma Surgery
Pediatric Surgery
Pediatrics
Pathology
Plastic and Reconstructive Surgery
Podiatry
Psychiatry
Psychology
Psychotherapy
Rehabilitation Medicine
Respiratory Medicine
Rheumatology
Therapeutic Spa Services
Urology
Women's Wellness Centre

2nd Floor
—Administration Office
—Blood Donor Centre
—Laboratory
—Medical Records Department

1st Floor
—Day Care Centre
—Diagnostic and Cardiac
—Catheterization Laboratory
—Intensive Care/Coronary Care Unit
—Operating Theatres

Grd. Floor
—Accident and Emergency/ Outpatient Services
—Admission Department
—Concierge Services
—Customer Care Services
—Diabetes Care Centre
—Diet Counseling Centre
—Imaging Department
—Insurance Service Oncology Centre
—Oncology Centre

Your BMD report will be ready within 45 minutes.

Gleneagles Intan Medical Centre Services

NEUROLOGICAL REHABILITATION PROGRAMME

Our team of therapists and physician understand that neurological injuries and diseases can often be devastating. This does not mean the beginning of a helpless and dependent existence. We provide a compassionate rehabilitation programme to help maximize recovery, prevent complications and assist the patient on the road to independence with confidence and dignity.

Time is precious. Early rehabilitation is very important for the best outcome, do not wait for days or even weeks before starting rehabilitation.

The types of neurological diseases that need rehabilitation services include:

Stroke
Head Injury
Parkinson's Disease
Multiple Sclerosis

Brain Tumour
Guillain Barre
Muscular Dystrophy
Demyelinating Disease

The rehabilitation team

We have a multidisciplinary and interdisciplinary team which provides rehabilitation for our patients. Our core team consists of a Rehabilitation Physician, Physiotherapists, Occupational Therapist and Speech language Therapists. Our team is complemented by other consultants including Counsellor, Psychologist, Prosthetics/Orthotist and Dietitian, depending on the individual patients requirement.

All the team members are dedicated and experienced in rehabilitating patients with neurological problems. We do care for your well being and together with you, we will ensure the success of your rehabilitation programme.

The Programme

Following an assessment, a treatment plan with realistic goals is recommended for the patient and family.

The goal-orientated programme is designed to accommodate the preferences or needs of the patients and include appropriate inpatient and outpatient care. The programme may include combination of activities from the following areas:

Neuromuscular

- To maintain and improve flexibility
- To gain strength
- To maintain/reduce tone
- To gain adequate dynamic balance in all functional activity
- To improve coordination
- To improve sensory motor integration

Mobility

- Wheelchair assessment and training
- Gait assessment and training (with/without aids)

Medical care

- Bladder training
- Bowel training
- Skin-care and pressure sore prevention
- Sexual Counselling

Activities of daily living

- Self-care
- Home management skills
- Life skills
- Home assessment and modification

Swallowing/diet

- Swallowing management
- Dietary advice

Communication

- Receptive and expressive communication
- Functional communication
- Alternative and augmentative communication

Cognitive

- Cognitive assessment and training
- Perceptual assessment and training

Psychosocial

- Counselling
- Social interaction
- Family/community adjustment and support

Community Reintegration (School, work-site and public area visits can be arranged)

- Educational skills
- Vocational skills
- Leisure/hobbies
- Sports

You and your family need to be actively involved right from the beginning and regular discussions regarding progress will be conducted with you. We also provide home visits to assess the patient's environment and recommend modification to optimize their quality of life and independence.

Referral

Patients who wish to enroll into this programme will need an assessment by a Rehabilitation Physician either as an outpatient or inpatient. For an appointment, please contact: Rehabilitation Centre: 03-42552833/2793.

Cost

The fee for the programme will vary from patient to patient depending on the intensity of the programme. We also have a package available for a specified duration of treatment. For further information, please contact the rehabilitation administrative assistant at the rehabilitation centre.

Other Services

- General Physiotherapy
- General Speech and Language Therapy
- General Occupational Therapy
- Spinal Cord Injury Rehabilitation
- Rheumatological Rehabilitation
- Paediatric Rehabilitation
- Amputation Rehabilitation
- Orthotics and Prosthetics
- Equipment and Aids

SPINAL CORD INJURY REHABILITATION PROGRAMME

SPINAL CORD INJURY REHABILITATION

Following spinal cord injury, it is very important for one to choose a good rehabilitation programme with skilled professionals to help oneself develop the skills needed to achieve maximum independence and good health throughout one's life. Almost all systems of the body are involved in spinal cord injury and if these are not looked into, complications will arise. Some of these problems are inability to move the limbs, pressure sores, bladder and bowel impairment, spasticity, autonomic, dysreflexia, pain, deformity, infertility, chest infection, depression and social issues.

THE TEAM

We work as a multidisciplinary and interdisciplinary team and the core team members include a Rehabilitation Physician, Physiotherapists, Occupational Therapists and Nurses, Other professionals involved include Dietitians, Urologists, Counsellors and Orthotists as required. The team members are all dedicated and experienced in managing spinal injury patients.

THE PROGRAMME

After an assessment, we would plan a goal-orientated programme based on the individual's conditions and needs. The programme can be designed to accommodate the preference or needs as outpatients or inpatients. The programme may include combinations from the following areas:

NEUROMUSCULAR

- To maintain and improve flexibility
- To gain strength
- To maintain/reduce tone
- To gain adequate dynamic balance in all functional activity
- To improve coordination
- To improve coordination
- To improve sensory motor integration

MOBILITY

- Wheelchair assessment and training
- Gait assessment and training (with or without aids)

MEDICAL CARE

- Bladder training
- Bowel training
- Skin care and pressure sore prevention
- Sexual counseling
- Pain control

ACTIVITIES OF DAILY LIVING

- Self-care
- Home management skills
- Life skills
- Home assessment and modification

PSYCHOSOCIAL

- Counselling
- Social integration
- Family/community adjustment and support

COMMUNITY REINTEGRATION (VISITS TO SCHOOL, WORK SITE, PUBLIC AREA CAN BE ARRANGED)

- Education skills
- Vocational skills
- Leisure/hobbies
- Sport

EDUCATION

- Patient and family
- Caregivers' training
- Support group

You and your family need to be actively involved right from the beginning and regular discussions regarding progress will be conducted with you. We also provide home visits to assess the patient's environment and recommend modification to optimize their quality of life and independence.

REFERRAL

Patients who wish to enroll into this prograame will need an assessment by a Rehabilitation Physician either as an outpatient or inpatient. For an appointment, please contact: Rehabilitation Centre: 03-42552833/2793

COST

The fee for the programme will vary from patient to patient depending on the intensity of the programme. We also have package available for a specified duration of treatment. For further information, please contact the rehabilitation administrative assistant at the rehabilitation centre.

OTHER SERVICES

- General Physiotherapy
- General Speech and Lanugage Therapy
- General Occupational Therapy
- Neurological Rehabilitation
- Rheumatological Rehabilitation
- Paediatric Rehabilitation
- Amputation Rehabilitation
- Orthotics and Prosthetics
- Equipment and Aids

WOMEN'S WELLNESS PROGRAMME

WOMEN'S WELLNESS CENTRE

As women of today face more challenges of career and family commitments, they need to take charge of their well-being by leading a healthy lifestyle. Gleneagles Intan Medical Centre extends this basic 'Wellness Programme' as a stepping stone to your total wellness.

The wellness paradigm in health care for women involves:

- Quality health care
- Affordable health care
- Continuum in health care

GIMC **Women's Wellness Centre** aims to create an awareness of the importance of:

- Annual Pap smear screening and regular breast examination
- Healthy Lifestyle

This Centre, with a female Resident Medical Officer is a place for you to reach out, and clarify any doubts you may have about your health, in order to overcome fears and be able to cope with life's challenges and difficulties; to begin each day with joy.

GIMC Cares

GIMC WOMEN'S WELLNESS CENTRE

Facts

1. Breast cancer has been rated as the number 1 most common cancer in women, and as the 2nd most common cause of deaths amongst women.
2. Cancer cervix ranks 2nd among cancers affecting women.
3. Annual Pap smear and regular breast examination aids early detection.
4. Early detection and prompt treatment limits the spread of cancer to the lymph glands and other parts of the body.

WOMEN'S WELLNESS CENTRE (WWC)
Women's Wellness Programmes (WWP)

1. Basic Gynaecological Screening **WWC-300**

- Consultation
- Physical/Breast examination
- Liquid-based Pap Test (ThinPrep) **RM95.00**

2. Breast Screening 1 **WWC-305**

- Consultation
- Physical/Breast examination
- Ultrasound breasts **RM108.00**

3. Breast Screening 2 **WWC-310**

- Consultation **RM223.00**
- Physical/Breast examination
- Ultrasound breasts
- Mammogram

4. Gynaecological Screening **WWC-315**

- Consultation
- Physical/Breast examination
- Liquid-based Pap Test (ThinPrep)
- Ultrasound abdomen and pelvis **RM280.00**

5. Menopause Screening **WWC-320**

- Consultation
- Physical/Breast examination
- Liquid-based Pap Test (ThinPrep)
- Mammogram
- Bone Mineral Densitometry (BMD)
- Menopause profile **RM505.00**

LABOUR DELIVERY UNIT

At Gleneagles Intan Medical Centre, we recognize that the birth of your baby is a significant event for you and your partner. Thank you for choosing Gleneagles Intan Medical Centre, as the centre to share this happy and memorable occasion with you.

The hospital has been designed and equipped with the following services:

- 8 delivery suites equipped with fetal monitoring, medical gases, attached bathroom and television. Your partner can be present during normal delivery if he desires.
- Fully equipped nursery and neonatal intensive care unit. Rooming in of babies with mothers is encouraged.
- Availability of the Obstetrician, Anaesthetist, Paediatrician, Neonatologist and Nursing Staff.
- A full range of support services including dietetics, physiotherapy, etc.
- 24 hours operating theatre services to cater for emergency cases.

TOUR OF LABOUR DELIVERY UNIT

Tours of the Labour Delivery Unit are regularly conducted upon request. Please contact the Front Office at Tel: 03-4255 2703 for more details.

BREASTFEEDING

GLENEAGLES INTAN MEDICAL CENTRE is committed to promote and support exclusive breastfeeding of babies born in GIMC from birth up to six months of age and continue up to two years with appropriate complementary feeds.

Breast milk is the ideal nutrition for the infant and we adopt the TEN STEPS TO SUCCESSFUL BREASTFEEDING as recommended by WHO and UNICEF. We abide by the National Code of Ethics For Infant Formula Products.

Our Glenie Mum's Club provides on-going support for all mothers. Further details can be obtained from our maternity ward staff.

NOTE/CHECK LIST

What to Bring

• *For yourself*

Bring comfortable clothing, casual shoes or slippers, supportive bras, personal toiletries

• *For your baby*

1 set of baby clothes, 1 toweling blanket, mittens and booties

When to Come to the Hospital

When you experience:

- Regular contractions/pain
- Waterbag leakage
- Any bleeding
- Reduced fetal movements

Our staff is available for advice 24 hours a day, so please feel free to ring 03-4255 2780/4255 2781 for more information if you are unsure.

When You Arrive

If you require immediate assistance upon arrival, so please have your partner notify the receptionist and remain in the car until assistance arrives.

Our receptionist will direct you to the Labour Delivery Unit on the 3rd Floor.

When You Arrive at Night

For security reasons the hospitals main entrance is closed from 10 p.m. till 7 a.m. Please use the night entrance to the Accident and Emergency Unit.

When to Register

If you have not pre-registered with the hospital your partner will be required to provide all the necessary information to our admission clerk.

1. If you arrive between 8 a.m.-10 p.m., the registration will be done at the admission counter at the hospital's main lobby.
2. If you arrive after 10 p.m. and before 8 a.m., the registration will be done at the Accident and Emergency Department.

Rooming-in

We encourage all our babies to be exclusively breastfed. In order to be successful in breastfeeding, we encourage 24 hours rooming-in with your baby. We believe you and your baby should remain together all the time to facilitate successful breastfeeding and bonding.

PARENTCRAFT COURSE (Ante-natal)

The parentcraft courses are designed to assist parents to cope with the physical and emotional changes during pregnancy and will also prepare for labour.

Programme Contents

Session 1
- Introduction
- Changes in pregnancy and the delivery process
- Pain management
- Overview on cord blood banking

Session 2
- Breathing techniques for labour and delivery
- Pre and Postnatal exercises

Session 3
- Common problems in infants
- Optimum nutrition for pregnant and lactating mothers
- Education on breastfeeding
- How to bath your baby
- Tour of the Nursery and Labour Room

DURATION OF PROGRAMME

3 consecutive Saturday from 2.00 p.m.-4.00 p.m.

COURSE FEE

RM 180.00 per couple. Course fees are non-refundable.

VENUE

Lectures: Training room, 8th Floor, Medical Consulting Suite.
Exercises: Physiotherapy Department, 4th Floor, Hospital Block.

POSTNATAL HOME VISITS

Postnatal home visit services are available and can be arranged upon request to support and help you cope in the first few months after birth, so that you don't feel stressed out. Experienced nurses/midwives will visit you to monitor you and your baby's progress in the privacy and comfort of your own home.

Our *raison d'etre* is to lesson the anxieties and heighten the joys of new parenting. Postnatal home visit services include.

FOR THE BABY

General Health Assessment

- Observation on baby (Temperature, Weight, Skin, etc.)
- Weigh your baby
- Care of baby cord
- Assist you in breastfeeding
- Assist in bathing baby
- Learn how to recognize your baby's different cries
- Counseling in handling common problems of baby and immunization.
- Wearing.

FOR THE MOTHER

General Health Assessment

- Observation (Temperature, Blood Pressure, Skin, Fundal Height, Breast and General Health).
- Examination of would (Abdominal or perineal).
- Check the height of fundus (uterus).
- Advise on diet.
- Advise on Postnatal exercise that could help you get back into shape.
- Hygiene and general care for yourself.
- Answers any queries you may have on mother and child care.
- Counseling on any postnatal problems..
  Cost—RM260 for visits/RM400 for 5 visits.

PROSTATE LASER CENTRE

Surgery for BPH works by removal of the unwanted benign prostate tissue which is causing obstruction to urine flow from the bladder. TURP (Transurethral Resection of Prostate) has been the most popular surgical technique to achieve this and remains very popular today. This involves slicing off pieces of obstructing prostate tissue with a cutting electrodiathermy tool. Bleeding is the main problem during and after surgery and it is customary practice to keep patients in hospital for 3-4 days for observation. Laser destruction of tissue depends on the interaction between the laser light and tissue. With our laser system, the green laser light is very efficiently absorbed by the red pigment of blood cells causing the tissue to heat up and vaporize whilst at the same time sealing the blood vessels to prevent bleeding, hence the term Photoselective Vaporization of the Prostate (PVP). The more red blood cells, the better the effect.

This technique is particularly suited to those large prostates rich in blood vessels which are prone to brisk bleeding during conventional TURP. Some laser treatment produces a layer of dead tissue which remains adherent and patients are unable to pass urine properly until this tissue sloughs off. With the Laser Scope® Green Light™ Laser System, obstructing prostate tissue can be instantaneously removed with minimal bleeding allowing almost all patients to pass urine normally within 24 hours. The very low risk of bleeding makes this method particularly suitable for anybody who are more prone to bleeding, especially those taking medication to prevent clotting of blood (antiplatlest such as Aspirin, Ticlid® or Plavix® and anticoagulants such as Warfarin).

We are a dedicated prostate disease centre offering professional, up-to-date evidence based service for all prostate diseases. We specialize in the use of the latest and least invasive technology for the treatment of BPH. We offer a one-stop service for consultation and investigations of all prostate diseases. We are set-up to carry out laser surgery for benign prostate disease without hospital stay and with minimal risk, blood loss and discomfort. We are integrated into the premier Gleneagles Intan Medical Centre which provides a comprehensive tertiary specialist care for any other medical conditions.

Our Services

- Ø Symptom or problem specific consultation
- Ø Well man health screening
- Ø Laboratory investigations
- Ø Outpatient endoscopic investigations
- Ø Ultrasound scan
- Ø Prostate biopsy
- Ø All outpatient treatment of prostate disease
- Ø PVP laser prostatectomy
- Ø Other non-laser prostate surgery
- Ø Other urological services

DIABETES CARE CENTRE

WHAT IS DIABETES?

About 9% of the Malaysian population is affected with diabetes. What is worrying is the fact that this number is increasing and a much younger population is affected.

Diabetes mellitus is characterized by high levels of blood sugar, resulting from defects in either insulin secretion or action, or both. The condition can lead to a host of acute and chronic complications, among which are heart attacks, strokes, blindness, kidney failure, nerve damage, impotence in men and blood vessel disease that may eventually lead to amputations.

Thankfully, research has shown that if blood sugar levels are kept as close to normal as possible, the risk of developing complications can be reduced substantially. Through the efforts of the patients and the help of health care professionals, many of these complications are preventable. Persons with diabetes can continue to live healthy, active and productive lives.

Whether you are newly diagnosed with diabetes or caring for someone with diabetes, we would like to offer our professional assistance to help you cope with diabetes.

Once diagnosed, a person will have to live with diabetes for life, as there is no cure for diabetes. Gleneagles Intan Medical Centre offers a holistic approach to diabetes management, with our team of Diabetes Physicians, Cardiologists, Neurologist, Nephrologist, Ophthalmologists, Rehabilitation Physician, Dietitian, Podiatrist, Diabetes Educator and many others.

Control of diabetes is dependent on lifestyle changes and adjustment, which may be overwhelmingly difficult and confusing for some to adjust to. Our team of experts will guide and advise you on the practical aspects of living and offer appropriate screening tests where appropriate.

Even when complications have already occurred, our Centre offers the appropriate rehabilitation programme and therapy to control, delay or halt the progression of complications.

DIABETES ANNUAL CHECK-UP

We offer an annual diabetes check-up which includes diabetes control assessment, heart, kidneys, eyes and nerve evaluation to assess the complication status. An extensive blood test including a cholesterol profile is also performed. At the end of this evaluation, you will be advised on appropriate changes that need to be made to further improve your diabetes control.

DIABETES EDUCATION

Our Centre provides regular diabetes lectures to the diabetic population and general public about good diabetes care. There will be updates on the latest treatment available for diabetics. You can also discuss with our diabetes educator about anything that concerns you—be it the correct method of taking medicine or taking injections. You can also join our diabetes support group, where you get to meet other diabetics and exchanges tips with one another.

MONITORING DIABETES CONTROL

Our Centre will help you to monitor your diabetic control and advise you on changes that may be required.

DIABETES COMPLICATIONS SCREENING

We offer diabetes complications screening with tests such as urine microalbuminuria, blood cholesterol and HbAlc. Our diabetes educator will also screen you for neuropathy (nerve complications of the feet) and if required refer you to one of our professionals for further evaluation.

DIABETES SCREENING

If you have any of the following risk factors, you should be screened for diabetes:

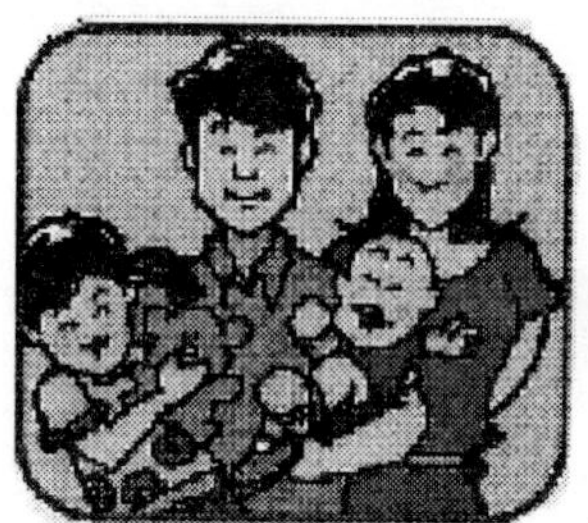

Close family member with diabetes

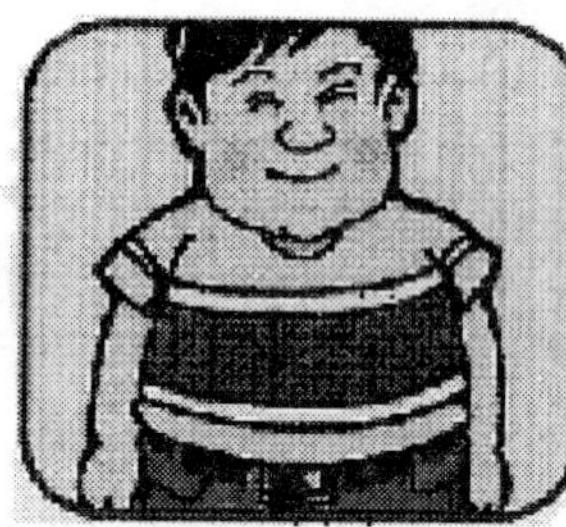

Overweight

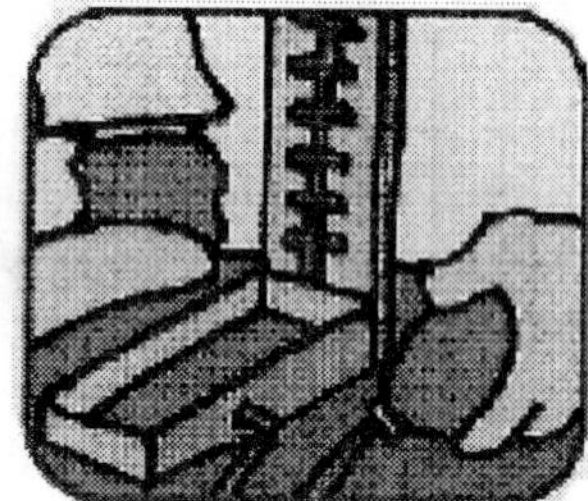

Hypertension

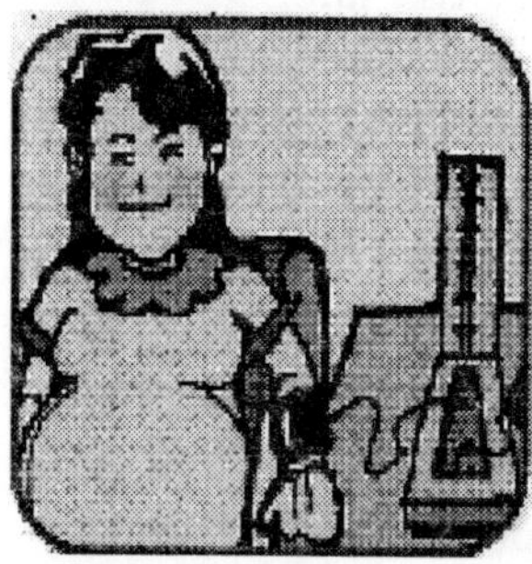

Diabetes during pregnancy

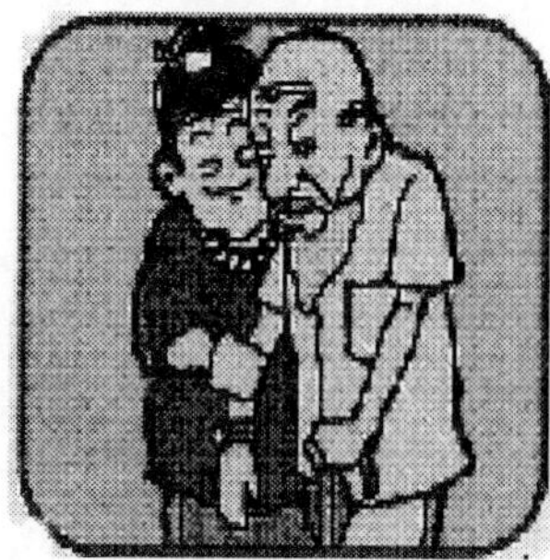

Age over 40 years old

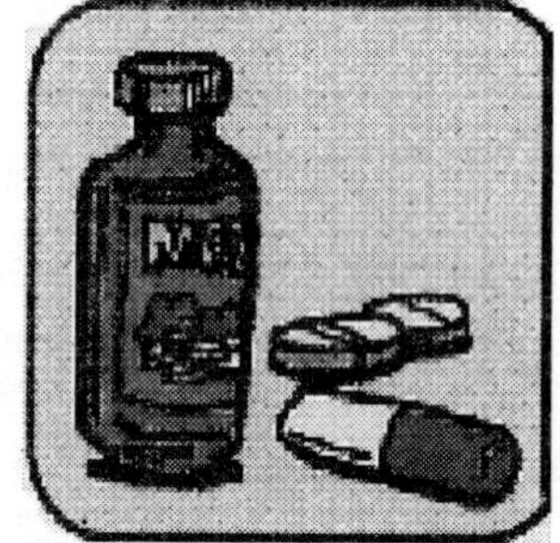

On certain medication such as steroids

We offer diabetes screening test at an appropriate time and interval of your life. Early detection means early control, which is good for you.

DIABETES RESOURCE CENTRE

Our Diabetes-friendly Centre also has a wide range of diabetes education materials that include pamphlets, audio-visuals and internet access to appropriate websites for the latest update and information on diabetes.

CORONARY CALCIUM SCORING

Coronary Artery Disease (Coronary Heart Disease) or coronary atherosclerosis is a common problem and cause of death among both men and women in America, Europe and South East Asia. Not only has this disease become more frequent, but it is affecting the younger people more and more.

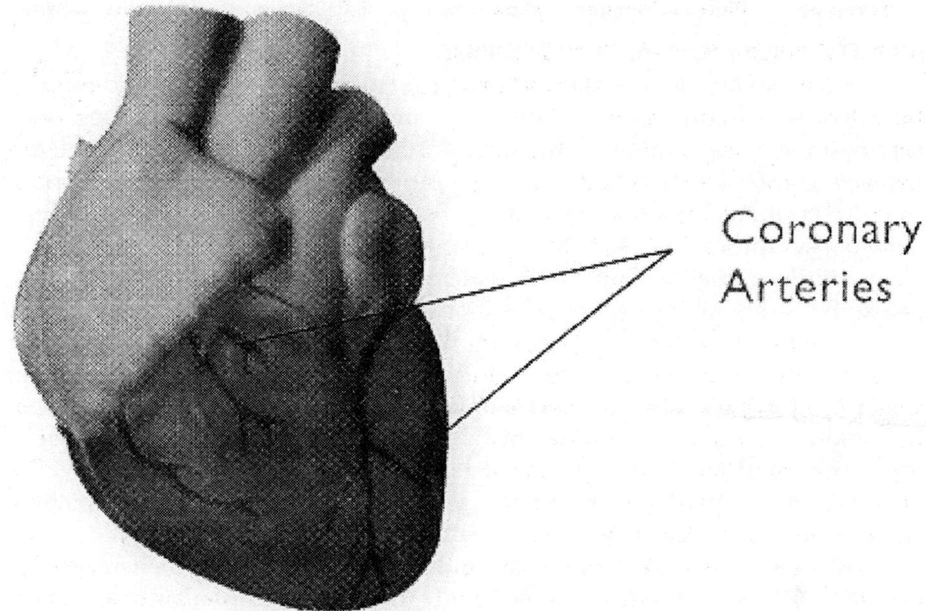

Atherosclerosis of the arteries, is a condition where fatty deposits build up on the insides of arteries causing narrowing of the arteries and overtime, blockage to the flow of blood. Atherosclerosis is the only process which results in the deposition of calcium within the walls of the arteries causing narrowing of the arteries. Calcification of the arterial bed is NOT a degenerative process but a very active metabolic process and similar to bone calcification in many ways. The interruption of the blood supply in the coronary arteries results in coronary heart disease. Patients are usually first diagnosed with coronary artery disease when they:

- Develop symptoms of chest pain,
- Display an abnormal response to stress testing, or
- Undergo coronary angiography

Coronary artery disease is not due to a single cause. Instead, it is linked to several coronary risk factors such as high levels of fat and cholesterol in the blood, lack of exercise, high blood pressure, diabetes, smoking stress and maximum in families.

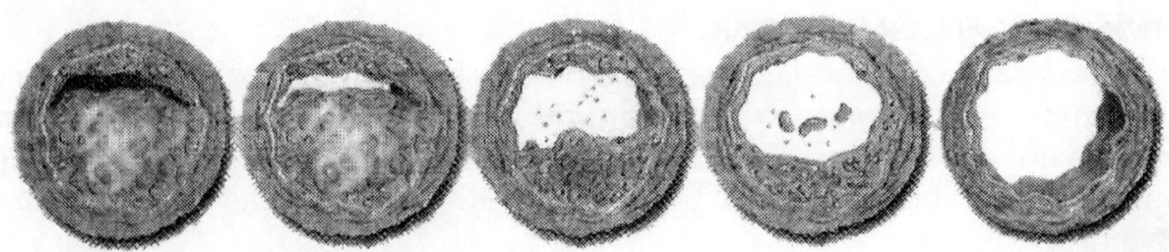

Occlusion Fibrous Plaques Atheromas Fatty Streaks Normal Artery

ABOUT CORONARY CALCIUM SCORING

Early in the atherosclerotic process, commonly called 'hardening of the arteries' calcium deposits are very small and difficult to detect with conventional x-ray imaging, but today with CT scanning, minute calcium deposits can be easily identified. Small deposits of calcium can be regarded as early coronary atherosclerosis and this may happen way before patients develop symptoms of heart disease.

While patients with high calcification score d not always have blocked vessels, a low score does not mean you are not at risk. Like all medical tests, it is not 100 per cent perfect as soft pockets of cholesterol could be embedded in the artery lining and too new to have accumulated calcium. However, research has shown that there is a direct link between the amount of calcium buildup in the artery and the amount of plaque in the arteries and hence the test can determine the patient's risk category. The atherosclerotic process of often relatively advanced when patients experience 'heart attack or chest pain'.

The test is within minutes and no stress involved. The patient lies flat on the CT examination table and the radiographer/nurse attach electrocardiograph (ECG) leads to the chest. The patient will be asked to take two or three deep breaths and hold them for about 10 seconds.

You Can Reduce The Risk Of Getting This Disease By Knowing the Facts And Doing What is Good For Your Heart.

WHAT IS CORONARY CALCIUM CT SCAN?

A Coronary Calcium CT scan is a non-invasive test similar to an X-ray used to take picture of the heart, detect and quantity and amount of calcium deposits in the coronary arteries. This test is used by physician to complement existing non-invasive modalities.

WHAT CAN BE LEARNED FROM THE SCAN?

- The presence or absence of coronary calcium.
- The degree and extent of calcification.
- The calcium score- a sum of the total size and density of the calcium deposits found in the coronary arteries and provide a "number evaluation" of the extent of the plaque.

WHAT A SCAN LOOKS LIKE?

Normal

No identifiable plaque

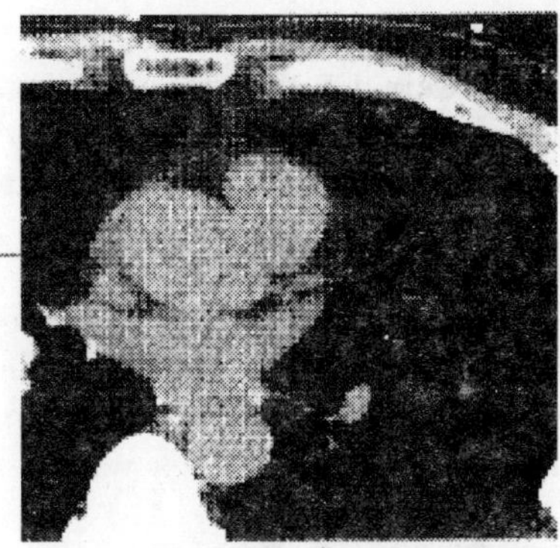

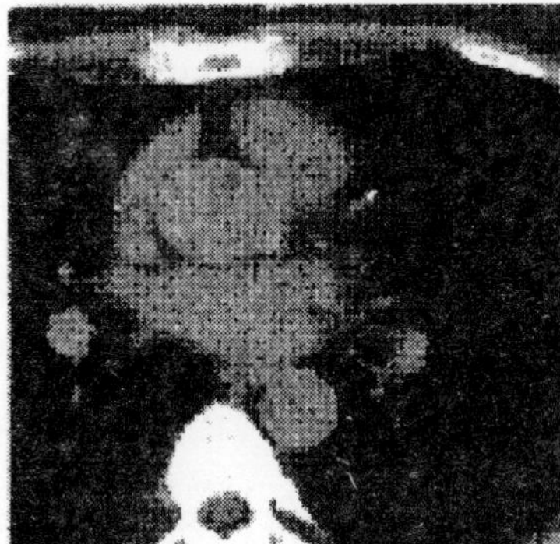

Moderate

Definite plaque burden

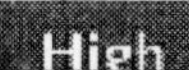

Extensive plaque burden

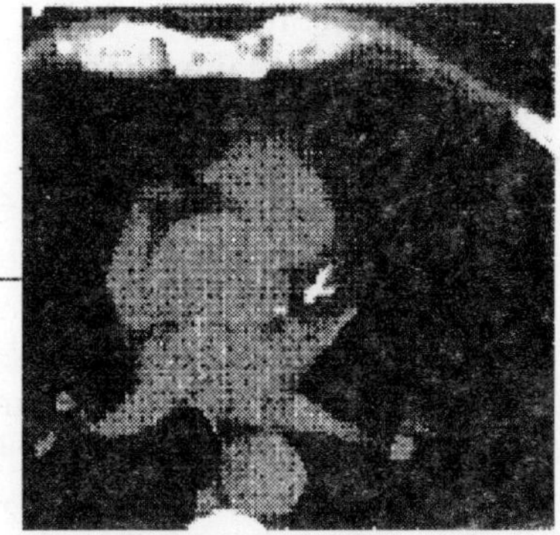

WHO WOULD BENEFIT FROM CORONARY CALCIUM SCANNING?

Suggested Patient Profile

- Male aged 40 to 65 with two or more risk factors.
- Female aged 45 to 70 with two or more risk factors.
- Asymptomatic/with risk factors.
- Symptomatic/with or no risk factors.

• *Risk factors*: High blood pressure, high cholesterol, cigarette smoking, diabetes, obesity, family history of heart disease, physical inactivity.

DIAGNOSTIC DEPARTMENT

DIAGNOSTIC LABORATORY

Our Diagnostic Cardiac Laboratory is situated on the 1st floor. It offers a wide variety of invasive and non-invasive procedures to test cardiac function with personalized attention during your evaluation.

INVASIVE PROCEDURE

Invasive procedures are carried out in our well-equipped Cardiac Catheterization Laboratory. Our centre is staffed with highly skilled and experienced cardiac technicians to assists the adult/pediatric cardiologists during the procedures which include:

1. Diagnostic Procedures

- Right and Left Heart Catheterization
- Coronary Angiogram

2. Therapeutic Procedures

- Percutaneous Translumina Coronary Angioplasty (PTCA)
- Percutaneous Balloon Valvuloplasty (Balloon diatation of stenotic heart valves)
- PDA Occlusion (Umbrella as well as coil embolisation techniques)
- Pacemaker Implant

NON-INVASIVE PROCEDURE

For non-invasive procedures we offer the whole range of investigations which include:

- Electrocardiogram (ECG)
- Stress ECG(Treadmill)
- Holter Monitoring (24 hours ECG)
- Echocardiogram M-Mode, 2-d, Doppler
- Stress Echo-Treadmill
- Stress Echo-Pharmacological
- Transoesophagael Echocradiogram (TEE)
- Respiratory Function Test (RFT)
- Spirometry

CARDIOTHORACIC SURGERY

Our operating theatres are specifically equipped for both paediatric and adult cardiothoracic surgery which include:

- By-pass surgeries for blocked/diseased coronary arteries

- Correction of tight valves
- Correction of "hole in the heart"
- Complex congenital heart disease
- Excision of aortic aneurysm
- Chest surgery for lung diseases.

Our surgeons, physicians, anaesthetists, perfusionists and technicians are on 24 hours standby for emergencies such as evaluation of suspected heart attacks which might require invasive procedures and it required emergency coronary by-pass operation.

SPECIAL PACKAGES

1. Coronary Angiogram	From RM 3,400
2. Right and Left Heart Catheterization	From RM 4,000
3. Open Heart Surgery	From RM 22,000

The above charges are on a case by case basis depending on the complexity of the case and exclusive of Government Service Tax.

IMAGING DEPARTMENT

Our Imaging Department is situated on the Ground Floor of the hospital building. The department is extensively equipped to offer a wide spectrum of diagnostic examinations for in-patients and out-patients.

Plain X-ray, Ultrasound, Magnetic Resonance Imaging (MRI), C.T. Scan, Bone Densitometry, Fluroscopy and interventional procedures are undertaken by a qualified highly skilled and experienced team.

Mammography examinations performed by a female radiographer are also available.

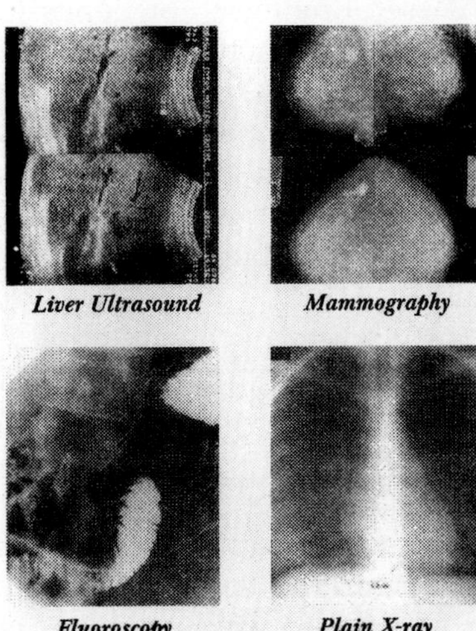

Liver Ultrasound *Mammography*

Fluoroscopy *Plain X-ray*

MAGNETIC RESONANCE IMAGING

Magnetic Resonance Imaging (MRI) utilizes a powerful magnet and radiofrequency pulses to generate images. There is no ionizing radiation. It is unsurpassed in the imaging of the brain and spine particularly for soft tissue details. It also provides excellent details of musculo-skeletal structures such as knees, hips and shoulders.

Magnetic resonance is inherently 'flow' sensitive so 'angiograms' or flow images of the blood vessels may be obtained without the injection of any contrast media.

Gleneagles Intan Medical Centre has an MRI machine with a high field superconducting magnet system.

MAMMOGRAPHY

Mammography is a very sensitive method for the early detection of breast cancer, and is recommended as a screening tool for women over 35 years. The machine for this procedure is a special X-ray unit dedicated to imaging the breast.

The mammography unit in this hospital is also able to perform aspiration biopsy and localization of breast lesions.

SPIRAL COMPUTED TOMOGRAPHY (C.T. SCAN)

This imaging modality is available in Gleneagles Intan Medical Centre.

In the latest refinement of this proven technology the patient moves through the system during continuous X-ray exposure.

C.T. is the workhorse of modern imaging, widely used now in the investigation of serious chest and abdominal disease processes. It is well established in the imaging of the head, neck and spine.

BONE DENSITOMETRY

Part of the process of aging is for bones to become more brittle, i.e. less dense particularly in post-menopausal women. This is referred to as osteoporosis. Hence the frequent fractures occurring in the elderly after a fall.

This machine gives an indication of the density of bone and the necessity for treatment if osteoporosis is present. The amount of radiation during the examination is negligible. It is quite safe and does not cause any inconvenience or pain.

16-SLICE CT SCANNER

WHAT IS CT SCAN?

- CT Scanning uses special x-ray equipment that produces cross sectional images of the body. The unit comprises a gantry, which is a large squarish machine with a wide hole in it and a table which the patient lies on.

- Conventionally, images were obtained slice by slice sequentially but with multidetector-CT in the spiral mode, large volumes of the body can be scanned rapidly and accurately. The digital information for the scanner is converted to images that can be viewed in any 3D orientation.

HOW SHOULD I PREPARE FOR THE PROCEDURE?

- You are required to arrive about half and hour before your appointment to register and to complete a medical history form.
- Before the examination, you will be require to change into a gown provided and to remove hairpins, jewellery, eyeglasses, hearing aids and any removable dental work that could obscure the images.
- You may also be aside to refrain from eating or drinking any thing for an hour or longer before the examination.
- If you are or may be pregnant, kindly inform the Doctor/ Radiographer.

WHAT WILL EXPERIENCE DURING THE PROCEDURE?

- You are required to lie still on the CT table. During the procedure, you will be moved up and down, as well as slide in the out from the centre of the hole as the images are being taken.
- Depending on the type of the study being done, contrast medium may be administered intravenously or orally. Some patients find the taste or the contrast medium mildly unpleasant but tolerable. The intravenous injection will produce a warm flush sensation and on occasion nausea, both of which will subside subsequently.
- Your examination may also require the administration of an enema and/or air, if the colon is the focus of the study.
- You will be alone in the room during the scan; however, the Radiographer/Radiologist can see, hear and speak with you at all times. For Pediatric patients, a parent/guardian who is not pregnant may be allowed in the room to comfort the patient and alleviate fear, but will be required to wear a lead apron to prevent radiation exposure.

WHAT ELSE SHOULD I KNOW?

- The test itself is relatively safe as the amount of the radiation is kept to an absolute minimum with the new technology.
- Many contrast iodine, which may cause an allergic reaction in some individuals. Please inform the Doctor/Nurse/ Radiographer if you:

- have had an allergic reaction to iodine
- have any other known allergies
- are asthmatic

- If you are, or think you may be pregnant, you should let your Doctor and the Radiographer known before the CT examination. Nursing mothers, before resuming breast feeding should wait for 24 hours after oral or an injection of contrast medium.
- Request for a scan can be made directly by our Consultation as well as our Resident Medical Officer, at our Executive Screening Centre/Women's Wellness Centre/Accident and Emergency Department.

HOW LONG DOES A CT SCAN TAKE?

- The picture-taking part of the test usually lasts less than 10 minutes. However, each examination may vary depending on the individual clinical requirements of the examination.

WHEN DO I GET THE RESULT?

- Your examination will be reviewed by a Radiologist. Your referring Physician will be informed immediately of any suspicious findings. You will receive a formal written report on the same day or within two (2) days depending on your clinical and diagnostic requirements.

WHAT ARE THE BENEFITS OF THE 16-SLICE CT SCANNER?

- The 16-slice CT Scanner captures multiple images of a patient's anatomy in a matter of seconds and presents information 3-dimensionally. This means the images of the body are now taken much faster, therefore reducing the examination time and increasing your comfort.
- The information provided is more detailed due to the ability of the scanner to produce thin-slice images; this allows early detection of certain diseases in a less invasive manner.

THE 16-SLICE CT SCANNER PROVIDES NON-INTERVENTIONAL ADVANCED CLINICAL APPLICATIONS, SUCH AS:

- Heart Examinations
  - o Coronary Artery and Calcium Scoring
- CE Coronary Angiography
- Lung Screening
- 'Fly-Through' Colon Examinations (Virtual Colonoscopy)
- Routine and Non-Routine Examinations of the:

- o head, neck and thorax
- o liver, spleen, pancreas and kidneys
- o abdomen and pelvis
- o blood vessels
- o oncology/cancer management
- o pulmonary emboli

HOW DO I SCHEDULE THE SCAN?

For further information and appointments, kidney contact our Imaging Department at (03) 4255 2719.

MAGNETIC RESONANCE IMAGING (MRI)

WHAT IS MRI?

MRI is a non-invasive technique which builds up pictures of an internal cross-section of the part of the body under investigations. It uses a magnetic field and radio waves with an advanced computer system to build up a series of images, each one showing a thin slice of the examined area. These images are very detailed and can show both the bones and soft tissues in the body, thus providing the Radiologists and Consultants with valuable diagnostic information. Utilizing the computer, the 'slices' can also be shown in multiple directions.

ARE THERE ANY RISKS OR RESTRICTIONS ASSOCIATED WITH THE PROCEDURE?

To date, MRI is considered a safe procedure. It does not involve the use of X-rays or radiation. However, because the MRI scanner uses a strong magnetic field, it can move objects in your body made of iron or steel. Therefore, you must inform your Doctor or the attending Technologist if you have any of the following implants:

- Pacemaker
- Metal Implants
- Aneurysm Clips
- Steel Surgical Staples or Clips
- Cochlear Implants

For female patients if you are or might be pregnant kindly inform your referring Doctor and the attending staff. MRI scanning may not be advisable during early pregnancy, except in specific cases or circumstances.

If you have tattoos in black or dark blue, you may experience a warming or slight heating effect directly on the site.

HOW DO I MAKE AN APPOINTMENT FOR AN MRI SCAN?

All MRI scans require an appointment and a referral letter from a Doctor. Details of the MRI investigation and your contact number shall be required whilst making an appointment.

Once the appointment is confirmed, you shall be informed of the date, time and special instructions, if any. If you are unable to attend, please inform the attending staff as soon as possible.

If you have any special needs, such as requiring the assistance of a wheelchair at the front lobby, higher waiting chairs or if you suffer from hearing or other impairments, please notify your Doctor and the attending staff at the department.

AM I REQUIRED TO MAKE ANY SPECIAL PREPARATIONS?

There are no special preparations necessary for the MRI scan. Unless specifically requested by your Doctor, there are no food or drink restrictions. You may also continue to take any medication prescribed by your Doctor, unless otherwise directed.

CAN I BE ACCOMPANIED BY A RELATIVE OR A FRIEND?

Yes, you may be accompanied and the same precautions and risks as mentioned above would apply to the accompanying person.

WHAT SHOULD I DO WHEN I ARRIVE FOR THE MRI SCAN?

Please go to the reception desk of the Imaging Department and there you will be assisted by an MRI Technologist or other staff. Before the test, you will be requested to fill in a questionnaire about your health, medial/surgical history and you will also be required to sign a consent form.

Prior to the scan, you will be shown to a private cubicle for you to change into a gown and remove any personal articles such as jewelleries, keys or watches. These items can be stored in a locker provided for you in the cubicle.

WHO WILL ATTEND TO ME?

You will be cared for by a team which includes a Technologist who will perform the actual examination. The Radiologist may look at the results on the computer screen during the scan, or may review a recording of the images later, before writing a report.

WHAT HAPPENS DURING THE MRI PROCEDURE?

You will be taken into the MRI room and made comfortable on the MRI table. You might be given a contrast which can help produce a more detailed image. The contrast medium would be injected into a vein in your arm and this may cause a warm feeling.

The table will be moved slowly to position the relevant part of your body within the 'tunnel'. The staff will proceed to the control room to monitor the scan. However, you will be able to communicate with him/her via an intercom and you will be monitored at all times. In addition, you will be provided with ear plugs and/or earphones as the scanner will make a tapping or knocking sound. If you feel uncomfortable or uneasy during the scan do alert the attending Technologist immediately.

Once the Radiologist or Technologist is satisfied with the scanning of each particular section, you will informed when a new scan is starting.

WILL IT BE UNCOMFORTABLE?

Apart from the noise generated by the scanner, you will not experience any discomfort. Most patients do not mind lying with their body in the 'tunnel'. However, if you suffer from claustrophobia please consult you Doctor and inform our staff prior to your appointment.

HOW LONG WILL IT TAKE?

The process of acquiring the images usually takes about 20-30 minutes. Unless there are any unforeseen emergency cases, your total time in the Department is likely to be about 45 minutes. However, you might have to stay for an additional 1 hour should an urgent Radiologist Report be required by your Doctor. Depending on the complexity of the case, the Radiologist may require more time to prepare a report and this shall be communicated to your earlier.

ARE THERE ANY SIDE EFFECTS?

There are no known side effects. You may return to your normal activities after the scan is completed.

AM I ALLOWED TO EAT AND DRINK AFTERWARDS?

Yes, unless you have any other medical investigation which requires you to fast.

If you have any other queries, please call the Department of Diagnostic Imaging and Interventional Services between 9 a.m. to 5 p.m., Monday to Friday and between 9 a.m. to 1 p.m. Saturday.

DIAGNOSTIC IMAGING AND INTERVENTIONAL SERVICES

The Department of Diagnostic Imaging and Interventional Services (Imaging Department) provides radiological examination for patients, using a range of X-ray equipment, Computed Tomography (CT Scan), Ultrasound and Magnetic resonance Imaging specialize in the interpretation of imaging results and complex examinations. They are supported by Technologists who are highly trained to carry out many of the X-rays and imaging procedures.

REHABILITATION UNIT

Gleneagles Intain's Rehabilitation Unit is dedicated to helping individuals with illnesses or disabilities to regain and improve their physical function. With their improved physical independence, it would enable them to participate fully in social, family and vocational pursuits. The rehabilitation team understands that injuries or illnesses which cause physical disabilities, affects the lives of not only the patients but their families as well.

We have an extensive range of rehabilitation services and programmes that are specifically to individual needs. The services include:

- Rehabilitation Medicine Consultation
- General Physiotherapy
- General Occupational Therapy
- General Speech and Language Therapy
- Spinal Cord Injury Rehabilitation
- Amputee Rehabilitation
- Neurological Rehabilitation
- Paediatric Rehabilitation
- Sports Rehabilitation
- Rheumatological Rehabilitation.

We operate as a multidisciplinary and interdisciplinary team comprising a Rehabilitation Physician, Physiotherapists, an Occupational Therapist and a Speech Therapist providing comprehensive rehabilitation to our patients. The patient and family forms part of the team. There is also an in-house prosthetics/orthotics service, where all prosthesis and orthosis can be made, modified and supplied here.

We offer a highly individualized treatment with sessions conducted on a one-to-one basis.

GENERAL PHYSIOTHERAPY

The physiotherapy services offered are directed towards evaluating, restoring and maximizing physical function or ability. Physiotherapy is needed for the following conditions:

- Musculoskeletal injury including pain, stiffness or weakness
- Sports injury
- Chest infection
- Bell's palsy
- Lymphoedema
- Antenatal and postnatal rehabilitation
- Bladder incontinence

OTHER SERVICES INCLUDE

- Neuromuscular therapy
- Electrotherapy
- Cryotherapy
- Chest physiotherapy

GENERAL OCCUPATIONAL THERAPY

The occupational therapy services offered will involve the patient in activities designed to promote the restoration and maximize the use of function with the aim of helping them participate in life in its fullest sense.

The services include:

- Training in activities of daily living and self maintenance tasks, for example feeding, dressing and home activities.
- Perceptual and cognitive assessment and training.
- Splinting for upper extremities.
- Home, school and work-site visit where assessment and modification of the environment will be done to ensure accessibility.
- Work simplification where energy conservation and joint protection techniques are being taught.
- Early stimulation and development assessment and training for paediatric age group.
- Neuromuscular training which include hand injuries, neurological and others.
- Vocational assessment and training.

GENERAL SPEECH AND LANGUAGE THERAPY

The Speech and Language Therapy service offers prevention, identification, assessment, diagnosis and treatment of communication disorders in both children and adults. The aim is to maximize the communication potential of the individual, using either speech or alternative/augmentative methods.

The Speech and Language Therapy service will benefit people with:

- Speech, articulation and phonological disorders
- Developmental language delay and/or specific language disorders
- Voice disorders
- Stammering/stuttering
- Craniofacial anomalies such as cleft lip and palate
- Hearing impairment
- Dysphagia (feeding or swallowing difficulties)
- Learning disabilities
- Autism

NEUROLOGICAL REHABILITATION

With regards to neurological problems, rehabilitation will help to maximize recovery, payment complications, and help the patients on to the road to independence with confidence and dignity. The types of neurological disease include:

- Stroke
- Head injury
- Parkinson's Disease
- Multiple sclerosis

- Muscular dystrophy
- Guillain Barre
- Tumour
- Demyelinating Disease

Our team comprises of a rehabilitation physician, physiotherapists, an occupational therapist and a speech therapist. We perform a comprehensive assessment and design a goal-orientated programme tailored to specific patients needs. The programme includes neuromuscular, mobility. Medical care (bladder, bowel management and skin care), activities of daily living, swallowing, communications, cognitive, psychosocial, community reintegration and education.

SPINAL CORD INJURY/DISEASE REHABILITATION

Spinal cord injury/disease often involves many organ systems with complications. Some of these problems include the inability to move the limbs, pressure sores, bladder and bowel impairment, spasticity, autonomic dysreflexia, deformity, pain, infertility, chest infection, depression and social issues. The rehabilitation team together with the patient and family, will plan a comprehensive, goal-orientated programme to suit their needs. This programme includes neuromuscular training, mobility, medical care (bladder/bowel management and pressure prevention), activities of daily living, psychological, community and social reintegration and spinal cord injury education. It will enable the individual to be as independent as possible and reintegrate back to the community.

PAEDIATRIC REHABILITATION

We offer a range of rehabilitation services to children with all types of disabilities including cerebral palsy, spina bifida, muscular dystrophy, arthrogyposis, head injury, rheumatoid arthritis and others. As there are a wide range of problems, the multi and interdisciplinary team will plan individualized programmes with the child and parents. The programme includes development assessment and training, activities of daily living training, neuromuscular training, mobility with wheelchair assessment and training, speech and swallowing training, school assessment and visit.

AMPUTATION REHABILITATION

Following any amputation, what happens now to the individual's life? At *Gleneagles Intan*, a team of well-trained and qualified staff will help the individual to regain independence. The Rehabilitation Physician, Physiotherapist, Occupational Therapist and Prosthetist will work together with the individual in a well tailored goal-orientated programme. This programme includes neuromuscular training, stump care, activities of daily living training, gait training with aids, assessment making, fitting and training with prosthesis and psychosocial aspects including vocational, driving assessment and training. The whole programme together with the prosthetic making, fitting, training and maintenance are conducted within the rehabilitation area.

OTHER SERVICES

- Rehabilitation Medicine Consultation
- Orthotic and Splinting
- Home Visit/Work-Site Visit/School Visit (Assessment and modification)
- Equipment and rehabilitation aids services

APPOINTMENT/ENQUIRIES

For further appointment and enquiries, please contact:

Rehabilitation Unit
4th Floor Hospital Building
Gleneagles Intan Medical Centre
Tel: 603-4255 2793/4255 2833

COSTS

It will be based on the type and duration of rehabilitation. There are packages for specialized areas which include neurological rehabilitation, spinal rehabilitation, amputee rehabilitation and paediatric rehabilitation. Please contact the rehabilitation staff for further details.

PAEDIATRIC REHABILITATION

The quality of life for many children can be severely restricted by their physical and/or cognitive disabilities. The multidisciplinary team at the Rehabilitation Centre in Gleneagles Intan Medical Centre (GIMC) understands the stresses the child and his/her family are under due to these disabilities. We believe that by offering our specialized services, through a comprehensive Paediatric Rehabilitation programme, we may help the child and his/her family cope with such stressors, and allow the child to lead a normal and healthy life.

Our rehabilitation team is trained to deal with various conditions, ranging from Down's Syndrome, Cerebral Palsy, Autism and other disorders which causes delayed development, to Spina Bifida, the muscular dystrophies and Attention Deficit Hyperactive Disorder (ADHD). We aim to help such children attain their full potential in all areas of development by providing advice and activities that create easy and enjoyable ways to learn.

OUR DEDICATED REHABILITATION TEAM

Our multidisciplinary interdisciplinary team consists of a rehabilitation physician, physiotherapists, occupational therapists and speech- language pathologists specializing in paediatric rehabilitation.

Depending on the child's specific requirements, GIMC's paediatricians, paediatric neurologists, clinical psychologists, psychiatrists, dietitians and orthotist/prosthetist complement the rehabilitation work performed by the Rehabilitation Centre's core team of specialists.

OUR COMPREHENSIVE REHABILITATION PROGRAMMES

Our rehabilitation programmes which are tailored specifically to meet the child's needs, cover the following areas:

• ***Sensory Processing and Integration***

- To provide sensory input in the form of movement, balance (vestibular), joint (proprioceptive), touch (tactile), auditory and visual training.
- To provide sensory motor integration.

• ***Communication***

- To develop child-specific speech and language skills, as well as functional skills of communication.
- To implement the use of alternative means of communications in order to augment the child's existing skills and reduce frustration.
- To facilitate the integration of all communication skills learnt.

• ***Neuromuscular Rehabilitation***

- To improve posture, provide gait training, improve and maintain the child's flexibility.
- To reduce stimulations which may have a negative impact on the child's condition.
- To improve visual-motor co-ordination.
- To provide advice on the various aids, adaptations and equipment available for the maintenance and improvement of the child's quality of life.

• ***Daily Living Activities***

- To provide advice and training on self-care and hygiene.
- To assess and provide modifications in the various environments in which the child interacts with peers and others, in order to reduce energy expenditure and maximize functional output.
- To instill survival instincts in the child, such as the correct techniques of falling.

• *Functional academics*

- To train sight reading and spelling, writing and drawing as well as counting.

• *Family sessions*

- To review the child's progress at regular intervals.
- To design and provide home programmes and ensure that the exercises and activities provided are performed properly.
- To provide a support group for the family where problems can be discussed.

• *Behaviour Management*

- To review and discuss with parents and care givers the common behavioral problems of the child and the relevant approach to managing the concerned behaviour.

• *Home and School Visits*

- To discuss the issues pertaining to the child's ability and functioning performance.
- To assess the home and schooling environment and its accessibility and feasibility to the child's conditions and to render advice on the modifications of these environments, to suit the child's needs, where necessary.

DIET COUNSELLING

WHAT IS DIETETICS?

It is the application of nutrition and nutritional care in health and disease. The person qualified to undertake diet counselling is the Dietitian.

WHAT DOES THE DIETITIAN DO?

The Dietitian will interpret a doctor's prescription and translate it into practical meals suitable to a person's lifestyle.

The Dietitian will also provide information on what food to buy, methods of food preparation and also suggest food substitutes that are equivalent in nutrients which is allowed within the dietary prescription.

THE IMPORTANCE OF DIET COUNSELLING

To facilitate recovery from illness and reduce the risk of developing disease-related complications.

Diet Counseling is individualized, i.e. a personalized diet plan will be tailored to suit your needs and lifestyle.

WHO WILL BENEFIT FROM DIET COUNSELING?

- Patients who have any medically-related dietary problem, e.g. diabetes, heart disease, renal disease, obesity, eating disorder, etc.
- Individuals with special dietary needs, e.g. pregnant mothers, growing children and the elderly.
- Healthy individuals without any medical dietary problems will also benefit from learning to adopt a healthy eating lifestyle.

PROCEDURE TO SEE A DIETITIAN

We would suggest you:

a. Obtain a referral letter from your doctor, together with relevant details of your medical history, or
b. If you are not sick but feel you can benefit from some dietary advice, call Dietetics Department, 603-4255 2715/4255 2733. Hospital Main Line. Tel.: 603-4257 1300 or Fax 603-4255 9233 for an appointment.

APPENDIX 3

PRINCE COURT MEDICAL CENTRE

INTRODUCTION

Prince Court Medical Centre is a 286 bed private medical facility located in the heart of Kuala Lumpur, Malaysia. Opened in 2007, Prince Court was born of a Malaysian vision to be the forerunner in the provision of clinical services and patient care delivery. We are supported by an international management team and the medical expertise of senior clinical specialists from the Medical University of Vienna (Austria).

Prince Court provides a comprehensive range of health care services anchored by our 5 Centres of Excellence;

- Heart and Lung
- Oncology
- Plastic Surgery, Cosmetology, Dermatology and Burns
- Urology, Nephrology and Men's Health, and
- Women and Children

We aim to deliver the best clinical outcomes to our patients through state-of-the-art equipment and our highly skilled personnel. We place high importance on patient safety, benchmarking them against international standards. We also offer dedicated hospitality services to cater to our customers' needs and comfort.

Having invested in advanced medical equipment and technology, Prince Court is privileged to be utilizing the Total Hospital Information System (THIS) software that seamlessly manages all patient information from admission to discharge. Through our collaboration with the Medical University of Vienna, we also aim to be at the forefront of establishing innovative Telemedicine, Telepathology, Teleradiology and Telecytogenetics services in Malaysia.

Our landscaped gardens, water features, charming ambience and soothing and therapeutic artworks create a conducive and comfortable environment for patients. Moreover, the futuristically designed architecture, incorporating abundant natural light and wide spaces, is recognized as a unique, positive and modern approach to health care.

NO NEED TO GO OVERSEAS FOR SUPERIOR TREATMENT

PRINCE Court Medical Centre was built with the aim of helping Malaysians receive superior medical treatment without having to travel abroad.

Another goal was to establish itself as the premier centre for medical tourism in Asia. To this end, there are already plans to expand the hospital and its services.

There is land for expansion at the current site of the hospital, which its chief executive officer Stuart Rowley hopes to develop in 2010.

- "Initially, to enable us to cater for medical emergencies, we want to have a helipad to fly in our patients. This would also be a requirement if we were asked to provide emergency and a burns services for the F1 Grand Prix," Rowley said.
- "In the second phase we would be planning for a medi-hotel, medical rooms, supporting services and a rehabilitation centre", he added.

The medi-hotel will cater to both the families of the medical tourist as well as patients who require less intensive care but need nursing supervision.

"The concept is on the drawing board", Rowley said.

The hospital has also set-up the centres of excellence that cover oncology, plastic surgery, cosmetology and burns, urology, nephrology and men's health, women and children's health and heart and lung.

It plans to develop each dedicated segment with state-of-the-art technology.

"Malaysia has the potential to become the leading health care tourism provide in Asia. We want to replace Thailand, India and Singapore as the place of choice," he said.

IF IMITATION is the best form of flattery, the chief of Kuala Lumpur's Prince Court Medical Centre, is probably blushing.

The hospital is only eight months old, not fully operational or officially launched, but requests are already coming in to replicate its model abroad.

Prince Court, which boasts services that one would find in a five-star hotel, has also started treating quite a number of medical tourists from as far as Australia, New Zealand and the UK.

Located on Jalan Kia Peng, the hospital did a soft-opening in October 2007 and it will only be fully operational next month.

Prince Court is owned by state-owned oil company Petrolium National Bhd (Petronas) and managed by Yarned Health Care Services Sdn Bhd and its partner the Medical University of Vienna International Hospital Operations GmbH.

"We have had a hospital in the Middle East which wants to replicate this model. We have had Thais, Cambodians and Mongolians come to see our facility," chief executive officer Stuart D. Rowley said.

Rowley said that the hospital which had planned to establish itself in Malaysia, then regionally before being recognized globally, was pleasantly surprised to see its current level of foreign patients touch 30 per cent.

A total of 710 inpatients and 80,000 outpatients have thus far, ought treatment at the hospital.

Based on the response so far, Rowley may achieve his goal to make the hospital "the best in Asia" within the next five years sooner than anticipated.

Prince Court is named so, given its location where historically, a number of royalty lived including the current monarch.

Built at a substantial cost, including land and equipment, the hospital expects to be operationally profitable by the end of the second year and achieve net profit in eight years.

"By the end of year two, our cash flow will be positive," Rowley said.

"By July 1, 2008, we will be fully operational and all our services will be offered from then," he said, adding that it has 53 clinics and 60 doctors/ specialists.

"We provide every possible clinical specialty with the exception of in-patient psychiatry," he said.

The hospital opened its door last October operating 12 beds. Today, it has 48 bed and all 300 beds will be available in October or November this year.

It will also have 800 nurses by then, up from 200 today.

The medical centre, which has six floors, and another three floors of parking space, measure some one million sq ft.

Its pull factors include it being the only private hospital offering a surgical robot for treatment in men's health, and later for gynaecology and cardiac surgery.

Its 10 operating theatres are said to be among the cleanest in the world with Laminar Flow ventilation which produces almost particle-free air at the operating table, thereby reducing significantly the risk of infection.

The hospital's emphasis on infection control is so stringent that it has 3,730 hand basins and 3,900 hands-free hygiene automatic dispensers and a fulltime professor of microbiology heading the infection control programme.

Rowley said that the hospital will soon have the country's first bladeless excimer/laser for Lasik (eye) surgery.

Other services in the hospital include valet parking, in-room check-in and check-out, 24-hour ala-carte dining service—basically anything one would find in a five-star hotel.

Its suites, which go for around RMl,000 a night, come with a separate bedroom for the family, two televisions, and two bathrooms, including toiletries.

EXECUTIVE HEALTH

HEALTH SCREENING

Health conditions such as heart disease, cancer, diabetes and kidney disorders often exhibit no symptoms. Regular health screenings make it possible for such health risks and conditions to be detected, prevented or properly treated. At Prince Court Medical Centre, we believe in the importance of preventive medicine to help you stay healthy.

Prince Court's one-stop Executive Health Screening Centre offers a range of the latest and most comprehensive health screening services. Conducted by our team of all female clinicians, screening is done in an exclusive environment which affords both comfort and privacy. You will receive a personalized medical report on the same day. Our clinicians will help you understand your results as well as answer any questions or concerns that you may have.

Our Executive Health Screening Centre offers a range of screening packages, from basic to comprehensive. Apart from our standard packages, we are able to custom design special screening programmes to cater to your every need.

Opening Hours

Mondays-Fridays	8.00 a.m.-5.00 p.m.
Saturdays	8.00 a.m.-1.00 p.m.
Sundays and Public Holidays closed	

What to bring

- NRIC
- Work Permit/Employee Pass or Passport (for foreigners)
- For those covered by insurance or employer medical benefits:
  - o Letter of Guarantee
  - o Authorization Letter/Chit from company
- Past Medical Records, recent Mammogram films and laboratory results
- And current medications (if applicable)

Preparations

- Fast 10 hours prior to tests. You may however, sip plain water.
- Postpone your routine morning medicine until your blood sample is taken; unless you have high blood pressure.
- If you are doing the Treadmill test, bring along an additional change of clothes and appropriate footwear.
- Pap smear should best be done 10 days after the last day of your menstruation.

EXECUTIVE HEALTH PACKAGES

Health Screening Profile 1

- Full Blood Count with PBF and ESR
- Lipid profile
- Liver function test
- Renal profile
- Glucose
- Bone metabolism profile
- Uric acid
- Urine test

Health Screening Profile 2

- Full blood count with PBF and ESR
- Unit ABO and RH typing
- Lipid profile
- Liver function test
- Glucose
- Renal profile
- Bone metabolism profile
- Free Thyroxine (FT4)
- Hepatitis B Screening
- Rheumatoid Arthritis (RA) Factor
- Alpha-feto-protein (AFP)
- VORL (RPR)
- Uric acid
- Urine test

Basic Screening Package (Men and Women) RM500.00

- Health Screening Profile 2
- Consultation and physical examination
- Vision Testing
- Pure Tone Audiometry (Hearing assessment)
- Resting electrocardiogram (ECG) with report by cardiologist
- Chest x-ray with report
- Cardiovascular Screening

Cardiovascular Screening Package

RM1,750.00

- Health Screening Profile 2
- Consultation and physical examination
- Stress ECG (Treadmill) with report by cardiologist
- Chest x-ray with report

- Coronary calcium score
- High sensitive CRP (for coronary risk factor)
- Free Tri-Iodothyronine (FT3)
- Thyroid Stimulating Hormone (TSH)
- Hepatitis C Screening
- Fitness Screening
- Diet Wellness Counselling

Well Man Screening Package **RM1,300.00**

Health Screening Profile 2

- Consultation and physical examination
- Vision Testing
- Pure Tone Audiometry
- Stress ECG (Treadmill) with report by cardiologist
- Lung Function Test
- Body fat analysis
- Chest x-ray with report
- Ultrasound Abdomen and PeMs
- DEXA (2 regions) (Bone screening for osteoporosis)
- Carcinoembryonic Antigen (CEA)
- Hepatitis C IgG Antibody
- Hepatitis A IgG
- HIV I and II Antibody
- Prostate Specific Antigen (PSA)

Well Women Screening Package **RM1,400.00**

Health Screening Profile 2

- Consultation and physical examination
- Vision testing
- Pure Tone Audiometry
- Stress ECG (Treadmill) with report by cardiologist
- Lung Function Test
- Body fat analysis
- Chest x-ray with report
- Ultrasound Abdomen and Pelvis
- Mammography
- DEXA (2 regions) (Bone screening for osteoporosis)
- Carcinoembryonic Antigen (CEA)
- Hepatitis C IgG Antibody
- Hepatitis A IgG
- HIV I and II Antibody
- Pap smear

Cancer Screening Package (Men) **RM1,950.00**

"Health Screening Profile 1

- Consultation and physical examination
- Chest x-ray with report
- Ultrasound Abdomen and PeMs
- Colonoscopy
- Free Thyroxine (FT4)
- Hepatitis B Surface Antigen
- Hepatitis B Surface Antibody
- Hepatitis C IgG Antibody
- Carcinoembryonic Antigen (CEA)
- CA-19.9 (for gastrointestinal cancer)
- Alpha-feto-protein (AFP)
- Prostate Specific Antigen (PSA)

Cancer Screening Package (Women) **RM2,200.00**

Includes Men's Gancer Package and:

- CA-125 (for ovarian cancer)
- CA-15.3 (for breast cancer)
- PAP Smear
- Mammography

Excluding Prostate Specific Antigen (PSA)

Pre-marital RM700.00 per person/RM1,300.00 per couple

Health Screening Profile 2

- Consultation and physical examination
- Vision testing
- Lung Function test
- Resting electrocardiogram (ECG) with report by cardiologist
- Chest x-ray with report
- Carcinoembryonic Antigen (CEA)
- Hepatitis C IgG Antibody
- Hepatitis A IgG
- HIV I and II Antibody
- Rubella IgG

CENTRE OF EXCELLENCE

PLASTIC SURGERY

A full range of plastic and reconstructive surgery services are available, providing patients with specialized care and treatment solutions. Surgical treatments range from simple skin lesion removal to complex craniomaxillofacial reconstruction.

Services and treatment offered include:

- Craniomaxillofacial surgery
- Cleft surgery
- Breast surgery
- Skin and related tissues surgery
- Hand and extremity surgery
- Flaps and microsurgery

COSMETOLOGY

We offer solutions for all your aesthetic, beauty and wellness needs. Every client is given individualized care with strict confidentiality. The Centre provides comprehensive packages using both surgical and non-surgical techniques.

Services and treatment offered:

- Non-surgical—lasers and intense light treatment, chemical peeling microdermabrasion, fillers; botox, and thread lift.
- Surgical—facelifts, eyelid blepharoplasty, rhinoplasty, pinnaplasty, facial implants and contouring, breast surgery and reduction, augmentations and lifts, liposuction, ifpoplasty, abdominoplasty and body contouring, body and extremity lifting (in combination with bariatric surgery), and hair replantation.
- Wellness and Fitness Programmes—slimming programmes, health and medical spa including massage therapy and beauty therapy.

DERMATOLOGY

An entire range of therapy for skin and dermatological problems is provided using advanced diagnostic tools and methods. Working closely with the Plastic Surgery Centre, it ensures comprehensive and seamless treatment of various skin diseases.

Services and treatment offered:

- Common inflammatory diseases and immune-mediated processes such as eczema, psoriasis, and lupus.
- Cutaneous infectious diseases such as bacterial, viral and fungal infections, and sexually transmitted diseases.
- Allergic-mediated processes such as rhinoconjunctivities and asthma, acute and chronic urticaria, food allergies, and drug allergies.
- Skin lesions and cancers.
- Phototherapy, and intense pulse light therapy.

BURNS

Our medical and allied personnel will provide treatment solutions to virtually all types of burn injuries. Our aim is to provide comprehensive burn care, ensuring the complete recovery of patients who will be sufficiently rehabilitated.

Services and treatment offered:

- Acute burns treatment—resuscitation, ventilator and respiratory support, wound dressing using biologic synthetic such as collagen, silver, hydrogel, hydrocolloid, surgery, dietary support, psychological support and social support.
- Chronic burns care—rehabilitation therapy including physiotherapy, occupational therapy, prosthesis and orthosis, and reconstructive burn surgery.

UROLOGY SERVICES

As well as its expertise in men's health and wellness, the Centre specializes in robotic surgery and renal transplantation services for its patients using the latest advanced technology.

The core services offered by the Centre include endoscopic procedures and treatments for:

- Benign prostatic enlargement
- Inflammation of the prostate
- Urinary tract infection
- Bladder, ureter and kidney stones
- Prostate, bladder and kidney cancers
- Pediatric hypospadias and antireflux surgery

Open urological procedures such as:

- Simple and radical nephrectomy
- Nephroureterectomy
- Partial nephrectomy
- Cystoprostatectomy
- Pyeloplasty
- Reimplantation of ureter for adults and children
- Transvaginal sling procedures for female urinary incontinence
- Surgery for Peyronie's disease
- Urethroplasty and substitution urethroplasty

Advanced Subspecialty procedures such as:

- Robotic radical prostatectomy, pyeloplasty and ureteric reimplantation
- Renal transplantation

- Artificial urinary sphincter-augmentation
- Penile prosthesis implants
- Penile curvarture correction
- Neurornodulation for incontinence
- Laparoscopic and minimally invasive surgery
- Laser surgery for stones and prostate enlargement

Apart from this, we also provide one stop Prostate Cancer diagnosis and management such as:

- Transrectal ultrasound biopsies
- Robotic Assisted Laparoscopic Prostatectomy (RALP)
- Low-dose Brachytherapy for localised disease
- Management of advanced prostate cancer

Nephrology Service

Diabetes, high blood pressure and other disorders contribute to chronic kidney disease. Early detection and treatment of kidney diseases can often keep chronic kidney diseases at bay, failing which patients may require dialysis or a kidney transplant to maintain life.

Other services provided are:

- Chronic kidney disease and end-stage renal failure
- Live donor and cadaveric renal transplantation
- Vascular access
- Chronic ambulatory peritoneal dialysis (CAPD)
- Haemodialysis
- Chronic transplant rejection
- Post-transplantation nephrotoxicity
- Chronic renal infections

Men's Health and Wellness Centre

We also provide a holistic approach to promote active aging through:

- Diet counselling
- A recommended exercise and fitness regime
- Assessment of cognitive functions and mental acuity
- Programme to stop smoking and alcoholism
- Screening for hypertension, diabetes, dyslipidaemia, obesity and osteoporosis
- Musculoskeletal assessment such as:
- Bone densitometry
- Biological markers of aging
- Assessment of quality of life
- Diagnostic and curative services for:
    - o Benign enlargement of prostate

    - o Prostate cancer
    - o Treatment of erectile dysfunction
    - o Incontinence
- Rehabilitation services will include:
    - o Physiotherapy
    - o Yoga
    - o Meditation
    - o Institutional services

Infertility treatment

Recognising that infertility can be emotionally stressful to those who wish to have children, we place importance on assisting those affected by this condition. Some of the procedures we offer are:

- Semen analysis and sperm function testing
- Evaluation of azoospermia and oligospermia
- Vasovasostomy
- Vasoepididymostomy
- Infertility
- Sperm analysis
- Testicular biopsy
- Treatment of varicocele

The following services are provided as daycare procedures:

- Transrectal biopsy of prostate
- Cystometogram (CMG)/Video CMG
- Diagnostic flexible cystoscopy
- Circumcision
- Diagnostic cystoscopy
- Retrograde stenting

HEART AND LUNG

The setting up of a Centre of Excellence (COE) for Heart and Lung demonstrates our commitment on diseases pertaining to these two major organs. Cardiovascular and respiratory diseases are the leading causes of death around the world, and this Centre has a mission to ensure that the best possible care is given to patients, as well as to engage the public in preventative measures against these diseases.

Our Centre of Excellence is fully equipped with both invasive and non-invasive diagnostic facilities to accurately identify the problem so that the appropriate treatment can be administered.

Besides that, we aim to conquer new frontiers in the management of heart and lung diseases and we will strive to do this through constant research and development.

What our Centre can do for you

If you have any established cardiovascular and respiratory problems, or you possess risk factors in potentially developing them, please make arrangements to see one of our specialists to discuss the proper care required. Early diagnosis, coupled with prompt and appropriate treatment, can alleviate suffering and even prolong and save lives.

What the Centre offers

- State-of-the-art facilities which include a dedicated non-invasive department, two invasive cardiac catherisation suites, electrophysiology, myocardial perfusion scans and pulmonary laboratories, as well as two 64-slice CT, 1.5Tesla MRI, and a PET Scanner
- Two dedicated operating rooms, and a fully equipped ten-bed Cardiothoracic Postoperative Intensive Care Unit to cater for patients undergoing heart and lung surgery.
- Dedicated interventional and non-interventional cardiologists and skilled surgeons to perform the entire spectrum of heart and thoracic surgery.
- A 24-hour primary Percutaneous Coronary Intervention (PCI) service for patients with acute heart attacks.
- An allied health care facility which provides cardiac and pulmonary rehabilitation, continuous medical evaluation, emotional counselling, dietary advice and lifestyle modification activities for risk prevention, will be part of our strategies to cater for a healthy life.

WOMEN AND CHILDREN

The Centre of Excellence (COE) for Women and Children is one of our five Centres of Excellence. Our medical consultants and nurses are here to provide care that you can rely on with confidence and our medical facilities are of international standards to ensure that you receive the best care possible.

We know that children often associate hospitals with needles, strange machines and at best, boredom. Here at Prince Court, we do our best to ensure that our hospital is a cheerful and lively place for them, making it conducive for healing. You may also bring along your child's favourite toys and video games to further lend a sense of comfort and familiarity to their environment.

For your comfort

Apart from modern equipment and treatment, we also provide our patients with pleasant surroundings to help accelerate the healing process. From concierge and butler services to food and beverage outlets that cater to all tastes, you can look forward to a pleasant and soothing environment.

Listed below are some of the services offered by the Centre for Women and Children. The list is by no means definitive, as new services continue to be added.

Obstetrics

- Ante-natal care
- Detailed fetal ultrasound scans
- Feto-maternal medicine
- Prenatal diagnosis
- All modes of delivery

Gynaecology

- General gynaecology-related services
- Gynaecological oncology (cancer therapy)
- Assisted reproduction (infertility treatment)
- Uroqynaecology
- Minimally invasive surgery (keyhole surgery)

Paediatrics

- General paediatrics
- Genetic counselling
- Neonatology
- Oncology
- Surgery (inclusive of cardiac surgery)
- The diagnosis and management of pulmonary diseases and inborn errors of metabolism (inherited genetic diseases)

Laboratory Services

The Centre is committed to providing comprehensive, rapid laboratory testing services that utilize the latest diagnostic tools. For patients, this translates to shorter waiting times, and more precise results.

MENTAL HEALTH

How Does Having Good Mental Health Help Me?

When you have good mental health, you will feel confident of yourself and will find life more enjoyable. You will also cope better under pressure and recover from a setback more quickly.

You are in good mental health if you:

- Have a strong sense of self-worth.
- Feel that your life is manageable and meaningful.
- Cope well under stressful situations.

- Are strong enough to regain a state of composure after a setback.
- Are able to balance the demands at home, at work and in your social life.
- Develop and maintain healthy relationships with family members, friends and colleagues.

However, having good mental health does not mean your life is now stress-free. We all encounter setbacks and crises from time to time. The good news is, you are better equipped to handle such situations if you have a healthy state of mind.

However, there may be times where you may feel overwhelmed. Look out for these warning signs that may indicate that your mental health may be affected: -

- You constantly feel overwhelmed by demands at home and at work.
- You feel that there is no solution or end to your problems.
- You have trouble sleeping at night.
- You lose interest in your usual recreational activities, and this persists over a prolonged period of time.
- You feel exhausted all the time.
- You feel like you could have a mental breakdown at any time.

If you experience any of the above, the following tips could help you regain good mental health.

Value Yourself

Realise that you are unique as an individual. Be confident of your abilities and resist the urge to underestimate yourself. Do your best, but don't keep blaming yourself if you make some mistakes along the way. Instead, learn from your mistakes and move on.

Know Your Strengths and Limitations

All of us have our strengths and Weaknesses. Recognizing and accepting them can help build your confidence and self-esteem.

Make a list of your strength and weaknesses. What are your skills and interests? What are the things you have difficulty with or make you feel frustrated when you carry them out? Ask your family and friends for their opinions of you. To get a clearer idea of yourself, include the qualities they mention in the list as well.

Stay Connected with Your Loved Ones

Develop and maintain strong afnd supportive relationships with your family and friends. Having people in our lives that we can rely on has an impact on our emotional well-being. Staying connected requires you to be open about your feelings with your loved ones. Whether it is to share a piece of good news or simply to tell them about your day, such openness strengthens the relationships you have with them. It also allows other people to become aware of what is bothering us.

Manage Your Time

Practice good time management to minimize stress and tension. Prioritize the tasks you need to do. Don't waste time worrying about aspects of the project which cannot be changed or are beyond your control.

In the midst of completing your tasks, do set aside time for yourself to do the things you enjoy, such as a carrying out a hobby or catching up with friends.

Set Realistic Goals

Whether it is at work or at play, setting realistic goals can help keep your spirits up and motivate you to move forward. Even the most complicated task seems less overwhelming when you break it down into smaller, more manageable steps.

Take Care of Your Body!

It is all too easy to neglect our body when we feel stressed or anxious. Being physically fit benefits your mental and emotional health as well.

Eat Healthily

A balanced diet is vital in helping us achieve good mental health. You can refer to the Healthy Diet Pyramid to ensure that you are selecting healthy foods in the correct portions for your meals.

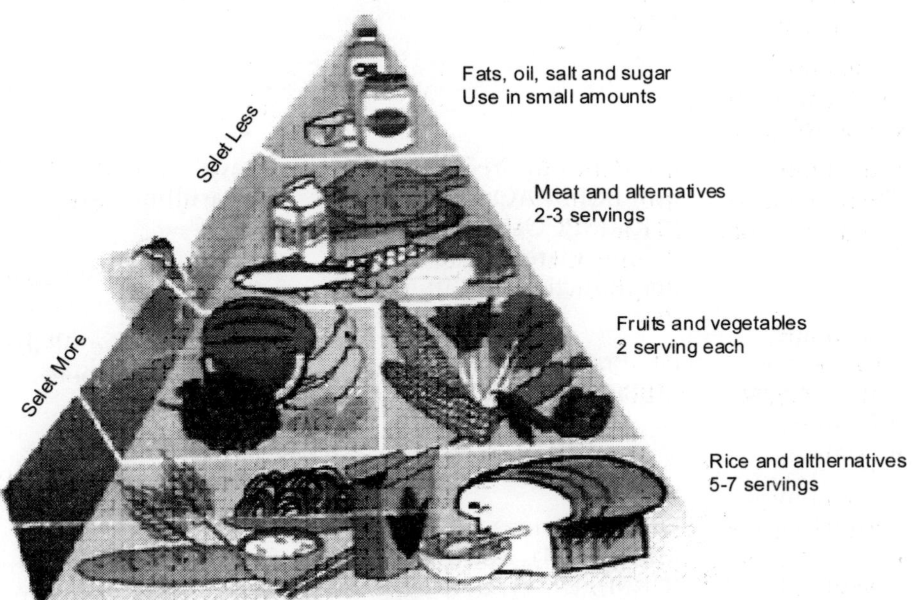

Get Active

Regular exercise does not only keep our bodies fit, it also helps regulate our moods and make us feel better. Do any form of exercise or a sport you enjoy for 30 minutes a day, 5 times a week to keep yourself physically active and emotionally uplifted!

Get Enough Rest

Ensure you get enough sleep so you will feel well rested upon waking up. Stressful situations can seem more difficult to solve when you feel tired. In contrast, you will feel more equipped to handle challenging situations if you have had sufficient rest the night before.

Take Up A Hobby

Taking up a hobby or learning a new skill, such as playing a musical instrument, stimulates your mind. Such activities are also a welcome break from the daily demands you face at home and at work.

CLINICAL DIRECTORY OF SERVICES

Centre of Excellence for Women and Children

Expertise	*Consultant's Name*	*Location*
1. Obstetric and Gynaecology	**Tel.: 603 2160 0000 Extn: 2143/2144** **Fax: 603 2160 0780**	
Clinical Director Centre of Excellence	Datuk Dr. Abdul Aziz Yahya MBBS (Mal), MRCOG (Lon), AM (Mal)	Level 6, Suite 6F-021 Consulting Room 6
Consultant Obstetrician & Gynaceologists		
Consultant Obstetrician & Gynaecologists	Dr. Paul Tay Yee Siang MB, BCh. BAO (Ireland), MD (UK), MRCOG (UK), DIP. Family Planning and Reproductive Health Care (UK)	Level 6, Suite 6F-016 Consulting Room 8
Consultant Obstetrician, Gynaecologist & Fertility Specialist	Dr. Prashant Nadkarni MBBS (Mal), FRCOG (UK)	Level 6, Suite 6F-018 Consulting Room 7
Consultant Obstetrician & Gynaecologist Consultant	Dr. Seri Suniza Sufian MBBS (UM), Masters O & G (UKM), Urogynaecology Clinical Research Fellow (Sheffield)	Level 6, Suite 6F-012 Consulting Room 9

Obstetrician & Gynaecologist	Dr. Tan Ngiap Hong MBBS (UM), Masters O & G (UKM), MRCOG (UK), MSc Prenatal Genetics and Fetal Medicine (Lon)	Level 6, Suite 6F-025 Consulting Room 5

2. Pediatrics **Tel.: 603 2160 0000 Extn: 2143/2144**
Fax: 603 2160 0780

Consultant Paediatrician and Geneticist	Dr. Choy Yew Sing MBBS (Mal), MRCP (UK), M. Med (Mal), AM (Mal)	Level 6, Suite 6F-032 Consulting Room 1
Consultant Paediatrician	Dr. Anthony James Mansul MBBS (Aus), MRCP (UK)	Level 6, Suite 6F-030 Consulting Room 3
Consultant Paediatrician	Dr. Adnan Adrian Goh MBBS (UM), MPaed (UM), MRCP (UK), FICM (Melb, Australia)	Level 6, Suite 6F-026 Consulting Room 4
Resident Consultant Paediatrician & Neonatologist	Dr. Anna Padmavathy Soosai MBBS (UM), MRCP (UK)	Level 6, Suite 6F-026 Consulting Room 4
Consultant Paediatrician & Neonatologist	Dr. Ananda Dharmalingam MB BCh, BAO, LRCPI, LRCSI, DCH, MRCPI (Paediatrics), MRCPCH (UK), AM	Level 6, Suite 6F-026 Consulting Room 4
Resident Consultant Paediatrician and Paediatric Intensive Care Specialist	Dr. Sharmila Kylasam MBBS (UM), MRCP (Paediatrics) (UK)	Level 6, Suite 6F-026 Consulting Room 4

Centre of Excellence for Heart and Lung

Expertise	*Consultant's Name*	*Location*

1. Cardiothoracic Surgery **Tel.: 603 2160 0000 Extn: 2140/2141/2142**
Fax: 603 2160 0680

Clinical Director Centre of Excellence	Dato' Dr. Ghandhiraj Somasundram DPTJ, MBBS AM (Mal), FRCS	Level 2, Suite 2D-022 Consulting Room 9

Consultant Cardiothoracic Surgeon	(Glasgow), CST STH (UK), M.D. (Vienna)	
Consultant Cardiovascular & Thoracic Surgeon	Dr. David Khoo Sin Keat MD (UKM), FRCS (Edinburgh), Fellowship in Advanced Cardiovascular and Thoracic Surgery (Mayo Clinic, USA)	Level 2, Suite 2D-022 Consulting Room 9

2. Cardiology **Tel.: 603 2160 0000 Extn: 2140/2141/2142**
Fax: 603 2160 0680

Consultant Interventional Cardiologist	Dr. Devan Pillay MBBS (Mangalore), Am (Mal), FRCP (Ireland), FESC (Europe), FACC (USA), FSCAI (USA), FNHAM (Mal)	Level 2, Suite 2D-019 Consulting Room 8
Consultant Interventional Cardiologist	Dr. Dewi Ramasamy MBBS (Mal), FRCP (Ire), FACC (USA), AM (Mal)	Level 2, Suite 2D-019 Consulting Room 8
Consultant Interventional Cardiologist	Dr. Yap Yee Guan BMedSci (Hons), MBBS (Nottm), MD (Lon), EC (Eur), FAMS CCT (UK) (Cardiology and Internal Medicine), FRCP (Glasgow), FRCP (Edinburgh), FESC, AM, FSCAI (USA), FAHA (USA)	Level 2, Suite 2D-017 Consulting Room 7
Consultant Interventional Cardiologist	Dr. Shanker Vinayagamoorthy	Level 2, Suite 2D-017 Consulting Room 7
Consultant Non-Interventional Cardiologist	Dr. Azani Mohd Daud MBBS (Newc), MRCP (UK)	Level 2, Suite 2D-017 Consulting Room 7
Consultant Non-Interventional Cardiologist	Dr. Norazlina Yusof	Level 2, Suite 2D-017 Consulting Room 7

Consultant Respiratory Medicine & Physician	Dr. Lim Kim Hatt MBBS (Mal), MRCP (UK), M.MED (Mal), FCCP (USA)	Level 2, Suite 2D-018 Consulting Room 22

Diagnostic Imaging

Expertise	*Consultant's Name*	*Location*
Radiology Services	**Tel.: 603 2160 3355** **Fax: 603 2160 0010**	
Director Radiology Services	Dr. Shahrin Merican MB BCh (Ireland), M.Med. Rad (UKM), FRCR (UK)	Level 1
Consultant Radiologist		
Consultant	Dr. Sumithra Ranganathan MBBS (Ind) M. Radiology (Mal) AM (Mal)	Level 1
Resident Consultant Interventional and General Radiologist	Dr. Liong Wei Chuen MD (HONS), M.MED, FRCR, CCT (UK)	Level 1

Centre of Excellence for Surgical Services

Expertise	*Consultant's Name*	*Location*
1. Surgical Services	**Tel.: 603 2160 0000 Extn: 2140/2141/2142** **Fax: 603 2160 0680**	
Director Surgical Services	Dr. Yunus Gul Bin Alif Gul LRCPI LRCSI MB BCh BAO (NUI), FRCS (Ireland), Certificate of Completion of Specialist Training (UK and Ireland)	Level 2, Suite 2D-026 Consulting Room 11
Consultant General, Laparoscopic and Colorectal Surgeon		

Consultant General, Upper GI and Laparoscopic Surgeon	Dr. Mohd Faisal Jabar B.Med. Sci (Hons), BM, BS, FRCS (Eng.)	Level 2, Suite 2D-023 Consulting Room 10
Consultant General and Vascular Surgeon	Dr. Tan Kong Hean MB BCh BAO (Hon) (Belfast), FRCS (Ireland), CCST (UK)	Level 2, Suite 2D-025 Consulting Room 21

2. Breast and Endocrine Surgery Tel.: 603 2160 0000
Extn: 2140/2141/2142
Fax: 603 2160 0680

Consultant Breast and Endocrine Surgeon	Dr. Harjit Kaur MBBS (Mangalore), MS (UKM), FRCS (Ireland), AM (Mal)	Level 2, Suite 2D-016 Consulting Room 6

3. Paediatric Surgeon Tel.: 603 2160 0000 Extn: 2140/2141/2142
Fax: 603 2160 0680

Consultant Paediatric Surgeon	Dr. Zuraidah Ibrahim MD (UKM), FRCS (Edinburgh)	Level 2, Suite 2D-027 Consulting Room 20

4. Ophthalmology (EYE) Tel.: 603 2160 0000 Extn: 2145/2146
Fax: 603 2160 0920

Head Department of Ophthalmology	Prof. Dr. Muhaya Haji Mohammad MD (UKM), FRCS (Edinburgh), M. Surgery (Ophth.) (UKM), M. Med (NUS), PHD (Ocular Immunology) (Lon), Fellowship in Uveitis (UK)	Level 3, Suite 3B-042 Consulting Room 1
Consultant Ophthalmologist and Vitreoretinal Surgeon	Dr. Barkeh Hanim Jumaat MBBS (Mal), M. Surgery (Ophth.) (UKM), FRCS (Edinburgh), M. Med (S'pore)	Level 3, Suite 3B-040 Consulting Room 2
Consultant	Dr. Tan Niap Ming MBBS (Mal), M. Surgery (Ophth.) (UKM), FRCS (Edinburgh), M. Med (Ophth) (S'pore)	Level 3, Suite 3B-040 Consulting Room 2

5. Otorhinolaryngology (ENT) Tel.: 603 2160 0000 Extn: 2145/2146
Fax: 603 2160 0920

Ophthalmologist Consultant ENT Surgeon	Dr. Kuljit Singh MBBS (Mangalore), M. Surgery (ORL-HNS), FAAO (USA)	Level 3, Suite 3B-036 Consulting Room 5
Consultant ENT, Head and Neck Surgeon	Dr. Koh Tat Ngee MB BCh (Ireland), FRCS (Sugery) (Ireland), FRCS (ENT) (Glasgow), FRCS (ENT) (Edinburgh)	Level 3, Suite 3B-038 Consulting Room 4
Consultant ENT, Head and Neck	Dr. Yeo Sek Wee MB BCh (Ireland), BAO LRCP/SI, FRCSI (Surgery), FRCSI (ORL), Fellowship in Head and Neck Surgery (Monash)	Level 3, Suite 3B-035 Consulting Room 3

6. Neurosurgeon Tel.: 603 2160 0000 Extn: 2140/2141/2142
Fax: 603 2160 0680

Surgeon Consultant Neurosurgeon	Dr. Jagdeep Nanra MB BCh. BAO. LRCPI, LRCSI, FRCSI, FRCS (Surgical Neurology)	Level 3, Suite 2D-036 Consulting Room 18
Visiting Consultant Neurosurgeon	Dr. Muruga Kumar MD (USM), FRCS (Edin.), FRCS (Glasgow) AM	Level 2, Suite 2D-036 Consulting Room 18
Consultant	Dr. Wong Fung Chu MBChB (Edinburgh), FRCS (Edinburgh), FRCSEd (Neurosurgery)	Level 2, Suite 2D-033 Consulting Room 16

7. Orthopaedic Surgery Tel.: 603 2160 0000 Extn: 2140/2141/2142
Fax: 603 2160 0680

Neurosurgeon Consultant Orthopaedic Surgeon	Dr. Badrul Shah Badaruddin MD (UKM), MS ORTH (UKM), AM (Mal), FAOI (Trauma) (Lon), CMIA (Niosh), Fellowship in Arthroplasty and Arthroscopy (Aus)	Level 2, Suite 2D-005 Consulting Room 23
Clinical Director Consultant Orthopaedic Surgeon	Dr. (Med) Cyril D Toma	Level 2, Suite 2D-038 Consulting Room 19
Consultant Orthopaedic Surgeon	Dato' Dr. Zulkharnain Ismail, DIMP MS Orth, MBBS (Malaya), Fellow in Joint and Tumour Reconstruction (Melb. Australia)	Level 2, Suite 2D-010 Consulting Room 3
Consultant Orthopaedic Surgeon	Dr. Mohd Asri Ghapar MD (UKM), MS Orth (UKM), BMed Sc (UKM), FAA (Monash)	Level 2, Suite 2D-033 Consulting Room 16
Resident Consultant Orthopaedic (Spine)	Dr. Deepak Ajit Singh MBBS (Mal.), Ms. Ortho (Mal.), FRCS (Edinburgh)	Level 2, Suite 2D-038 Consulting Room 5

8. Anaesthesiology Tel.: 603 2160 0000 Extn: 2701/2227
Fax: 603 2160 0010

Surgeon Consultant Anaesthesiologist and Intensive Care Specialist	Dr. Syed Rozaidi Wafa MD (UKM), M.Med (Anaes) (UKM)	Level 2, Suite 2 G&H
Consultant Anaesthesiologist and Intensive	Dr. Anuradha Pathmanathan MD (UKM), M. Med. (Anaest)	Level 2, Suite 2 G&H

Care Specialist Consultant Anaesthesiologist	Dr. Ghazaime Ghazali MD (USM), FCARCS (Ireland), Fellow in Neuroanaesthesia (Toronto)	Level 2, Suite 2 G&H
Consultant Anaesthesiologist and Intensive Care Specialist	Dr. Sekar KPK Shanmugam MBBS (Mal), M. Anaest (Mal.), Fellowship Intensive Care (Adelaide)	Level 2, Suite 2 G&H
Consultant Anaesthesiologist	Dr. Kattayat Mohandas MBBS, DA, MD (Anaes), FFARACS, FANZCA, AM	Level 2, Suite 2 G&H

Centre of Excellence for Medical Services

Expertise	*Consultant's Name*	*Location*
Medical Services	**Tel.: 603 2160 0000 Extn: 2140/2141/2142** **Fax: 603 2160 0680**	
Head, Medical Services Director Endoscopy Services Consultant Internal Medicine Physician and Gastroenterologist	Dr. Ryan Ponnudurai MB BCh, LRCP and SI (NU Ireland), BAO, Board Certification Int. Med. And Gastroenterology (USA), Am (Mal)	Level 2, Suite 2D-033 Consulting Room 16
Consultant Internal Medicine Physician and Endocrinologist	Dr. Faridah Ismail BSc (St Andrews), MB CHb (Glasgow), M. Med (UKM)	Level 2, Suite 2D-012 Consulting Room 4
Consultant Metabolic Medicine (Endocrinology) and Chemical Pathologist	Dr. Leslie Charles Lai Chin Loy MBBS (Lon), MSc (Lon), MD (Lon.), FRCP (Edinburgh), FRCPath (UK), FAMM (Mal)	Level 2, Suite 2D-012 Consulting Room 4

Consultant Internal Medicine Physician and Gastroenterologist	Dr. L. Sanker V MBBS, FRCP, AM	Level 2, Suite 2D-028 Consulting Room 13
Consultant Neurologist	Dr. Vimalan Ramasundram MBBS (Mal), M. Med. (Mal)	Level 2, Suite 2D-012 Consulting Room 4
Consultant Neurologist	Dr. Dulia Shanaz Merican MB BCh. LRCPSI (IRE), MRCP (UK) MRCP (IRE)	Level 2, Suite 2D-038 Consulting Room 19
Consultant Neurologist	Dr. Hj Hamidon Basri B.Sc. (UKM), MD (UKM), MMED (UKM), AM (Mal)	Level 2, Suite 2D-038 Consulting Room 19
Consultant Psychiatric	Dr. Rabin Gonzaga MBBCh, LRCP and SI (NU Ireland), BAO, MRCPsych (UK)	Level 2, Suite 2D-010 Consulting Room 3

Laboratory Services

Expertise	*Consultant's Name*	*Location*
Laboratory	**Tel.: 603 2160 0757/0754** **Fax: 603 2160 0760**	
Consultant Histopathology and Cytopathologist	Dr. Norizan Annuar KMN, MBBS (Mal), DCP (Lond.), AMM	Level 4
Consultant Microbiology	Prof Dr. Ngeow Yun Fong	Level 4
Consultant Haematologist	Prof Dr. Elizabeth George MBBS (Mal.), FAMM, DCP (Lon), FRCPA (Aust.), MD (S'Pore), FRCPE (Edinburgh)	Level 2, Suite 2D-012 Consulting Room 4

Centre of Excellence for Urology, Nephrology and Men's Health

Expertise	*Consultant's Name*	*Location*
Urology	**Tel.: 603 2160 0000 Extn: 2147** **Fax: 603 2160 0930**	
Clinical Director Centre of Excellence Honorary Consultant IUN, HKL	Dato' Dr. Sahabudin Raja Mohamed DSPN, KMN, MBBS, M. Surgery, SCFP (Bristol), FICS, AM	Level 2, Suite 2B-040 Consulting Room 1
Consultant Urologist Consultant Urologist	Dr. Chua Chong Beng B. Med. Sci. (Hons.), BMBS, DM (Nottingham), FRCS (Ed.), FRCS Urology (UK)	Level 2, Suite 2B-041 Consulting Room 2
Consultant Internal Medicine Physician and Nephrologists	Dr. Tharmaratnam Rasanayagam MBBS (Mangalore), M. Med. (UKM)	Level 2, Suite 2B-041 Consulting Room 2

Centre of Excellence for Plastic Reconstructive, Cosmetology, Dermatology and Burn

Expertise	*Consultant's Name*	*Location*
1. Plastic Reconstructive and Cosmetology	**Tel.: 603 2160 0000** **Extn: 2150/2382** **Fax: 603 2160 0940**	
Clinical Director Centre of Excellence Consultant Plastic and Reconstructive Surgeon	Dr. Mohd Nasir Zahari MBBS (Melb), FRCS (Edin), MS (UKM)	Level 2, Suite 2D-008 Consulting Room 1

Consultant Plastic and Reconstructive Surgeon	Dr. Eileen Fong Pek Siew MBBS (Mal), FRCS (Edinburgh), AM (Mal), FAMS (Plastic Surgery) Dip. Plastic Surgery (UK)	Level 2, Suite 2D-009 Consulting Room 2

2. Dermatology **Tel.: 603 2160 0000 Extn: 2150**
Fax: 603 2160 0940

Consultant, Dermatology	Dr. Guru Ratnavelu MBBS, DVEN, DDERM (London)	Level 2, Suite 2D-009 Consulting Room 2

Executive Health Services

Expertise	Consultant's Name	Location
Executive Health	**Tel.: 603 2160 8888** **Fax: 603 2160 0088**	
Head Executive Health Services	Dr. Rohini Van K Van Hoboken MBBS (Mangalore)	Level 1

ROOM CHARGES

Room Types	*Established Rate*	*Corporate Rate*
Private Rooms (Single)	RM 380.00	RM 300.00
Suites	RM 1,000.00	RM 1,000.00
Double Room (2 bedded) available in Paediatric Ward only	RM 200.00	RM 200.00
ICU/CCU/Burns ICU—with ventilator	RM 600.00	RM 600.00
ICU/CCU/Burns ICU-without ventilator	RM 300.00	RM 300.00
Neonatal ICU (NICU)—with ventilator	RM 500.00	RM 500.00
Neonatal ICU (NICU)—without ventilator	RM 300.00	RM 300.00
Delivery Room	RM 300.00	RM 300.00
Nursery	RM 80.00	RM 80.00
Nursery with Special Care	RM 120.00	RM 120.00

3 meals, 2 snacks, tea and coffee are provided in the private rooms, suite and 2 bedded rooms. The private rooms also come complete with a TV, Fridge, Safe and a Sofa Bed at no additional cost. Basic toiletries, towels, bathrobes and slippers such are also provided. The 2 bedded rooms are also equipped with TV, fridge and basic toiletries.

MEDI-ASSIST4U

In Corporation with Narayana Hrudayalaya Institute of Cardiac Sciences

MediAssist4U HEALTH SCREENING

MediAssist4U is a one stop community health screening centre which provides the public with the latest in medical technology complete with specialist consultation and trained staff. It offers both convenience and privacy at its ground floor location in Brickfields, Kuala Lumpur.

Services by specialist doctors include:

- Full Cardiac Screening
- Eye Examination
- Women's Wellness and Health
- Dermatology
- Orthopaedics

Because we understand everyone has a different lifestyle and needs, we have a wide range of health screening programmes for you to choose from. We offer one-on-one attention, time for questions and discussion, personal follow-up and testing.

What to expect

- Physical examination and appropriate tests
- Consultation with a doctor
- Information on maintaining a healthy lifestyle
- A full written report

MediAssist4U provides an affordable "snapshot" of the internal functioning of your body. We provide the latest and most comprehensive health screening services available today. Understanding what goes on within your body is essential to prevent untoward medical conditions arising without warning signs or symptoms.

Aims of Health Screening

- To identify pre-existing health problems
- To assess your risk factors for disease

- To provide recommendations on your lifestyle that will encourage a longer and healthier life

Regular health screening especially for those with high-risk lifestyles will facilitate early detection and prevention of life threatening disease.

Risk Factors

Anyone with the following risk factors is an ideal candidate for medical screening:

- Smoking
- Diabetes
- Hypertension (Increased Blood Pressure)
- Obesity
- Stress
- Diet
- Sedentary Lifestyle
- Family history of heart disease or stroke

Package I: GENERAL EXECUTIVE SCREENING RM 49.00

- Laboratory Investigations
- Consultations

Blood Screening (30 Tests)

Full Blood Counts
Hb
RBC (RCC)
WCC (TWDC)
5 Part Differential Count
Platelet Count
PCV
MCH/MCV
MCHC

Blood Film Comment

ESR
Renal Function Test
Sodium
Potassium
Chloride
Urea
Calcium
Creatinine

Liver Function Test
Total Protein
Albumin
Globulin
Total Bilirubin
ALP
AST (SGOT)
ALT (SGPT)
GGT

Lipid Profile
(Coronary Risk Factor)
Total Cholesterol
HDL Cholesterol
LDL Cholesterol
Triglycerides
Total Chol/HDL Chol

Urine FEME

Phosphate
Uric Acid

Diabetic Screen
Fasting Blood Sugar
Random Blood Sugar

RPV (VDRL)

ABO Blood Group + Rhesus

Package 2: EXECUTIVE HEALTH SCREENING RM 99.00

- **Laboratory Investigations**
- **Consultations**
- **Electro Cardiogram (ECG)**

Blood Screening (60 Tests)
Full Blood Counts
Hb
RBC (RCC)
WCC (TWDC)
5 Part Differential Count
Platelet Count
PCV
MCH/MCV
MCHC

Blood Film Comment

ESR
Renal Function Test
Sodium
Potassium
Chloride
Urea
Calcium
Creatinine
Phosphate
Uric Acid

Diabetic Screen
Fasting Blood Sugar
Random Blood Sugar

Free Thyroxine (free T4)

HIV I and II Antibodies (HIV)

Liver Function Test
Total Protein
Albumin
Globulin
Total Bilirubin
ALP
AST (SGOT)
ALT (SGPT)
GGT

Lipid Profile
(Coronary Risk Factor)
Total Cholesterol
HDL Cholesterol
LDL Cholesterol
Triglycerides
Total Chol/HDL Chol

Urine FEME

RPV (VDRL)

ABO Blood Group + Rhesus

Hepatitis B surface Antigen (HBsAg)
Hepatitis B surface Antibody (HBsAb)

Rheumatoid Factor (RF)
TAG-ONS

Package 3: CARDIAC ASSESSMENT (Non-invasive Diagnosis)
RM 149.00

- Electro Cardiogram (ECG)
- ECHO Doppler
- Tread Mill Test (TMT)
- Consultation with Cardiologist

WHAT IS A HEART ATTACK?

A heart attack (also called myocardial infarction) is when part of the heart muscle is damaged or dies because it isn't receiving oxygen. Oxygen is carried to the heart by the arteries (blood vessels). Most heart attacks are caused by a blockage in these arteries. Usually the blockage is caused by atherosclerosis, which is the buildup of fatty deposits (called plaque) inside the artery. This buildup is like the dirt that blocks a drainpipe and slows the flow of water.

Heart attacks can also be caused by a blood clot that gets stuck in a narrow part of artery. Clots are more likely to form where atherosclerosis has made an artery more narrow.

What are the symptoms of a Heart Attack?

Symptoms may include:

- Pressure or crushing pain in your chest, sometimes with sweating, nausea or vomiting
- Pain that extends from your chest into the jaw, left arm or left shoulder.
- Tightness in your chest.
- Shortness of breath for more than a couple of seconds.

Why go for Periodic Heart Check-up?

Most victims of heart attack do not know about their heart disease until a heart attack.

Risk Factors

Heart disease is not due to a single cause. Instead it is linked to several coronary risk factors such as: Diabetes, Hypertension (Increased Blood Pressure), Obesity, Smoking, Stress, Diet, Sedentary Lifestyle, Age, Heredity (Family History of heart attack), and Lack of Exercise.

Prevention of Heart Attack

Most heart attacks are caused by Coronary Artery Disease (CAD). You can prevent a heart attack:

- Know your risk factors for CAD and heart attack and take action to lower your risks.

- Make lifestyle changes.
- Conduct Cardiac Screening (ECG/ECHO/TMT)
- Consult a cardiologist for advise and treatment

Package 4: ULTRASOUND (Non-invasive Diagnosis) RM 25.00

- Scanning
- Consultation

WHAT IS ULTRASOUND?

Ultrasound is a very high frequency sound wave that images the internal organs. It is a safe and non-invasive procedure. Pelvic ultrasound is done trans-abdominally or trans-vaginally. For trans-abdominal scan, a full bladder helps with visualization of the uterus and ovaries.

Why it is done?

- Check what is causing pelvic pain.
- Check the cause of bleeding.
- Check the size and shape of the uterus and the thickness of the uterine lining.
- Check for uterine fibroids and its growth.
- Check the size and shape of the ovaries.
- Check the condition and size of the ovaries during treatment for infertility.
- Confirm a pregnancy and if it is in the uterus, age of the pregnancy, or to find a tubal pregnancy/multiple pregnancy.
- Find an intrauterine device (IUD).

How is it done?

- The test is done in an ultrasound room by a doctor who specializes in performing and interpreting imaging tests.
- Clothes over the area of interest are removed.
- You will need to drink 4 to 6 glasses of juice or water about an hour before the test.

What's the procedure like?

For a pelvic scan, you lie on your back on an examination table with your lower abdomen exposed and a mineral-based cool gel applied to your skin. The transducer is pressed against your lower belly and moved back and forth.

How does it feel?

The gel may feel cool when it is applied. You will feel light pressure from the transducer as it passes over your abdomen. The ultrasound is not uncomfortable.

Are there any risks or side effects from this procedure?

There are no known risks from having an ultrasound test.

Package 5: PAP SMEAR SCREENING **RM 19.00**

- Laboratory Investigations
- Consultation

WHAT IS A PAP SMEAR?

A Pap smear is a simple test to check for signs of cancer of the cervix. The cervix is part of your uterus (womb). During a Pap smear, a sample of cells from your cervix is taken to be tested.

Why does the Pap smear do?

A Pap smear checks for changes in the cells of the cervix. It is a screening procedure to find early warning signs that cancer might develop in the future.

How effective is the Pap smear?

Regular Pap smears can help prevent 90 per cent of the most common type of cervical cancer.

When should I have Pap smear?

Every woman from the beginning of sexual activity upto 65 years is advised to have a yearly Pap smear.

How do I prepare for a Pap smear?

A Pap smear is not carried out when you are bleeding or having your periods. Do not douche or use vaginal creams for 48 hrs prior to the test. A Pap smear is also not carried out when there is an ongoing infection.

Would it be painful?

It is not a painful examination. The most important aspect of this examination is that you have to be relaxed. Breathing in and out slowly during the procedure helps make it more comfortable.

Who are at higher risk for cervical cancer?

- Women with more than one sexual partner or whose partner has more than one partner.
- Women who were sexually active at a young age.
- Women who have a history of genital warts.
- Women who smoke.

Package 6: EXECUTIVE HEALTH SCREENING/CARDIAC ASSESSMENT
RM 239.00

- Laboratory Investigations
- Consultations

Electro Cardiogram (ECG)
ECHO Cardiogram Screening
Treadmill Stress Test (TMT)
Blood Screening (60 Tests)

Full Blood Counts
Hb
RBC (RCC)
WCC (TWDC)
5 Part Differential Count
Platelet Count
PCV
MCH/MCV
MCHC
Blood Film Comment

ESR
Renal Function Test
Sodium
Potassium
Chloride
Urea
Calcium
Creatinine
Phosphate
Uric Acid

Diabetic Screen
Fasting Blood Sugar
Random Blood Sugar

Liver Function Test
Total Protein
Albumin
Globulin
Total Bilirubin
ALP
AST (SGOT)
ALT (SGPT)
GGT
Lipid Profile
(Coronary Risk Factor)
Total Cholesterol
HDL Cholesterol
LDL Cholesterol
Triglycerides
Total Chol/HDL Chol

Urine FEME
RPV (VDRL)
ABO Blood Group + Rhesus
Hepatitis B surface Antigen (HBsAg)
Hepatitis B surface Antibody (HBsAb)
Free Thyroxine (free T4)
Rheumatoid Factor (RF)
Alpha Feto Protein (AFP)

Hepatitis A Antibody (HAV 1gG) HIV I and II Antibodies (HIV)
TAG-ONS

GENTING INTERNATIONAL CONVENTION HALLS

Grand Ballroom and Convention Hallsa

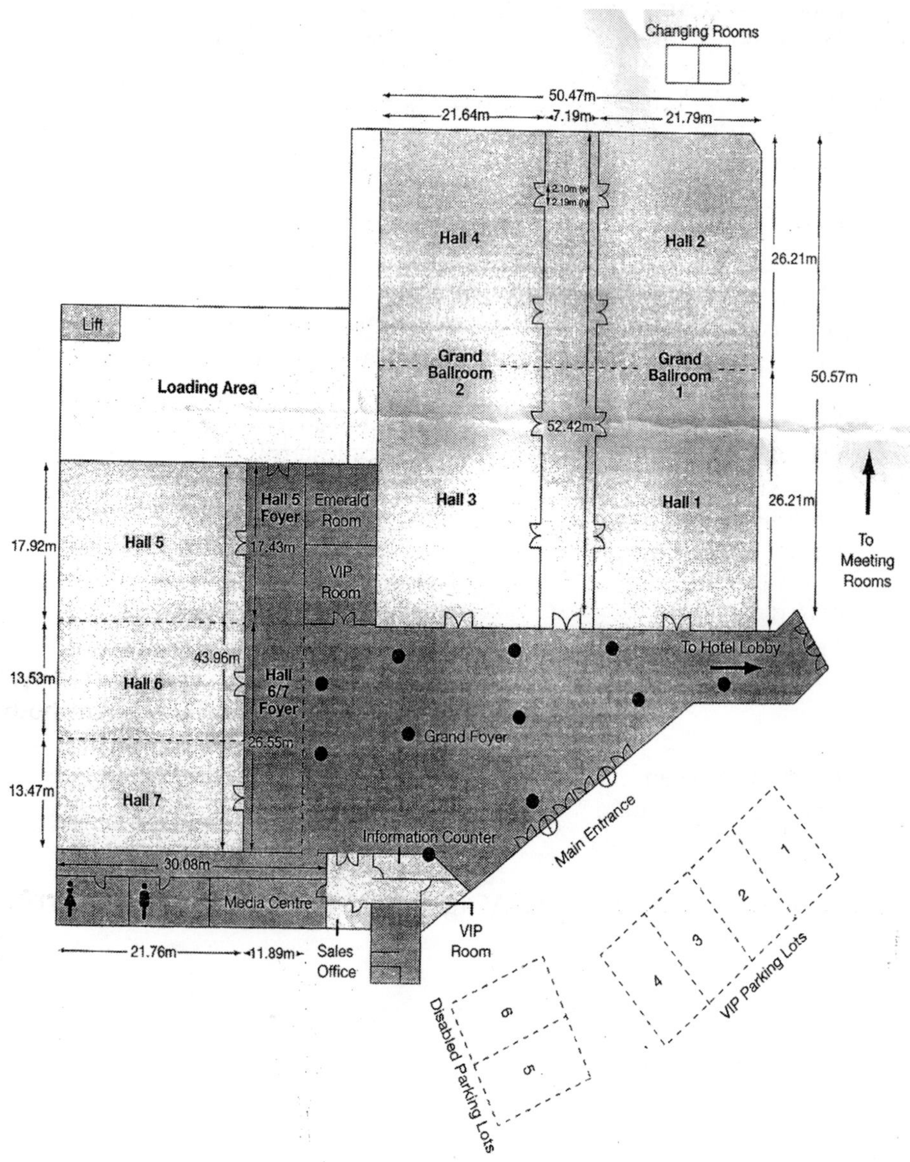

SEATING CAPACITY

Venue	*Ceiling Height*	*Approx. Area (m)*	*CAPACITY* Theatre (m^2)	*Classroom*	*Hollow*	*Buffet*	*U-Shape*	*Banquet Sit Down*	*Cocktail Reception*
Grand Ballroom (1-4)	6.7	9,705	4,200	1,200	220	1,600	320(D) 220(S)/	2,000	3,100
Grand Ballroom (1-2)	6.7	4,188	1,200	600	140	550	140(S)/ 220(D)	650	800
Grand Ballroom (3-4)	6.7	4,194	1,200	600	140	550	220(D) 140(S)/	650	800
HALL									
Hall 1	6.7	2,088	450	200	60	250	40	220	320
Hall 2	6.7	2,100	450	200	60	250	40	220	320
Hall 3	6.7	2,091	450	200	60	250	40	220	320
Hall 4	6.7	2,100	450	200	60	250	40	220	320
Hall 5	4.3	1,965	300	120	40	100	25	90	150
Hall 5 (include foyer)	4.3	2,063	350	150	50	150	30	140	200
Hall 6	4.3	1,875	300	120	40	100	25	80	150
Hall 7	4.3	1,871	300	120	40	100	25	80	150
Halls 5,6	4.3	3,840	550	200	60	220	60	200	300
Halls 6,7	4.3	3,746	500	200	60	220	60	200	300
Halls 5,6,7	4.3	5,711	1,000	400	100	550	80(S)/ 120(D)	600	800
Halls 5,6,7 (include foyer)	4.3	5,928	1,200	550	150	650	100(S)/ 140(D)	700	1,000

Grand Ballroom and Convention Hallsa

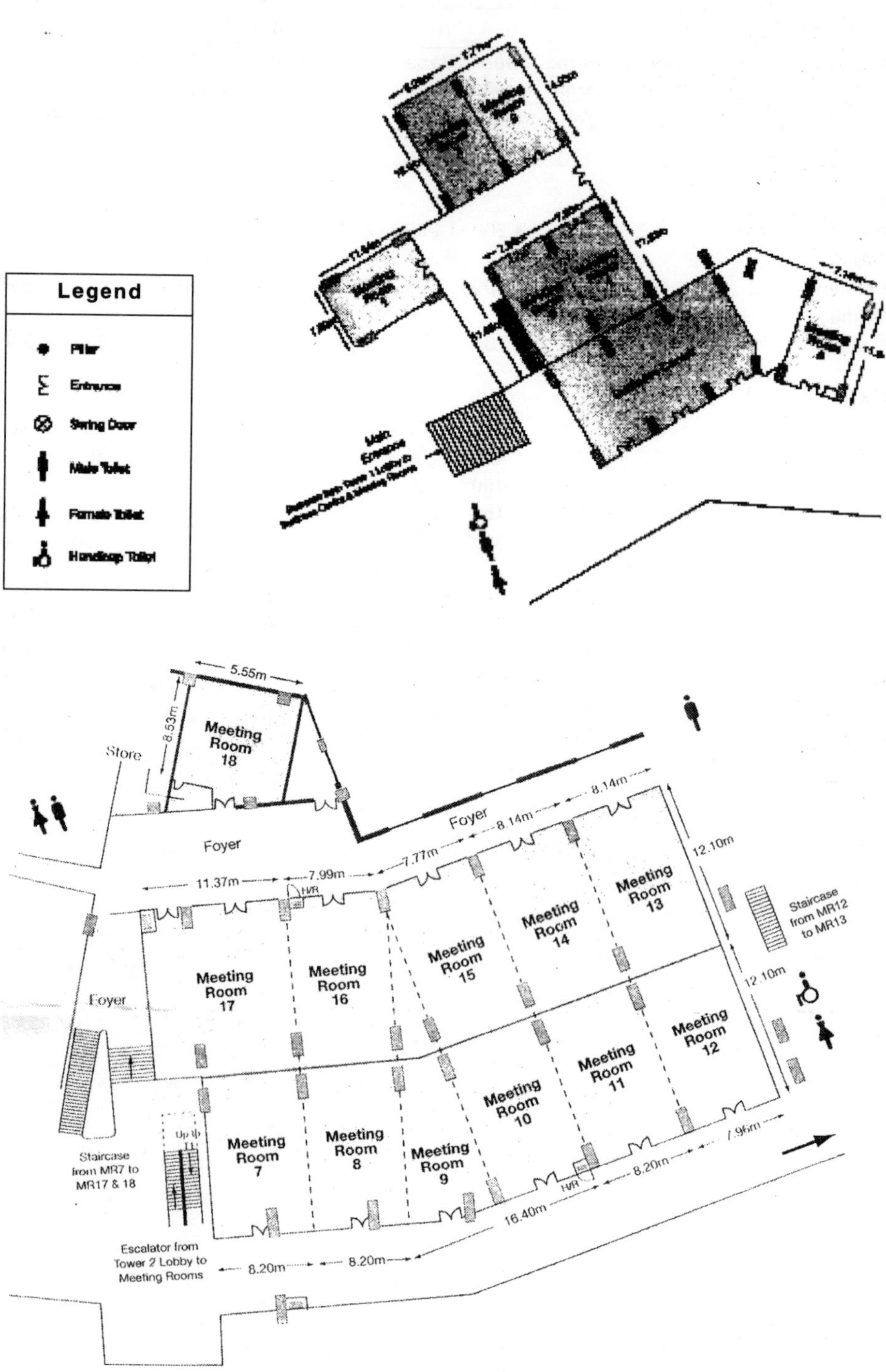

SEATING CAPACITY

Venue	*Ceiling Height*	*Approx. Area (m)*	*Theatre (m^2)*	*Classroom*	*Hollow*	*Buffet*	*U-Shape*	*Banquet Sit Down*	*Cocktail Reception*
			CAPACITY						
MR1	3.2	331	60	20	20	20	15	40	50
MR2	2.6	476	80	30	26	30	22	50	70
MR3	2.6	488	80	30	26	26	22	50	70
MR4	3.2	335	80	30	26	30	22	50	70
MR5	3.2	335	80	30	26	30	22	50	70
MR6	2.3	349	80	30	26	30	22	50	70
MR7	2.3	381	100	36	30	30	24	50	80
MR8	2.3	381	100	36	30	30	24	50	80
MR9	2.3	263	50	18	20	20	16	20	30
MR10	2.3	381	100	36	30	30	24	50	80
MR11	2.3	381	100	36	30	30	24	50	80
MR12	2.3	381	100	36	30	30	24	50	80
MR13	2.7	385	100	36	30	30	24	50	80
MR14	2.7	385	100	36	30	30	24	50	80
MR15	2.7	470	120	40	30	40	30	60	90
MR16	2.7	385	100	36	30	30	24	50	80
MR17	2.7	385	100	36	30	30	24	50	80
MR18	2.7	329	80	30	20	30	24	40	80
Combination of	**Seating**	**Capacity**							
MR4,5	3.2	671	180	60	50	80	30	100	150
MR7,8	2.3	761	220	60	64	60	36	90	110
MR7,8,9	2.3	1,025	250	80	40	80	40	100	120
MR8,9	2.3	644	180	40	30	50	26	60	80
MR7,8,9,10	2.3	1,406	350	120	46	110	50	150	170
MR8,9,10	2.3	1,025	250	80	40	80	40	100	120
MR9,10	2.3	644	180	40	50	50	26	60	80
MR7,8,9,10,11	2.3	1,789	400	140	50	140	60	180	200
MR8,9,10,11	2.3	1,406	350	120	46	110	50	150	170
MR9,10,11	2.3	1,025	250	80	40	80	40	100	120
MR10,11	2.3	761	220	60	64	70	40	90	110
MR7,8,9,10,11	2.3	2,167	550	200	60	180	100	250	270
MR8,9,10,11	2.3	1,786	400	140	50	150	60	220	240
MR9,10,11,12	2.7	1,406	350	120	46	110	50	150	170
MR10,11,12	2.7	1,142	300	80	40	90	40	120	140
MR11,12	2.7	761	220	60	36	70	40	90	110
MR13,14	2.7	769	220	60	36	70	40	90	110
MR13,14,15	2.7	1,240	330	110	40	100	50	130	150
MR14,15	2.7	855	250	80	40	70	40	100	120
MR13,14,15,16	2.7	1,624	380	130	46	130	50	200	220
MR14,15,16	2.7	1,240	330	110	46	100	50	130	150
MR15,16	2.7	855	250	80	40	70	40	100	120
MR13,14,15,16,17	2.7	2,009	500	180	50	160	60	220	240
MR14,15,16,17	2.7	1,624	380	130	46	130	50	200	220
MR15,16,17	2.7	1,240	330	110	46	100	50	130	150
MR16,17	2.7	769	220	60	36	70	40	90	110

Index